Milestones in Drug Therapy
MDT

Fluoroquinolone Antibiotics

Edited by A.R. Ronald and D.E. Low

Springer Basel AG

Editors

Allan R. Ronald
Faculty of Medicine
The University of Manitoba, Room C5124
409 Tacho Avenue
Winnipeg, Manitoba, R2H 2A6
Canada

Donald E. Low
Microbiology Laboratory
Mt. Sinai Hospital, Room 1487
600 University Avenue
Toronto, Ontario M5G 1X5
Canada

Library of Congress Cataloging-in-Publication Data

Fluoroquinolone antibiotics / A.R. Ronald, D.E. Low (editors).
p. cm
Includes bibliographical references and index.
ISBN 978-3-0348-9437-1 ISBN 978-3-0348-8103-6 (eBook)
DOI 10.1007/978-3-0348-8103-6
1. Quinolone antibacterial agents. I. Ronald, Allan R. II. Low, Don E.

RM666.Q55 F577 2003
616.9'2061–dc21 2002043611

Bibliographic information published by Die Deutsche Bibliothek

Die Deutsche Bibliothek lists this publication in the Deutsche Nationalbibliografie; detailed bibliographic data is available in the internet at http://dnb.ddb.de

ISBN 978-3-0348-9437-1

Originally published by Birkhäuser Verlag, Basel - Boston - Berlin in 2003
Softcover reprint of the hardcover 1st edition 2003

Printed on acid-free paper produced from chlorine-free pulp. TFC ∞
Cover illustration: Quinolone structure-side effect relationship (see. p. 7)

ISBN 978-3-0348-9437-1

9 8 7 6 5 4 3 2 1 http://www.birkhauser-science.com

Contents

List of contributors

Anastasia Antoniadou, Athens University School of Medicine, 4th Department of Internal Medicine, Sismanoglio General Hospital, 1 Sismanogliou St., 15126 Maroussi, Athens, Greece; e-mail: cfk@hol.gr

Vincent C.C. Cheng, Division of Infectious Diseases, Department of Microbiology, Queen Mary Hospital, The University of Hong Kong, Pokfulam Road, Pokfulam, Hong Kong SAR, China; e-mail: cccqmhhk@netvigator.com

Nicholas S.Y. Chew, Department of Infectious Diseases, Mater Misericordiae Hospital, Eccles Street, Dublin 7, Ireland; e-mail: mtbdude@hotmail.com

Anthony W. Chow, Division of Infectious Diseases, Department of Medicine, University of British Columbia and Vancouver Hospital Health Sciences Centre, 2773 Heather Street, Vancouver, BC, Canada V5Z 3J5; e-mail: tonychow@interchange.ubc.ca. Present address: UCSD, 3717 Nobel Dr, Apt 1327, San Diego, CA 92122, USA

Ron Dagan, Pediatric Infectious Disease Unit, Soroka University Medical Center, P.O. Box 151, Beer-Sheva 84101, Israel; e-mail: rdagan@bgumail.bgu.ac.il

John Embil, Infection Control Unit, Health Sciences Centre, MS 673-820 Sherbrook Street, Winnipeg, MB, R3A 1R9 Canada; e-mail: jembil@hsc.mb.ca

Helen Giamarellou, Athens University School of Medicine, 4th Department of Internal Medicine, Sismanoglio General Hospital, 1 Sismanogliou St., 15126 Maroussi, Athens, Greece; e-mail: hgiama@ath.forthnet.gr

Pak-Leung Ho, Division of Infectious Diseases, Department of Microbiology, Queen Mary Hospital, The University of Hong Kong, Pokfulam Road, Pokfulam, Hong Kong SAR, China; e-mail: plho@hkucc.hku.hk

James R. Johnson, VA Medical Center and Department of Medicine, University of Minnesota, Minneapolis, MN, USA; e-mail: johns007@umn.edu

Eugene Leibovitz, Pediatric Infectious Disease Unit, Soroka University Medical Center, P.O. Box 151, Beer-Sheva 84101, Israel; e-mail: eugenel@bgumail.bgu.ac.il

Donald E. Low, Department of Microbiology, Mount Sinai Hospital, 600 University Ave., Rm. 1487, Toronto, Ontario, Canada M5G 1X5; e-mail: dlow@mtsinai.on.ca

Zhenkun Ma, Medicinal Chemistry, Cumbre Inc., 1502 Viceroy Drive, Dallas, TX 75235-2304, USA; e-mail: zhenkun.ma@cumbre.net

Manuel W. Mah, Infection Prevention and Control, Peter Lougheed Centre, 3500-26th Avenue NE, Calgary, AB, T1Y 6J4 Canada; e-mail: manuel.mah@CRHA-health.ab.ca

Lionel A. Mandell, McMaster University, Henderson Hospital, 5th floor, 40 Wing, 711 Concession St., Hamilton, Ontario L8V 1C3, Canada

Thomas J. Marrie, Department of Medicine, University of Alberta, 2F1.30 Walter C. Mackenzie Health Sciences Center, 6440 112th Street, Edmonton, Alberta, Canada T6H 2B7; e-mail: tom.marrie@ualberta.ca

Ziad A. Memish, Departments of Medicine and Infection Prevention and Control, King Fahad National Guard Hospital, P.O. Box 22490, Riyadh 11426, Saudi Arabia; e-mail: memish@ngha.med.sa

Lester A. Mitscher, Medicinal Chemistry Department, Kansas University, 4010 Malott Hall, 1251 Wescoe Hall Drive, Lawrence, KS 66045-7582, USA; e-mail: lmitscher@ku.edu

Ayman M. Noreddin, Microbiology, Health Sciences Centre, MS673-820 Sherbrook Street, Winnipeg, Manitoba R3A 1R9, Canada

Geoffrey L. Ridgway, Department of Clinical Microbiology, University College London Hospitals, Grafton Way, London WC1E 6DB, UK; e-mail: geoff.ridgway@uclh.org

Allan R. Ronald, Faculty of Medicine, The Unversity of Manitoba, Room C5124, 409 Tacho Avenue, Winnipeg, Manitoba, R2H 2A6, Canada; e-mail: aronald@ms.umanitoba.ca

Gerard Sheehan, Department of Infectious Diseases, Mater Misericordiae Hospital, Eccles Street, Dublin 7, Ireland

Sarah A. Wyllie, Department of Clinical Microbiology, University College London Hospitals, Grafton Way, London WC1E 6DB, UK; e-mail: wylliewolf@po139org.freesurf.co.uk

George G. Zhanel, Microbiology, Health Sciences Centre, MS673–820 Sherbrook Street, Winnipeg, Manitoba R3A 1R9, Canada; e-mail: ggzhanel@pcs.mb.ca

Preface

Since the introduction of ciprofloxacin in 1987, fluoroquinolones have expanded far beyond their early role in the treatment of urinary tract infections. Clinical applications beyond genitourinary tract infections include upper and lower respiratory infections, gastrointestinal infections, gynecologic infections, sexually transmitted diseases, and some skin and soft tissue infections. Their ease of administration, favorable pharmacokinetic properties, excellent tolerability, and efficacy give them enormous potential for use and misuse alike. Quinolones have few common adverse effects, most notably nausea, headache and dizziness. Less frequent but more serious adverse events include prolongation of the corrected QT interval, phototoxicity, liver enzyme abnormalities, arthropathy, and cartilage and tendon abnormalities. While possessing many of the favorable properties of intravenous agents, most fluoroquinolones offer the convenience of oral administration, thus contributing to decreased health-care costs through increased outpatient therapy and shortened hospital stays. With the recent introduction of agents such as gatifloxacin and moxifloxacin, the traditional Gram-negative coverage of fluoroquinolones has been expanded to include Gram-positive organisms, most importantly *Streptococcus pneumoniae*.

Several issues have arisen over the last few years with the widespread acceptance and use of these agents: the emergence and dissemination of resistance, the need for extensive clinical experience before we can feel confident about the safety of new agents, and the need for head-to-head clinical trials to define the optimal role of each agent. During the last decade we have seen the emergence and dissemination of resistance to the main pathogens for which these agents have been targeted, including *Escherichia coli*, *Klebsiella* spp., *Pseudomonas aeruginosa*, *Neisseria gonorrhoeae*, *Salmonella enterica*, and *Streptococcus pneumoniae*. If we had known what we know now regarding the pharmacokinetics and pharmacodynamics parameters of these antimicrobials when they were first introduced, we may have been able to prevent or slow the emergence of resistance by more appropriate use, especially with regards to agriculture.

The approval of trovafloxacin by the Food and Drug Administration (FDA) in 1998 was met with great excitement by many clinicians based on its utility as monotherapy for numerous indications. In comparison with other available fluoroquinolones, trovafloxacin offered enhanced activity against anaerobic and Gram-positive organisms. In June, 1999 the FDA made a formal statement outlining recommendations for the cautious use of trovafloxacin in specific patient populations. Postmarketing experience revealed several cases of liver toxicity associated with the use of trovafloxacin, although similar findings had not been documented in earlier studies. The experience magnified the limitations of information gained through clinical trials.

Finally, we have seen the introduction of a number of new fluoroquinolones during the last 5 years. However, most of the clinical trials have been designed for equivalency and have included comparator agents in other classes. There are few studies which have been able to define the most optimal clinical indication for each of these agents.

The new fluoroquinolones should currently rarely be prescribed as first-line agents and should always be employed judiciously. Inappropriate use of agents from this important class of antibiotics will likely worsen current problems with fluoroquinolone resistance.

Allan R. Ronald
Donald E. Low

August 2002

Fluoroquinolone Antibiotics
ed. by A.R. Ronald and D.E. Low

The history of quinolones

Gerard Sheehan and Nicholas S.Y. Chew

Department of Infectious Diseases, Mater Misericordiae Hospital, Eccles Street, Dublin 7, Ireland

The first quinolone emerged in the early 1960s, with the isolation of 7-chloro-1-ethyl-1, 4-dihydro-4-oxoquinoline-3-carboxylic acid, a by-product of the commercial preparation of chloroquine. This compound was found to have anti-bacterial activity and was subsequently modified to produce nalidixic acid, a 1, 8-naphthyridine [1] (see Fig. 1).

Nalidixic acid was introduced into clinical practice 2 years later after relatively limited clinical trials. Adequate studies of its use in urinary tract infections (UTI) were carried out only after its introduction and marketing, reflecting a less stringent regulatory environment.

Oral absorption of nalidixic acid was low with peak serum concentrations of <0.5 μg/ml and it was therefore unsuitable for the treatment of systemic infections. However, urinary concentrations of the drug were high and so its clinical utility was largely confined to UTIs [2]. Along with nitrofurantoin and methenamine, it was sometimes classified as a urinary antiseptic, and remains today as a useful, inexpensive agent for both upper and lower urinary tract infection. *In vitro* sensitivity to nalidixic acid was defined as an minimum inhibitory concentration (MIC) of 10 μg/ml or less, intermediate sensitivity as 11–50 μg/ml, and resistance determined as >100 μg/ml. *In vitro*, nalidixic acid demonstrated excellent activity against enterobacteriaceae, but little or no activity against *Pseudomonas aeruginosa*. Of 125 enterobacteriaceae isolated from women with clinical UTIs, 117 demonstrated exquisite sensitivity with MICs <15 μg/ml. Conversely, 25 of 25 isolates of *P. aeruginosa* from such

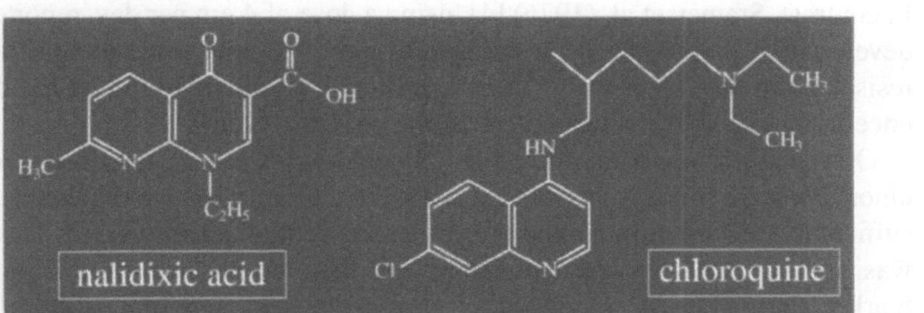

Figure 1. Structure of chloroquine and nalidixic acid

patients were highly resistant, with MIC >100 µg/ml. In the same study, 25 of 25 isolates of *Enterococcus faecalis* from these patients were highly resistant with MICs >100 µg/ml. Nalidixic acid was also shown to have poor activity against other Gram-positive bacteria [3, 4].

Nalidixic acid was well tolerated and widely accepted for the therapy of urinary tract infections in the 1960s and 70s. A randomised controlled trial in patients with upper tract infection comparing nalidixic acid to cephalexin showed a lower relapse rate in patients receiving nalidixic acid [5]. This was the earliest evidence that antimicrobial agents with mechanisms of action other than cell wall disruption may be superior in the hypertonic milieu of the upper urinary tract. Unfortunately, no studies of nalidixic acid as single dose or short course therapy were done for lower urinary tract infections. Nalidixic acid's incomplete absorption was associated with high faecal concentrations, and it was found to be useful for shigella dysentery, but never widely used for this indication. Its lack of anaerobic and Gram-positive activity made it attractive as a selective agent in the bowel as prophylaxis for neutropenic patients. In the early 1980s, it was shown to be equivalent to co-trimoxazole for this indication, but was never widely used, as the new fluoroquinolones, norfloxacin and ciprofloxacin superseded it.

After its introduction into widespread clinical use, several significant adverse effects were noted, including headaches, gastrointestinal and visual disturbances, photosensitivity reactions and more frequent convulsions in seizure prone patients. Less frequent side-effects included drowsiness, toxic psychoses and haemolytic anaemia in patients with glucose-6-phosphate dehydrogenase deficiency. Its short half-life necessitated six hourly administrations, so that either amoxycillin or co-trimoxazole was often chosen in preference. Concern arose regarding the emergence of resistance on therapy, especially in those with complicated UTI. Ronald et al. (1966) [3] studied nalidixic acid in a highly selected group of 50 patients at a referral centre, many of whom had failed previous antimicrobial agents but the majority of whom were without demonstrable structural abnormalities of the urinary tract. Most received nalidixic acid 500 mg qid for 6 weeks. Persistence of bacteriuria occurred in 22 out of 50 patients. Thirteen of the 50 patients had an initially sensitive organism but failed to clear it and developed a highly resistant strain. In contrast, Stamey et al. (1976) [4], using a dose of 4 gm per day, reported the development of resistance on therapy in only 7% and minimal selection of resistance in the faecal flora. These conflicting results may reflect the difference in dosage or the select nature of the patients studied.

Other early compounds (see Fig. 2) such as rosoxacin, oxolinic acid and cinoxacin were found to be active against most Gram negative organisms, with sufficient concentrations in the prostate, and urethral secretions [6]. Their use was limited to urinary tract infections and they did not achieve a significant market share. The development of pipemidic acid with the addition of a 7-piperazine side chain in the late 1960s allowed better penetration of the bacterial cell wall, conferring improved activity against *P. aeruginosa* as well as

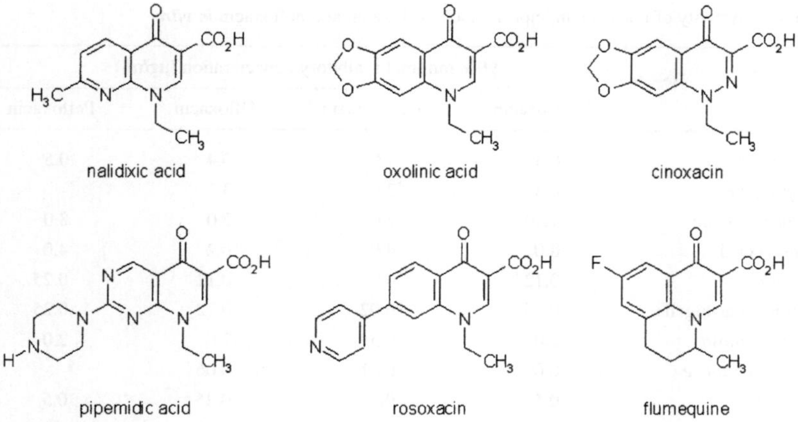

Figure 2. First generation quinolones

some Gram-positive bacteria. Another early modification was the addition of a 6-fluorine group giving flumequine, first introduced in the early 1970s. This compound was found to have better action against Gram-positive bacteria [7].

By the late 1970s, norfloxacin was developed, combining both the 7-piperazine and 6-fluorine group in its structure. It was launched in 1984 and is regarded as the first modern fluoroquinolone. It proved highly active against enterobacteriaceae, *Haemophilus influenzae*, *Pasteurella multocida*, *Aeromonas hydrophila*, neisseria spp. and *P. aeruginosa.* It was marginally active against streptococci and staphylococci, and was not active against anaerobes, *C. trachomatis, mycobacteria or mycoplasma* (see Tab. 1) [8]. It had an oral bioavailability of 50%, with high faecal concentrations. Volume of distribution was high and exceeded total body water content but the peak serum concentration was marginal at 1.5 µg/ml. Thus norfloxacin was considered adequate for systemic infections due to highly sensitive organisms but only reliably effective against *P. aeruginosa* in the urinary tract. Nevertheless, this was a significant advance as *P. aeruginosa* was increasingly recognised as a significant nosocomial urinary pathogen. Previously, the only oral antipseudomonal agent for UTI had been indanyl-carbenicillin. Norfloxacin was effective as an oral agent for both simple and complicated urinary tract infections [9], as well as the prevention and treatment of travellers' diarrhoea, the treatment of bacterial enteritis and enteric fever and the prophylaxis of Gram-negative infections in neutropenic patients. It was also effective in the treatment of uncomplicated gonococcal infections, including those caused by penicillinase producing *N. gonorrhoeae* (PPNG). In the 1980s, norfloxacin was widely used for urinary tract infections and gonococcal urethritis. The introduction of norfloxacin signified the beginning of a period of rapid development of other oral second-generation quinolones including pefloxacin,

Table 1. Activity of norfloxacin, ciprofloxacin, ofloxacin and pefloxacin *in vitro*

Species	90% minimal inhibitory concentration (μg/ml)			
	Norfloxacin	Ciprofloxacin	Ofloxacin	Pefloxacin
S. aureus	6.3	1.0	0.4	0.5
S. pyogenes	6.3	2.0	3.1	-
S. pneumoniae	16.0	2.0	2.0	8.0
enterococci	8.0	4.0	6.2	4.0
E. coli	0.12	0.03	0.12	0.25
salmonella/shigella	0.06	0.02	0.12	0.25
P. aeruginosa	2.0	0.5	2.0	2.0
N. gonorrhoeae	0.06	0.01	0.06	-
C. jejuni	0.5	0.12	0.25	0.5
H. influenzae	0.06	0.01	0.03	0.06
B. fragilis	>128	8.0	8.0	16.0
M. tuberculosis	8.0	1.0	1.3	8.0
C. trachomatis	25.0	1.6	0.8	-

enoxacin, fleroxacin, ciprofloxacin and ofloxacin. Of these, only ciprofloxacin and ofloxacin became widely established for the treatment of infections at sites other than the urinary tract. Ciprofloxacin, released in 1987, was the first quinolone to become available intravenously.

In comparison with the first generation quinolones, ciprofloxacin had improved activity against a broad spectrum of Gram-positive and Gram-negative bacteria, mycobacteria, mycoplasma and legionella spp. It also showed good oral bioavailability, allowing for a stepdown from intravenous to oral therapy in hospitalised patients with serious systemic infections, a significant cost containment benefit. However, antimicrobial resistance later became a concern, particularly with *Staphylococcus aureus,* enterococcus spp. and *P. aeruginosa.*

Ciprofloxacin was the first orally available antimicrobial agent with reliable activity against *P. aeruginosa* at sites other than the urinary tract. Its low toxicity made it a more attractive option than aminoglycosides. Its reliable oral absorption meant that it could be less costly than third generation cephalosporins or extended spectrum penicillins and its lack of anaerobic activity minimized the disturbance of the normal gastrointestinal flora. The incidence of diarrhoea due to *Clostridium difficile* superinfection was thought to be lower than with other broad-spectrum agents. It was also an alternative agent for atypical pulmonary infection, with reliable activity against legionella, mycoplasma and chlamydia. Serum peak concentration was 1.5 μg/ml with a half-life of 3.3 h and a high volume of distribution of 348 litres, reflecting excellent intracellular penetration [10, 11].

Unexpected drawbacks included rare case reports of failures and deaths due to septicaemia from *Streptococcus pneumoniae* and *Streptococcus pyogenes.*

The susceptibilities of these organisms were borderline, especially in relation to serum levels. Other disadvantages that emerged included significant drug interactions. Oral iron and sucralfate virtually abolished ciprofloxacin absorption [12, 13]. Dairy products and antacids were also shown to significantly reduce oral bioavailability. Its concomitant use with non-steroidal anti-inflammatory drugs (NSAIDs) increased the risk of seizures in patients with epilepsy. The use of theophylline and ciprofloxacin together caused a doubling of theophylline levels. These concerns later extended to other second and third generation quinolones. Chondrotoxicity of ciprofloxacin (and other quinolones) was observed in immature animals, effecting articular cartilage and the epiphyseal growth plate. Use of ciprofloxacin in paediatrics and pregnancy was restricted, although retrospective reviews of nalidixic acid use in children prior to the 1980s revealed no cases of chondropathy or arthropathy. In adults, there were cases of tendinitis manifesting as arthralgia and rarely tendon rupture occurring as late as several months after treatment with ciprofloxacin and later other quinolones.

Ofloxacin was initially developed in the mid 1980s and approved by the United States Food and Drug Administration (FDA) in 1990, and challenged ciprofloxacin for market share throughout the 1990s. In comparison with ciprofloxacin, ofloxacin was more rapidly absorbed from the gastrointestinal tract, with higher serum concentrations and a longer half-life [10, 11, 13–17]. Most enterobacteriaceae, enteropathogens and fastidious Gram-negative bacteria were highly susceptible, with MICs less than 2 µg/ml. However the MICs of *P. aeruginosa* were generally lower for ciprofloxacin, which has remained the quinolone of choice for infections due to this organism. Obligate anaerobes

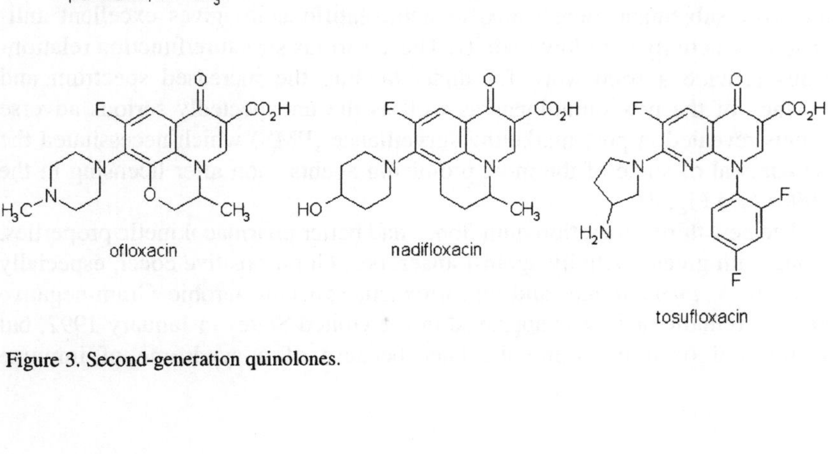

Figure 3. Second-generation quinolones.

are usually resistant to ofloxacin, whereas, chlamydia, legionella, mycoplasma and many mycobacteria are susceptible (see Tab. 1) [14, 15, 17]. Both ciprofloxacin and ofloxacin were effective in the treatment of septicaemia, infections of the skin and soft tissues, urinary tract, intra-abdominal, pelvic and respiratory tract infections, as well as gonococcal and non-gonococcal urethritis and prophylaxis and treatment of spontaneous bacterial peritonitis secondary to cirrhosis.

In the early 1990s, the area under the concentration-time curve (AUC) to MIC ratio (AUIC), was shown to be the most important predictor of outcome in a study of critically ill patients receiving ciprofloxacin [18]. This seminal work was part of an improved understanding of the pharmacodynamics of antimicrobial agents in general. The 1990s also brought a clearer understanding of the mechanisms of action and structure function relationships of quinolones [19]. The constant structural feature is a bicyclic aromatic core consisting of two fused six-membered rings, with variations in substituents explaining differences in spectrum of activity, potency and adverse effects. The R1 moiety influences anti-bacterial potency and theophylline interaction, with a cyclopropyl substituent optimal for activity, present in ciprofloxacin and in all the new third generation agents other than levofloxacin and trovafloxacin. A carboxylic acid group at position 3 and a carbonyl group at position 4 is present in all fluoroquinolones and is important in binding the DNA/DNA gyrase complex, in cell entry and for the interaction with magnesium, aluminium and iron. The R5 substituent influences Gram-positive activity with an amino group optimal, as found with sparfloxacin. However it also influences phototoxicity and genetic toxicity. The C6 position has a fluoro substituent in all of the second and third generation agents, hence the ‘fluoro’ nomenclature. The R7 substituent controls gamma-amino-butyric acid (GABA) binding and hence adverse events in the central nervous system (CNS), especially convulsions. It is also important for NSAID potentiation of CNS adverse events and the interaction with theophylline. Variations in R7 also influence anti-bacterial potency and spectrum as well as pharmacokinetics. Position 8 influences anti-anaerobic activity, but also phototoxicity, which is greatest with a halogen substituent, as with fluoro for sparfloxacin and chloro for clinafloxacin. A methoxy substituent here (moxifloxacin, gatifloxacin) gives excellent anti-anaerobic activity with low toxicity. These various structure/function relationships provide a framework for understanding the increased spectrum and potency of the new quinolones as well as the unexpectedly serious adverse events revealed in post-marketing surveillance (PMS) which necessitated the withdrawal of some of the most promising agents soon after licensing in the 1990s (see Fig. 4).

The new third generation quinolones had better pharmacokinetic properties, along with greater activity against anaerobes, Gram-positive cocci, especially resistant *S. pneumoniae*, and ciprofloxacin resistant aerobic Gram-negative bacilli. Temafloxacin was approved in the United States in January 1992, but withdrawal occurred 4 months later because of a syndrome of immune

R_1 controls theophylline interaction and genetic toxicity

R_2 no side effects associated with this position

R_5 influences phototoxicity and genetic toxicity

F no side effect reported from this group

R_7 controls GABA binding, theophylline interaction

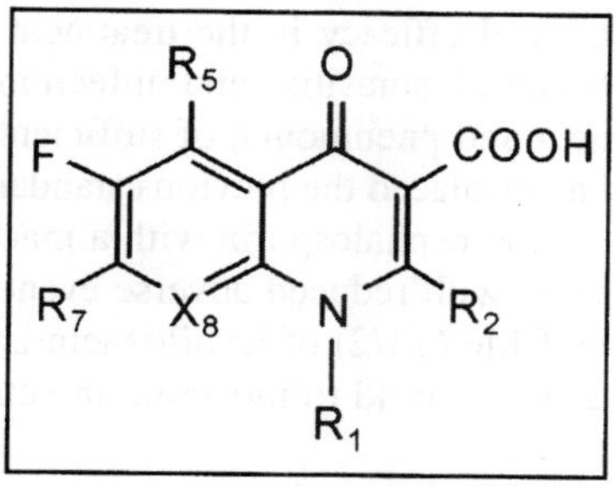

Figure 4. Quinolone structure-side-effect relationship.

haemolytic anaemia sometimes with multi-organ failure that became known as the "Temafloxacin Syndrome" [20]. One hundred and fourteen cases were spontaneously reported to the FDA, during a period when an estimated 189,000 prescriptions were issued. Most had haemolysis (95) and/or multi-organ dysfunction (90), consisting of renal or hepatic abnormalities or coagulopathy. The typical presentation was of fever, jaundice, nausea, vomiting, abdominal pain, myalgia, and back pain, with resolution occurring within days or weeks following discontinuation. Dialysis was required by 34 patients, CNS complications developed in four of these, and two patients died. In a total of ten patients, the syndrome developed after exposure to only one dose. The syndrome may have been due to an immune-complex mediated haemolytic anaemia.

Four other major adverse reactions were associated with third generation quinolones, namely convulsions, phototoxicity, prolonged electrocardiographic Q-Tc interval, and hepatotoxicity [21, 22]. Hepatotoxicity caused trovafloxacin to be suspended. One hundred and forty trovafloxacin-treated patients developed hepatic problems, 14 of which were severe, and eight required transplantation. Cardiotoxicity associated with grepafloxacin, and phototoxicity caused by clinafloxacin caused both to be withdrawn. Phototoxicity has been described for all quinolones, but derivatives with a halogen atom at position 8 show the highest potential for such reactions. Fleroxacin, sparfloxacin, clinafloxacin and lomefloxacin belong to this group of fluoroquinolones. Prolongation of the Q-Tc interval emerged as a class effect of concern, especially for sparfloxacin and grepafloxacin. The new 8-methoxy quinolones, moxifloxacin and gatifloxacin, are without evidence of these adverse effects. Postmarketing surveillance of moxifloxacin in Germany has revealed no additional concerns to date. They are more potent against both penicillin-susceptible and multidrug-resistant *S. pneumoniae*, while retaining activity against enterobacteriaciae.

Ciprofloxacin, ofloxacin and levofloxacin have maintained excellent safety profiles. Levofloxacin, the levo isomer of ofloxacin, has achieved a dominant role in the therapy of community acquired pneumonia and has demonstrated clinical efficacy in the treatment of genitourinary and skin infections, acute bacterial sinusitis, and infections of the head and neck. For community acquired pneumonia, of sufficient severity to require admission to hospital, it has displaced the previous standard of a combination of a second or third generation cephalosporin with a macrolide, giving an equivalent or superior efficacy, with reduced adverse events, costs and duration of hospitalisation. The half-life (T1/2) of levofloxacin is nearly 8 h, and it can be administered once daily for mild to moderate infections and twice daily for more serious infections.

The adverse drug reaction rate (ADR) associated with individual fluoroquinolones was reviewed in a 5-year PMS in Japan and in European and international data from approximately 130 million prescriptions [23]. The ADR was 1.3% to 2% for levofloxacin, compared to rates of 2–10% for other fluoroquinolones. Gastrointestinal effects were the most common adverse events for all fluoroquinolones. Levofloxacin had a low rate of hepatic reactions (1/650,000). Levofloxacin, ofloxacin, and moxifloxacin had the lowest potential of inducing CNS adverse events. Cardiovascular problems were seen in 1/15 million levofloxacin prescriptions compared to 1–3% of sparfloxacin patients having QTc prolongation of greater than 500 ms. Ofloxacin and levofloxacin had a very low phototoxic potential.

Quinolones have evolved in the last five decades from a small, relatively unimportant group of drugs used predominantly for UTIs to a class with multiple applications and broad-spectrum antimicrobial cover (see Tab. 2). In the wake of the September 11th 2001 terrorist attack, ciprofloxacin became a focus of media attention, as the prophylactic antimicrobial agent of choice for the prevention of pulmonary anthrax [24]. Studies in macaques showed that it was effective and possibly superior to penicillin and other agents. It was prescribed for 60 days for this purpose. There was a worldwide run on stocks and debate raged about national reserves of the agent and about production outside

Table 2. Examples of fluoroquinolones in clinical use

Generation	FDA approval	Generic name	Trade name/manufacturer
First		Nalidixic acid	NegGram®/Sanofi
Second	1986	Norfloxacin	Noroxin®/MSD
	1987	Ciprofloxacin	Ciproxin®/Bayer
	1990	Ofloxacin	Floxin®/Ortho
	1991	Enoxacin	Penetrex®/Aventis
	1992	Lomefloxacin	Maxaquin®/Searle
Third	1996	Levofloxacin	Levaquin®/Ortho
	1996	Sparfloxacin	Zagam®/Aventis
	1999	Gatifloxacin	Tequin®/BMS
Fourth	1997	Trovafloxacin	Trovan®/Pfizer
	1999	Moxifloxacin	Avalox®/Bayer

of its patent. The growth of quinolones is likely to continue and they are likely to remain a central part of the anti-bacterial armamentarium for many decades into the 21st century.

Important lessons from the experience of the past decade surely include that we cannot be confident about the utility or superiority of an agent in development based solely on the results of *in vitro* studies, knowledge of chemical structure and clinical trials to phase III. The latter generally have been powered to show equivalence to standard therapy with regard to efficacy. Larger sized trials are desirable to detect important differences in efficacy for specific clinical syndromes. Of greater importance, larger sized trials might have better detected adverse events. However some of these were so uncommon that the past decade has shown us the vital importance of post marketing surveillance for all new drugs.

References

1 Lescher GY, Froelich ED, Gruet MD, Bailey JH, Brundage (1962) RP 1-8 naphthyridine derivatives. A new class of chemotherapeutic agents. *J Med Pharm* 5: 1063–1068

2 Jameson RM (1965) Tissue concentration of nalidixic acid and its use in pyelonephritis. *BMJ* 2: 621

3 Ronald R, Turck M, Petersdorf R (1966) A critical evaluation of nalidixic acid in urinary tract infections. *NEJM* 20: 1081–1089

4 Stamey T, Bragonje J (1976) Resistance to nalidixic acid. A misconception due to underdosage. *JAMA* 236: 1857–1860

5 Preiksaitis JK, Thompson L, Harding GK, Marrie TJ, Hoban DJ, Ronald AR (1981) A comparison of the efficacy of nalidixic acid and cephalexin in bacteriuric women and the effect on fecal and periurethral carriage of enterbactericeae. *J Inf Dis* 143(4): 603–608

6 Maigaard S, Frimodt-Moller N, Hoyne U, Madsen PO (1979) Rosoxacin and cinoxacin distribution in prostate, vagina and urethra. An experimental study in dogs. *Invest Urol* Sep: 149–152

7 Felmingham D, O'Hare MD, Robbins MJ, Wall RA, Williams AH, Cremer AW, Ridgway GL, Gruneberg RN (1985) Comparative *in vitro* studies with 4-quinolone antimicrobials. *Drugs Exp Clin Res* 11(5): 317–329 (abstract)

8 Mandell L, Bergeron M, Marrie T, Nicolle L, Scheifele D, Shafran S (1988) Committee on antimicrobial agents, Canadian Infectious Diseases Society. Norfloxacin: a new quinolone. *CMAJ* 139: 305–307

9 Sheehan GJ, Harding GK, Haase DA, Thomson MJ, Urias B, Kennedy JK, Hoban DJ, Ronald AR (1988) Double-blind, randomized comparison of 24 weeks of norfloxacin and 12 weeks of norfloxacin followed by 12 weeks of placebo in the therapy of complicated urinary tract infection. *Antimicrob Agents Chemother* 32: 1292–1293

10 Oates JA, Wood AJ (1991) Fluoroquinolone antimicrobial agents. *N Engl J Med* 324: 384–394

11 Sanders C (1988) Ciprofloxacin: *in vitro* activity, mechanism of action and resistance. *Rev Infect Dis* 10: 516–553

12 Frost RW, Lasseter KC, Noe AJ, Shamblen ECLettieri JT (1992) Effects of aluminium hydroxide and calcium carbonate antacids on the bioavailability of ciprofloxacin. *Antimicrob Agents and Chemotherap* 36(4): 830–832

13 Garrelts JC, Godley PJ, Peterie JD, Gerlach EH, Yakshe CC (1990) Sucralfate significantly reduces ciprofloxacin concentrations in serum. *Antimicrob Agents and Chemother* 34(5): 931–933

14 Sanders CC (1992) Review of preclinical studies of ofloxacin. *Clin Inf Dis* 14: 526–538

15 Sanders WE (1992) Oral ofloxacin: A critical review of the new drug application. *Clin Inf Dis* 14: 539–554

16 Lettieri JT, Rogge MC, Kaiser L, Echols RM, Heller AH (1992) Pharmacokinetic profiles of

ciprofloxacin after single intravenous and oral doses. *Antimicrob Agents and Chemother* 36(5): 993–996
17 Blondeau JM (1999) Expanded acitvity and utility of the new fluoroquinolones: A review. *Clin Ther* 21: 3–40
18 Forrest A, Nix DE, Ballow CH, Goss TF, Birmingham MC, Schentag JJ (1993) Pharmacodynamics of intravenous ciprofloxacin in seriously ill patients. *Antimicrob Agents Chemother* 37: 1073–1081
19 Zhanel GC, Walkty A, Vercaigne L, Karlowsky JA, Embil J, Gin AS, Hoban DJ (1999) The new fluoroquinolones: a critical review. *Can J Infect Dis* 10: 207–234
20 Blum MD, Graham DJ, McClosky CA (1994) Temafloxacin syndrome: review of 95 cases. *Clin Infect Dis* 18: 946–950
21 Carbon C (2001) Comparison of side-effects of levofloxacin *versus* other fluoroquinolones *Chemotherapy* 47 Suppl 3: 9–14
22 Chemotherapy 2001;47 Suppl 3: 3–8; discussion 44–8 History of quinolones and their side-effects. Rubinstein E. Department of Internal Medicine and Unit of Infectious Diseases, Tel Aviv University School of Medicine, Tel Aviv, Israel. unit@netvision.net.il Fluoroquinolone de
23 Chemotherapy 2001;47 Suppl 3: 38–43; discussion 44–8 Latest industry information on the safety profile of levofloxacin in Japan. Yagawa K. Drug Safety Administration Department, Daiichi Pharmaceutical Co., Ltd., Tokyo, Japan
24 Friedlander AM, Welkos SL, Pitt MLM et al (1993) Postexposure prophylaxis against experimental anthrax. *J Infect Dis* 167: 1239–1242

Fluoroquinolone Antibiotics
ed. by A.R. Ronald and D.E. Low

Structure-activity relationships of quinolones

Lester A. Mitscher[1] and Zhenkun Ma[2]

[1] *Medicinal Chemistry Department, Kansas University, 4010 Malott Hall, 1251 Wescoe Hall Drive, Lawrence, KS 66045-7582, USA*
[2] *Cumbre Inc., 1502 Viceroy Drive, Dallas, TX 75235-2304, USA*

Introduction and history

The first of the antiinfective agents belonging to the quinolone class was discovered 50 years ago. Since that time many thousands of analogs have been prepared and nearly two dozen examples have found clinical use. New agents are still being introduced at a significant pace and research continues to be intensive in this area. With the passage of time and the accretion of more and more evidence, a deeper understanding of how these agents work and the structural characteristics required for significant activity and freedom from toxicity has been achieved. The purpose of this chapter is to provide a summary view of the present state of the art. It is important, however, to bear in mind that several surprises have upset our confidence in the generality of conventional wisdom. This has occurred already several times in this therapeutic area and constitutes a warning against uncritical reliance on overinterpreted or generalized beliefs.

The structural and historic relationships between the various clinically used quinolones is set forth in cartoon form in Figure 1. The structures and approximate dates of introduction of these molecules are presented in Figure 2. For comparative purposes, the names and abbreviated antimicrobial spectra of the commercially significant quinolones are tabulated in Table 1. From all this it is apparent that the 4-quinolone and the 1,8-naphthyridine ring systems were intermingled from the outset. This continues to date. The mainline connects nalidixic acid with moxifloxacin and interest in the field became particularly notable with the discovery of norfloxacin. The early agents are of relatively minor modern significance because of limited therapeutic value (primarily against urinary tract infections) and the ease with which bacteria become resistant to them. With the discovery of norfloxacin, potency was enhanced and the spectrum was broadened sufficiently to approximate that of many fermentation-derived agents of continuing interest. With its discovery, the inclusion of C-6 fluorine and C-7 cyclic amines became standard in the field. Norfloxacin was still restricted, however, primarily to the treatment of urinary tract infections caused by Gram-negative microorganisms because oral admin-

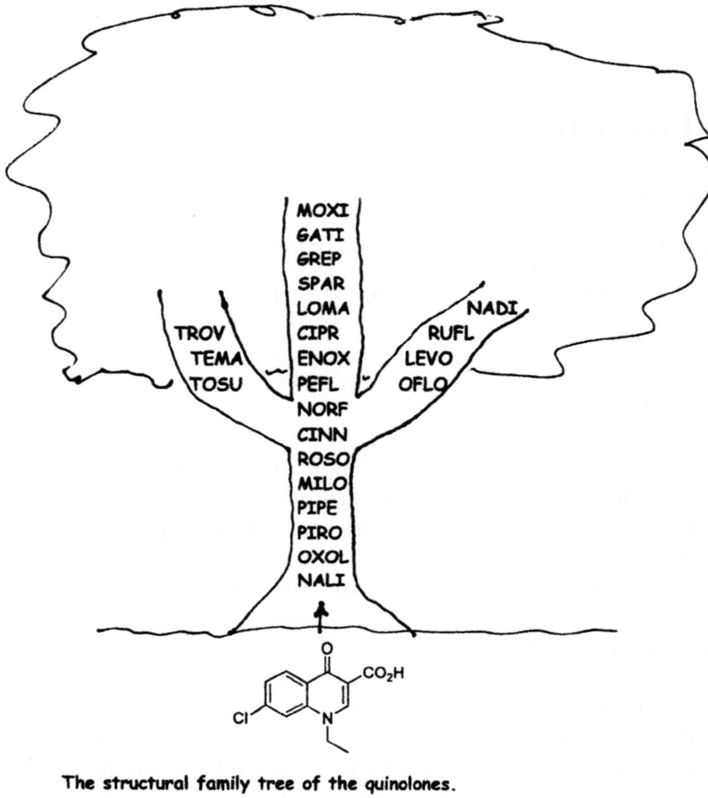

Figure 1. Structural and historical relationships between clinically useful quinolone antiinfective agents.

istration produces comparatively low serum concentrations. With the subsequent discovery of ciprofloxacin and ofloxacin, broad-spectrum general-purpose orally active antiinfective agents were in hand against which resistance develops comparatively slowly. Subsequent developments have resulted in molecules with a shift in emphasis towards treatment of streptococcal infections (levofloxacin, gatifloxacin, clinafloxacin and moxifloxacin, for example), anaerobic (trovafloxacin, gatifloxacin, moxifloxacin, clinafloxacin and sitafloxacin, for example) and resistant microorganisms.

In Figure 1 one can discern two offshoots and a modification in the mainline, each of which required the use of novel chemistry (as did the discovery of ciprofloxacin) and whose members can be used for a wide variety of serious systemic infections. The key structural changes that produced these molecules are the introduction of an N-cyclopropyl group starting with ciprofloxacin and continuing with sparfloxacin, grepafloxacin, gatifloxin and

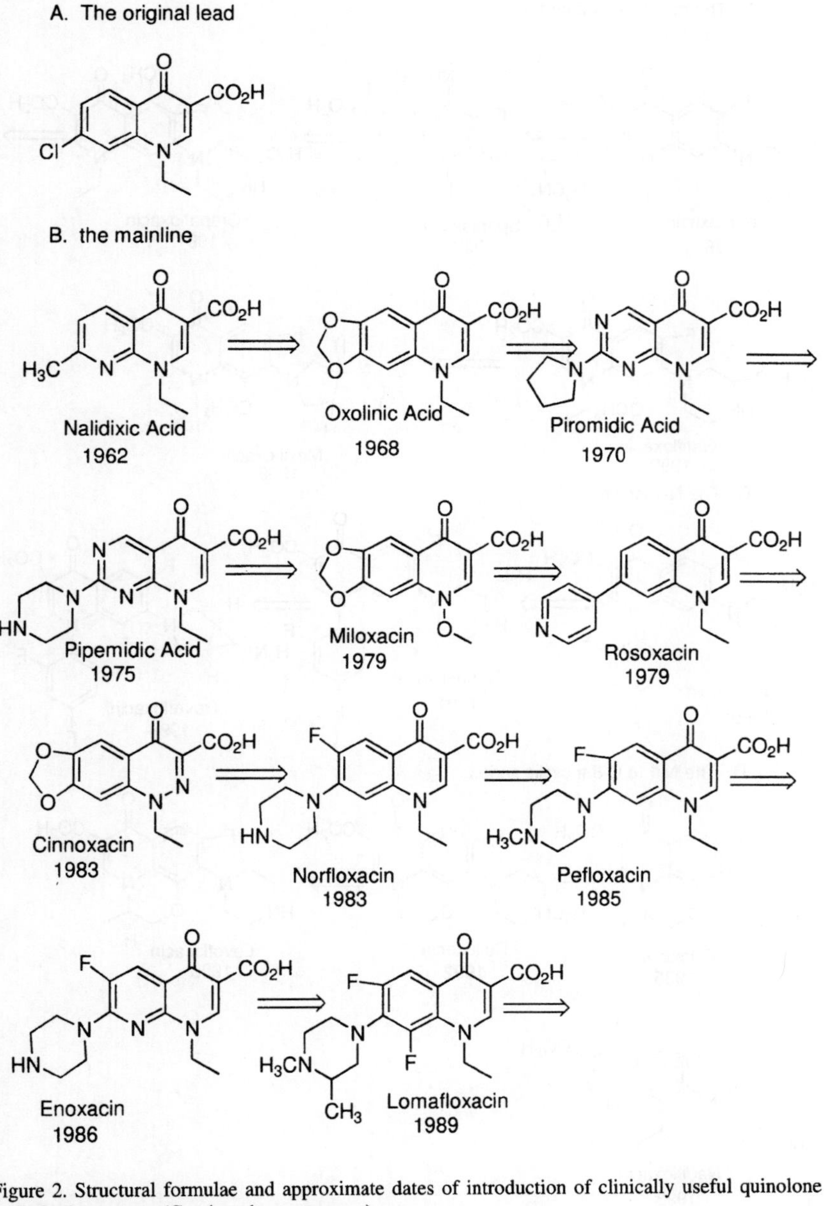

Figure 2. Structural formulae and approximate dates of introduction of clinically useful quinolone antiinfective agents. (Continued on next page)

moxifloxacin; and bridging N-1 to C-8 which lead first to ofloxacin then to levofloxacin, rufloxacin and nadifloxacin. Most recently the N-aryl group has also appeared starting with tosufloxacin then continuing on to temafloxacin

B. The mainline (continued)

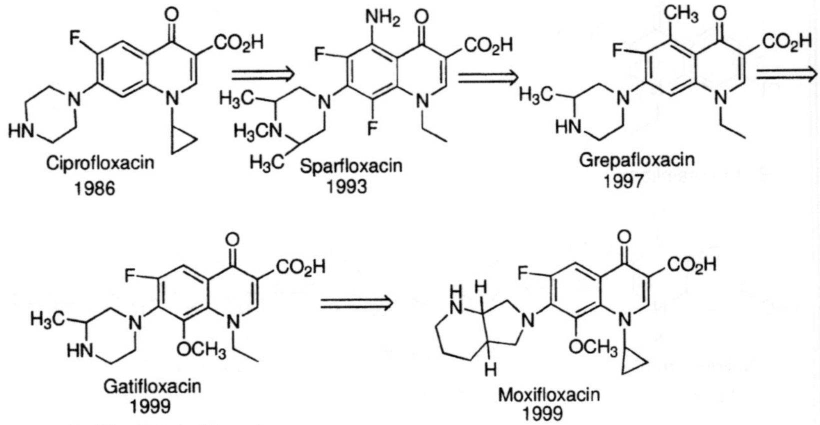

C. The N-1 Aryl branch

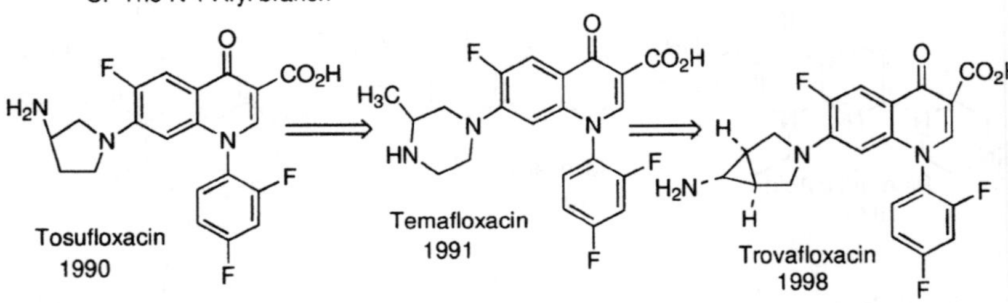

D. The N-1 to C-8 tricyclic series

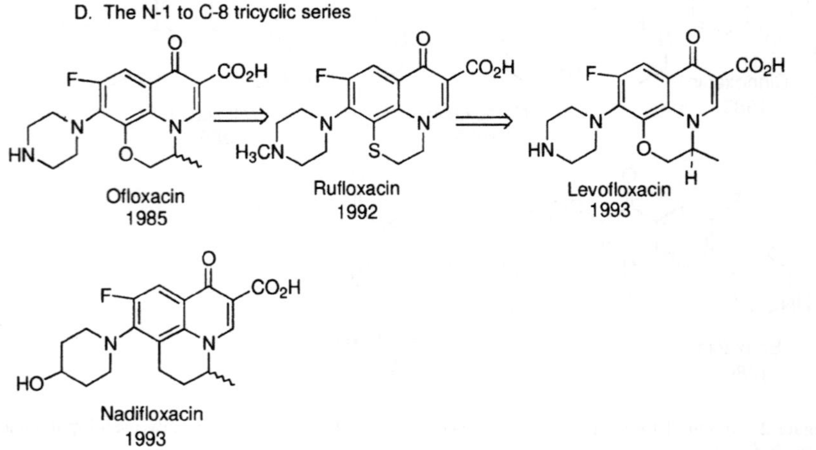

Figure 2. (Continued.)

and trovafloxacin. All three of these series violate the previous consensus that N-1 should be substituted with a small, non-polar substituent.

Table 1. Commercially significant quinolone antiinfective agents with abbreviated *in vitro* antimicrobial spectra

Quinolone	*S. aureus*	*S. pyogenes*	*E. coli*	*Ps. aeruginosa*
Nalidixic acid	>100	>100	6.3	>100
Oxolinic acid	>100	>100	0.2	6.3
Pirimidic acid	50	>100	25	>100
Pipemidic acid	50	>100	1.6	6.3
Miloxacin	6.3	100	0.4	12.5
Rosoxacin	0.4	12.5	0.2	6.3
Cinnoxacin	>100	>100	3.1	>100
Norfloxacin	0.8	1.6	0.025	0.2
Pefloxacin	0.2	0.8	0.025	0.4
Enoxacin [1]	0.39	4.0–8.0	0.05	0.39
Ciprofloxacin	0.1	0.39	0.012	0.05
Lomafloxacin	1.0	8.0	0.12	1.0
Sparfloxacin	0.05	0.39	0.0125	0.39
Grepafloxacin [2]	0.1	0.39	0.1	0.78
Gatifloxacin [3]	0.05	0.16	0.02	0.72
Moxifloxacin [4]	0.03	0.25	0.015	>32
Tosufloxacin	0.05	0.25	0.02	0.2
Temafloxacin [5]	0.06	1.0	0.06	1.0
Trovafloxacin [6]	0.03	0.12	0.02	0.5
Ofloxacin [7]	0.25	2	0.05	2
Levofloxacin	0.12	0.5	0.008	0.12
Rufloxacin [8]	0.78	2.0–8.0	0.78	12.5
Nadifloxacin [9]	0.024	-	0.39	3.13

As will be seen in a later section, the second millenium may see the appearance of novel agents lacking the C-6 fluorine or the 2-pyridones in which the N-1 nitrogen has been exchanged with the C-4a carbon. These latter families are yet to realize their clinical promise but are under intensive investigation. Their potencies are high and they promise to deal with infections resistant to the lesser active present agents.

A brief review of reviews

The first review of the quinolone antiinfectives was that of Albrecht [10] whose conclusions were based upon examination of the properties of the first several hundred analogs. In general, it was asserted that the N-1 substituent should be non-polar, aliphatic and small. No useful alterations were reported at carbons 2–4, little work involved carbons 5 and 8. Changes at carbon 6 were restricted to CH and its bioisosteres (N and S, for example) while significant structural variations were allowed at C-7. Work in the next decade indicated that the restrictions imposed by these teachings on C-1 were premature. Introduction of the cyclopropyl moiety as a profoundly useful change and the finding that N-1 could be bridged to C-8 in the form of a suitably substituted six-membered ring and, further, that the chirality of the group attached to N-1 was important were also key events from a chemical viewpoint. Albrecht had no such examples to draw from and his conclusions actually taught away from some of these useful alterations. More than a dozen reviews of quinolone properties have appeared in the last decade [11–27] and these considerably expand our understanding of the influence of structure and activity in this series and encompass these new beliefs. The reviews appearing in 1990 include primarily the advances of the decade of the 1980s. In the last decade, this trend continues with particular note being the introduction of N-1 aryl substituents. These molecules were unanticipated by Albrecht and were only slightly forecast by the reviews of 1990. Three such substances have now seen clinical use.

Newer substituents such as the tert-butyl moieties at N-1 saw considerable exploration without, however, producing clinically useful examples. Continued examination of novel ring systems, with emphasis on N-1 involvement, saw the double bioisosteric interchange leading to the very potent 2-pyridones. These have seen very extensive evaluation and will be covered by a section of its own in the following.

Near the close of the decade it was found that the nearly ubiquitous C-6 fluorine moiety could be dispensed with if the rest of the ring system were appropriately substituted. This important development reinforces the gathering conviction that there is "cross-talk" through the fused aromatic ring system such that substituent effects are often non-additive and so re-optimization of structures could pay useful benefits.

The realization that the antimicrobial spectrum of the quinolones often involves action against both bacterial DNA gyrase and topoisomerase IV and that toxicity involves action against mammalian topoisomerase II requires the simultaneous manipulation of structure-activity relationships against all three of these enzymes. This makes a difficult job even more difficult. Finding the best compromise among these contending cellular targets suggests that the future will see the introduction of special purpose quinolones rather than a continuing quest for perfection in the form of a single "utopiafloxacin".

Introduction of new targets for (fluoro)quinolones

When the quinolones were first discovered their cellular target was completely unknown so that advances were made entirely empirically. Ultimately, several bacterial and human topoisomerases were discovered and some of these were shown to be the targets of the quinolones. These enzymes have yet to be crystallized although an X-ray structure is available for a large fragment [28]. Thus the specific molecular mode of action of these drugs is as yet based upon hypothesis. These hypothetical proposals have proven to be useful to chemists and have led to the semi-rational design of novel agents of significant value. It was long a puzzle to chemists that it was so hard to develop truly broad spectrum quinolones. An important piece helping to rationalize this conundrum fell into place early in the decade of the 1990s when bacterial topoisomerase IV was discovered [29]. It quickly became apparent that many of the available agents showed activity against both of these enzymes and that whereas anti Gram-negative activity often depended strongly upon activity against DNA gyrase, activity against Gram-positives often particularly involved potency against bacterial topoisomerase IV. A number of the clinically useful molecules possess different blends of action against all three of these enzymes (including human topoisomerase II).

The action of the topoisomerases involves separation of the two strands of double-helical DNA preliminary to enzymic action leading to replication and transcription. The act of separation produces conformational strain (over winding) that can be relieved by cutting the strands, holding on to the cut strands, opening a molecular gate through which the uncut portion of the DNA molecule is passed, and then resealing the molecule in its new, strain free, conformation. Energy in the form of ATP is consumed in this process. DNA gyrase operates within a given DNA molecule whereas topoisomerase IV separates the intertwined (catenated) daughter molecules following replication. The action of both enzymes is essential for access to a cell's DNA and its appropriate functioning. Quinolones bind to form a non-functional ternary complex involving enzyme, substrate and drug that can neither dissociate back to its components nor progress to final products. The consequences are rapidly lethal to the cell. The selective toxicity of quinolones is a consequence of the fact that mammals do not have DNA gyrase but rather have a similarly functioning isoenzyme, mammalian topoisomerase II. The latter enzyme is much less sensitive to the action of the quinolones.

Resistance to the quinolones is due to protein-mediated expulsion of the drugs from bacterial cells and to alterations in the structure of either of the target bacterial enzymes. No indications exist as yet that bacteria are able to inactivate these drugs by altering their structures through enzymatic action.

It is apparent that some quinolones also possess significant activity against human topoisomerase II and that this can lead to unacceptable toxicity. The problem of finding agents with negligable activity against this enzyme but potent activity against the two bacterial enzymes is not going to be easy.

Structure-activity relationships of classical quinolones

The structure-activity relationships of classical quinolones, including both the 4-oxo-1,4-dihydroquinoline and 4-oxo-1,4-dihydronaphthyridine systems, have been extensively reviewed in the past [10–27]. The ring and numbering systems for these two classes are illustrated in Figure 3. In this section, we will emphasize recent developments in this area. Readers should refer to the

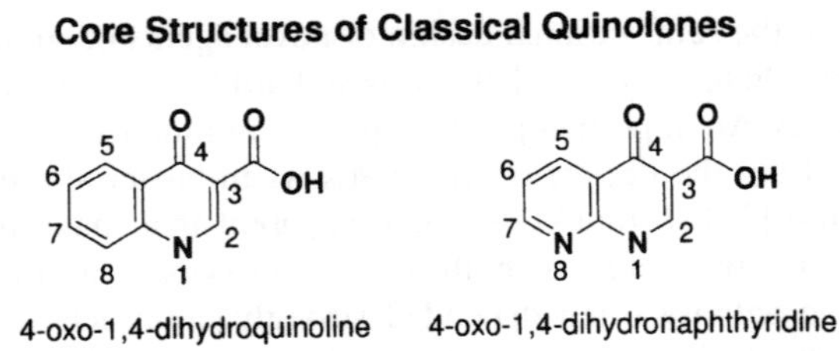

Figure 3. The core structures and numbering systems for the classical quinolone antiinfective agents.

original reviews synopsized in section 2 for more detailed information relating to the structure-activity relationships developed in the early era. The structure-activity relationships of some non-classical quinolones, including 2-pyridones and non-fluorinated quinolones, will be discussed in a separate section below.

Historically, for clarity of discussion, the structure-activity relationships associated with each atom of the core ring systems of the quinolones has been discussed independently. We will continue with this tradition but the reader should keep in mind that the structure-activity relationships for moieties at a particular position are often influenced by substituents at other positions in the molecule. Thus an optimal group at one particular position is meaningful only when it is discussed in context of functional groups at other positions in the molecule. The cause of this phenomenon is usually attributed to the fully aromatic character of the central ring system. Thus electronic influences are readily transmitted through the molecular framework to distant atoms.

Modification of N-1 position

Structure-activity relationship studies in the early era suggested that the optimal groups to be attached to the N-1 position were relatively hydrophobic and relatively small [10]. Only ethyl and a few bioisosteric replacements (such as the methoxy group of miloxacin) were present in the quinolone drugs of the classic era. A few representative examples of the best N-1 moieties known today are ethyl, cyclopropyl, and 2,4-difluorophenyl groups [15]. The N-1 substituent is believed either to be interacting with a hydrophobic pocket in the drug-DNA-enzyme ternary complex, or to be forming a tail-to-tail hydrophobic interaction when the drug binds to DNA gyrase or topoisomerase IV. Recent publications continue to support these notions. Compounds with a hydrophilic group or compounds with bulky substituents at the N-1 position are usually significantly less active than their counterparts with a smaller, hydrophobic N-1 substituent [30–33].

Some novel N-1 groups have been explored recently. The data in Table 2 illustrates that attaching a cis-fluoro group to the cyclopropyl moiety provides a series of analogues with similar antibacterial activity to that of their non-flu-

Table 2. Comparison of *in vitro* MIC and cytotoxicity for quinolones with variation at the N-1 position

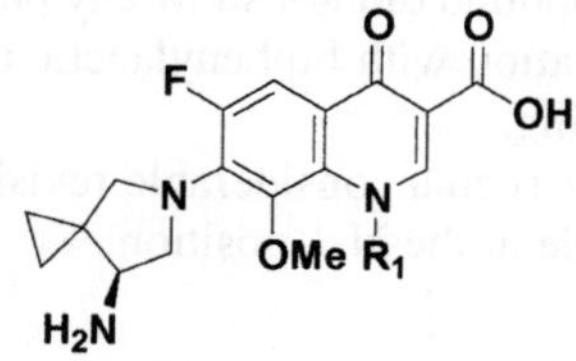

R1	MIC (μg/ml)						Micronucleus test (150 mg/kg)	Ref
	Sa Cip-R	Sa Cip-S	Ef	Spy	Ec	Pa		
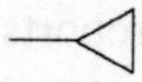	0.015	-	0.12	0.06	<0.004	0.12	Positive	[35]
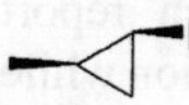	0.008	0.25	0.12	0.06	<0.004	0.12	Negative	[35]
Levofloxacin	0.12	4	1	1	0.008	0.12	-	[35]

orinated counterpart. However, these compounds were less cytotoxic in the micronucleus test in the bone marrow of mice than were their non-fluorinated analogues (Tab. 2) suggesting that they might be safer [34].

Another interesting modification to the N-1 position results from introducing an amino group into the N-1-difluorophenyl functionality or its pyidinyl equivalent. This modification results in a series of analogues with potent antibacterial activity and improved toxicity profiles [35–38]. Table 3 summarizes data for two of these compounds. The N-1 3-amino-2,4-difluorophenyl ana-

Table 3. Comparison of *in vitro* MIC for quinolones with variation at the N-1 position

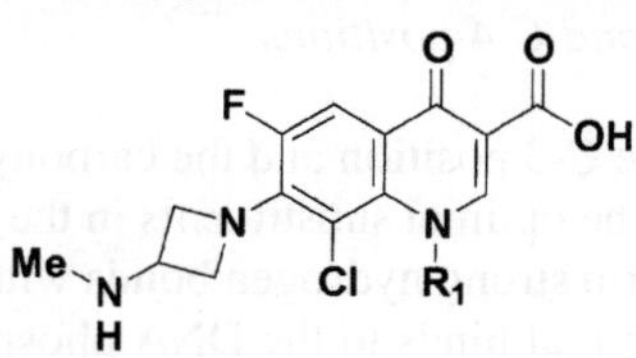

R1	MIC_{90} (μg/ml)					Ref.
	Sa	MRSA	Sp	Ec	Pa	
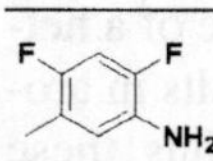	0.025	0.78	0.025	0.025	0.78	[35]
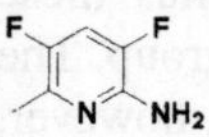	0.05	6.25	0.10	0.025	1.56	[36]
Ciprofloxacin	1.56	>100	6.25	0.05	6.25	[36]

logue was highly efficacious in murine subcutaneous and respiratory tract infection models. The compound did not show any phototoxicity or convulsive activity upon co-administration with biphenylacetic acid in mice. The pyridyl analogue was less interesting.

Thus the last decade has seen a considerable revision of thought relating to the groups that are tolerable at the N-1 position.

Modification of C-2 position

Classically only small substituents (such as the position 2-nitrogen atom of cinnoxacin) or, alternatively, only when a larger group is cyclized to the N-1 or C-3 position, are consistent with significant activity. There are a few recent reports detailing attempts at modification of the C-2 position. One such report describes the attachment of a methyl or a phenyl group to the C-2 position while leaving the N-1 position unsubstituted. The authors report that these compounds showed interesting activity against both Gram-positive and Gram-negative bacteria although this was slightly weaker than with norfloxacin [39]. The unexpected activity of these compounds is clearly against the conventional wisdom based upon previous work. Table 3 illustrates that when a sulfur substituent is linked to the N-1 position to form a four-membered ring, compounds with potent activity can be obtained [40–41]. The stereochemistry of the bridge substituent appears to be very important to the antibacterial activity. The (–)-isomer of the fluoromethyl analogue showed two to 64-fold better activity than the (+)-isomer. This suggests that the C-2 position is in comparatively close contact with a significant molecular feature in the ternary complex and is reminiscent of the situation with analogous isomerism of ofloxacin derivatives.

Modification of the C-3 and C-4 positions

The carboxyl group at the C-3 position and the carbonyl group at the C-4 position were established as the optimal substituents in the classical era. These two groups are believed to form strong hydrogen bonds with DNA bases or to coordinate to a Mg (II) cation that binds to the DNA phosphate backbone. Both of these theories have current adherents. Additional studies indicate that replacement of the carboxylic acid with certain functional groups that allow the formation of an anion at physiological pH can also provide compounds with potent antibacterial activity. Such groups usually require the presence of a heterocycle fused to the C-2 and C-3 positions such that enolizaton results in aromaticity and this serves as the driving force for the deprotonation. Thus, these groups can be regarded functionally as surrogates for the carboxyl group. The resulting ring system is also planar in this region. The ring system, however, can attack DNA through intercalation so these compounds are too toxic to find use as antibacterial agents.

Table 4. Comparison of *in vitro* MIC for quinolones with variation at the C-2 position

R1, R2	MIC (μg/ml)					Ref.
	Sa	MRSA	Ef	Ec	Pa	
$—CH_3$	0.05	1.56	0.2	0.025	0.2	[41]
$=CH_2$	0.05	0.39	0.2	0.12	0.39	[41]
$—CH_3F$	0.1	1.56	0.39	0.05	0.39	[40]
$—CH_3F$ (+)-isomer	0.2	50	3.13	0.1	0.78	[40]
$—CH_3F$ (–)-isomer	0.05	0.78	0.2	0.0125	0.2	[40]
Ciprofloxacin	0.1	12.5	0.39	0.012	0.05	[41]

Some unconventional modifications in which the carboxyl group is replaced with an unrelated functionality, such as an alkyl group, have also resulted in some potent gyrase inhibitors. However, the selectivity between DNA gyrase and mammalian topoisomerase II has been diminished by these modifications so one presumes that these substances will be toxic to mammals. Other modifications, such as replacement by esters, amides or a primary alcohol function show some activity *in vivo*, but not *in vitro*, indicating that these moieties must be converted by metabolism to a carboxy group and so these are thought of as prodrugs.

Altogether, then, modifications at the C-3 or C-4 position have been unrewarding.

Modification of the C-5 position

Most of the potent quinolones are unsubstituted at this position. Certain relatively small groups such as amino, hydroxyl and methyl have been shown to enhance antibacterial activity with certain substituent combinations at other positions. For example, both sparfloxacin and grepafloxacin possess such molecular features and have found clinical application. The precise role of the C-5 substituent is unclear since widely different hydrophobic and hydrophilic groups with and without hydrogen-bonding capabilities are allowed at this position. No significant recent developments have appeared involving this position.

Modification of the C-6 position

The original quinolones were often unsubstituted at the C-6 position and were weakly active compared to present day analogs. Introduction of a fluorine substituent to the C-6 position significantly enhanced the antibacterial activity and pharmacological properties of quinolones. Since the introduction of norfloxacin, for example, in 1983, the dominant position of the fluoroquinolones has been firmly established. All analogues introduced commercially since that time retain this molecular feature. It has become almost an article of faith that a fluorine at the C-6 position is essential in order to maintain potent antibacterial activity for quinolones and this is underscored by the class name fluoroquinolones now almost universally used to characterize these important drugs. The dominant position of the fluoroquinolones is further demonstrated by noting that the majority of the quinolones in present clinical development are fluoroquinolones. However, this landscape has been challenged recently by the potential "reintroduction" of non-fluorinated quinolones. It was recently demonstrated that the beneficial properties of a fluoro group are totally dependent on the nature of the other substituents in the molecule. With certain structural combinations, the non-fluorinated quinolones are actually more advantageous. This observation further emphasizes the caution that the structure-activity relationships of a particular group are quite often dependent on the nature of other contributing groups in the molecule. Several non-fluorinated quinolones are currently in various stages of development and this topic will be discussed in detail in a later section. One rationalizes this striking development by assuming that the favorable molecular contribution of the C-6 fluorine atom to bioactivity and pharmacokinetics can also be provided by suitable contributions of other functions in the molecule. When these are present, one has gotten all the mileage available and the addition of a fluorine atom to C-6 does not contribute to a measurable further increase.

Table 5 illustrates that the effect of an amino group at the C-6 position is dependent upon the structure of the C-8 group present [42]. When the C-8 position is unsubstituted, 6-amino analogues are significantly less active than the corresponding 6-fluoro compounds. However, when the C-8 position is occupied by a methyl group, the 6-amino analogue is almost as active as the corresponding 6-fluoro compound. The 6-nitro analogues are much less active than the amino

Table 5. Comparison of *in vitro* MIC for quinolones with variation at the C-6 position

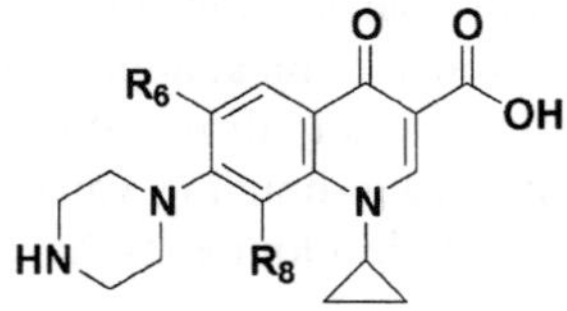

R6	R8	MIC (μg/ml)				Ref.
		Sa ATCC6538	Sf LEP Br	Ec ATCC8739	Pa ATCC9027	
—F	—H	0.06	0.5	0.015	0.06	[42]
$—NH_2$	—H	2	32	0.25	4	[42]
—F	$—CH_3$	0.06	1	0.03	2	[42]
$—NH_2$	$—CH_3$	0.5	4	0.03	2	[42]
$—NO_2$	$—CH_3$	4	16	16	64	[42]

Table 6. Comparison of *in vitro* MIC for quinolones with variation at the C-4 and C-6 position

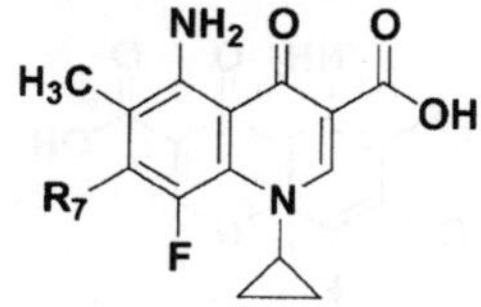

R7	MIC (μg/ml)				Ref.
	Sa 6538	Sa 241	Ec 851E	Pa 1012E	
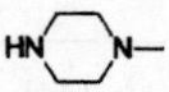	0.25	16	0.031	1	[43]
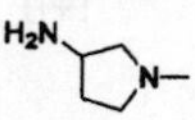	0.25	8	0.13	1	[43]
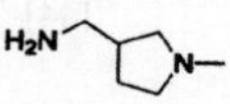	0.031	8	0.063	1	[43]
Ciprofloxacin	0.13	128	0.016	0.13	[43]

analogues. Table 6 shows that compounds with a methyl group at the C-6 position, in combination with other modifications at the C-5 and C-8 positions, are as potent as ciprofloxacin, particularly against Gram-positive bacteria [43].

Modification of the C-7 position

Position 7 is the most extensively studied among all the positions of the quinolones. Variation at this position often results in significant changes to the physicochemical properties and antibacterial potency of the resulting molecule. Unlike any other position, great structural variability is allowed here with maintenance of potent activity. Thus, modification of this position has been widely utilized by quinolone researchers to optimize potency and to manipulate the pharmacokinetic profile after a potent core with appropriate substitutions at other positions has been established. Given the interdependence of functional groups noted in various places earlier, this may now be considered to be a risky practice. Nonetheless, it has recently been recognized that modification of this position can also help to improve the selectivity of inhibition between eukaryotic topoisomerase II and DNA gyrase and thus enhance apparent safety [44]. Table 7 illustrates that introduction of methyl groups in the C-7 piperazine ring dramatically reduces the eukaryotic topoisomerase II mediated DNA cleavage activity, while the gyrase activity was relatively unchanged. Commercial drugs with this type of substituent include lomafloxacin, sparfloxacin, grepafloxacin, and gatifloxacin. In this context, temafloxacin would appear to be an exception.

Table 7. Structure of the C-7 group and activity for inducing DNA gyrase and eukaryotic topoisomerase II mediated DNA cleavage

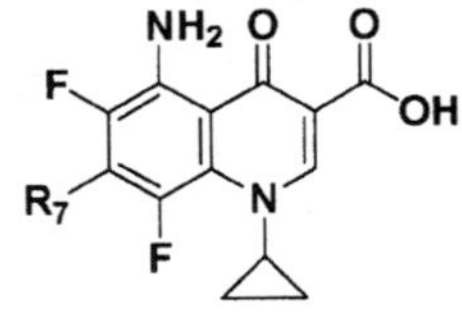

R7	MIC (µg/ml)		Ref.
	Calf thymus topo II CC_{50} (µM)	*E. coli* DNA gyrase cleavage endpoint CC_{50} (µM)	
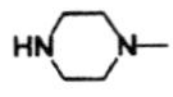	83	0.52	[44]
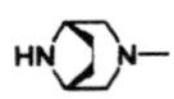	75	0.48	[44]
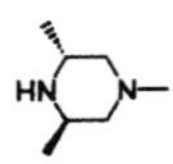	658	0.48	[44]
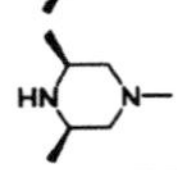	>2000	0.48	[44]

Although the C-7 position can be substituted with a comparatively wide range of moieties with retention of potency, the optimal substituents are most frequently basic amino derivatives of piperidine, piperazine or pyrrolidine. Almost all the quinolones in contemporary clinical use or in clinical development possess a C-7 substituent of this general type. However, it is important to remember that the optimal structure at this and at other positions are dependent on the core quinolone structure as well as on the other substituents around the molecule. Table 8 summarizes the effect of variations in the N-1 substituent upon C-7 structure-activity relationships [45]. From the data it is apparent that activity against Gram-positive and Gram-negative bacteria follow different trends. The methylaminopyrrolidine moiety is always the best group for activity against Gram-positive bacteria regardless of the N-1 structure, while piperazine is often the best group for activity against Gram-negative bacteria. A pyrrolidine group, however, tends to give balanced activity between both Gram-positive and Gram-negative organisms. The molecular rationale for this effect is obscure but surely depends heavily upon the fact that anti Gram-positive activity depends more upon inhibition of the action of topoisomerase IV and anti Gram-negative activity depends primarily upon inhibition of the action of DNA gyrase. It can be assumed that the drug-binding pocket in these two enzymes is similar but not identical. This would rationalize these findings.

A significant amount of work has been directed to the modification of the C-7 position recently for the purpose of improving Gram-positive activity and

Table 8. Comparison of *in vitro* MIC for quinolones with variation at the C-7 position

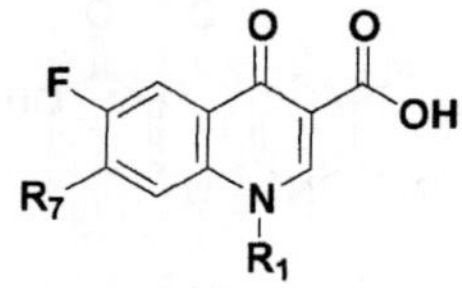

R1	R7	MIC (μg/ml)				Ref.
		Sa H-228	Spy C203	Ec Vogel	Pa U1-18	
	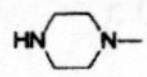	0.8	0.4	0.05	0.2	[45]
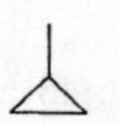	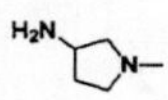	0.4	0.8	0.05	0.2	[45]
	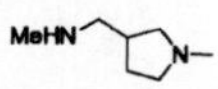	0.2	0.1	0.2	0.8	[45]
	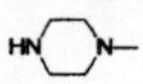	0.4	0.4	0.1	0.2	[45]
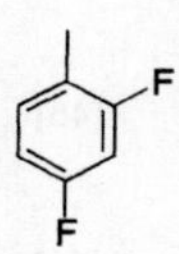	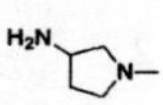	0.05	0.1	0.03	0.2	[45]
	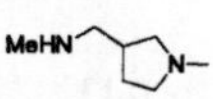	0.1	0.1	0.2	0.8	[45]
	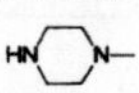	3.1	>3.1	0.1	0.8	[45]
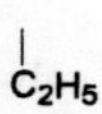	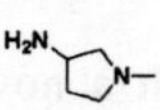	1.6	0.8	0.4	0.8	[45]
	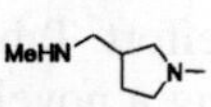	1.6	0.4	3.1	>3.1	[45]
	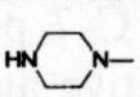	0.8	1.6	0.2	0.4	[45]
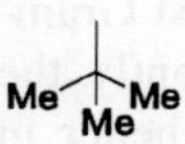	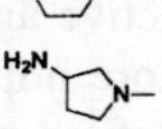	0.4	0.4	0.2	0.4	[45]
	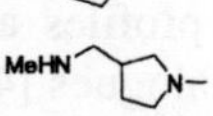	0.2	0.2	0.4	1.6	[45]
	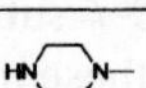	>3.1	>3.1	0.8	1.6	[45]
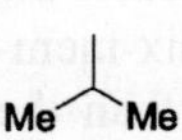	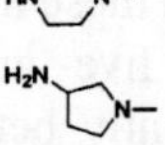	3.1	>3.1	0.8	1.6	[45]
	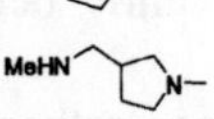	3.1	3.1	3.1	>3.1	[45]
	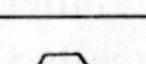	3.1	>3.1	0.4	1.6	[45]
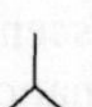	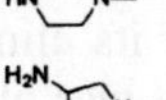	3.1	1.6	0.4	1.6	[45]
	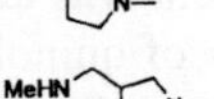	0.8	1.6	0.8	3.1	[45]
Sparfloxacin		0.05	0.1	0.025	0.8	[45]

Table 9. Comparison of *in vitro* MIC for naphthyridones with a novel C-7 substituent

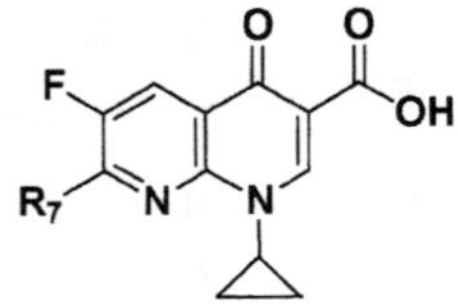

R7	MIC (μg/ml)				Ref.
	Sa Cip-S	Sa Cip-R	Ec 3190Y	Pa 1912E	
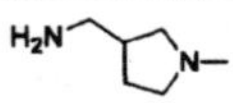	0.031	16	0.031	0.5	[46]
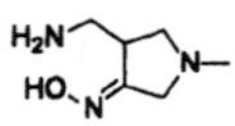	0.031	8	0.031	2	[46]
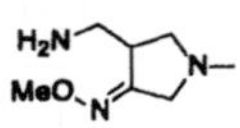	<0.008	4	<0.008	0.25	[46]
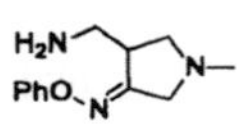	0.016	<0.008	0.031	2	[46]
Ciprofloxacin	0.13	64	0.016	0.13	[46]

overcoming quinolone-resistance. Many compounds with a novel C-7 substituent have consequently been identified through this effort. Table 9 summarizes the findings with a series of naphthyridones having a novel oxime-substituted (aminomethyl) pyrrolidine group attached to the C-7 position [46]. Some of these oxime-containing compounds are highly active against Gram-positive bacteria, including quinolone-resistant strains. More importantly, the oxime derivative provides improved pharmacokinetic profiles and better *in vivo* efficacies than do the corresponding non-oxime analogues [46].

2-Aminomethyl-1-azetidine represents another novel C-7 substituent that provides potent antibacterial activity [10]. It is clear that in these molecules the four-membered ring analogues are more active than the five- and six-membered ring analogues and that the R-isomer is significantly better than the S-isomer [47].

Some unconventional substituents with a C–C linkage rather than a N-C linkage at C-7 have also been explored recently. It will be recalled that this feature was present in nalidixic acid but only rosoxacin, of its clinical descendants, retained this type of linkage and that its substituent was also aromatic. Table 11 summarizes the relevant properties of a series of quinolones substituted with various aminoalkyl groups at the C-7 position [48]. The aminocyclopropyl analogue is the most potent compound and the activity decreases with the increase in size of the ring. These compounds showed less cytotoxic-

Table 10. Comparison of *in vitro* MIC for quinolones with a novel C-7 structure

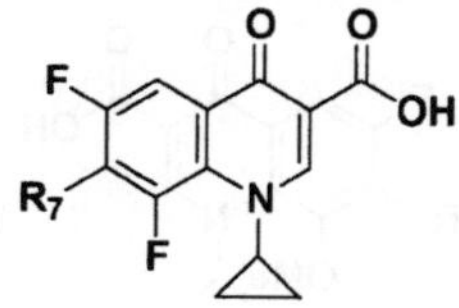

R7	MIC (μg/ml)			Ref.
	Sa 209P	Ec NIHJ	Pa 12	
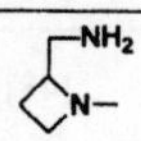	0.05	0.0125	0.1	[47]
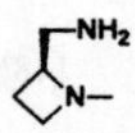	0.025	<0.003	0.1	[47]
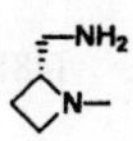	0.78	0.2	6.25	[47]
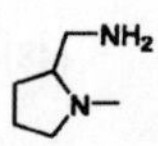	0.1	0.025	0.39	[47]
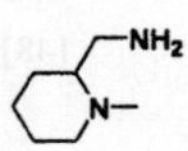	0.1	0.1	1.56	[47]
Sparfloxacin	0.05	0.0125	0.39	[47]

ity than ciprofloxacin and little differentiation between the susceptible and MRSA activities.

Table 12 presents the properties of another group of compounds with C–C linked substituents attached to the C-7 position [49]. As one can see from the table that the most potent compounds in the series are about two dilutions weaker on average than sparfloxacin.

Modification of the C-8 position

The C-8 position allows some useful structural variations provided that the groups involved are relatively small and hydrophobic. The most commonly studied groups at this position are –H, –F, –Cl, -Me, and -OMe. The effect of these groups on antibacterial potency and on some side-effects is profound. The data in Table 13 indicates that the contribution of the C-8 group to antibacterial activity is dependent upon the substituent at the N-1 position [50]. When the N-1 group is cyclopropyl, the relative rank order from the most potent to the least potent is C–OMe > C–F > N. When the N-1 group is 2,4-difluorophenyl, the relative rank order is N > C–F > C–OMe. Table 14

Table 11. Comparison of *in vitro* MIC and cytotoxicity for quinolones with an aminoalkyl substituent

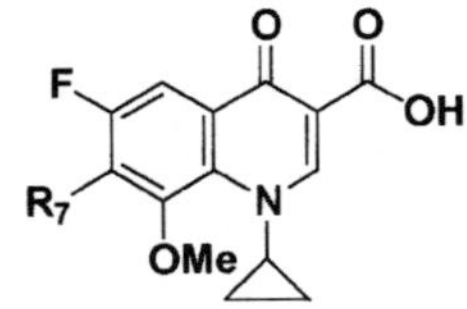

R7	MIC (μg/ml)				Cytotoxicity (μg/ml)	Ref
	Sa 209P	MRSA	Ec NIHJ	Pa CSJ		[48]
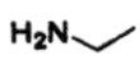	12.5	50	0.39	6.25	615	[48]
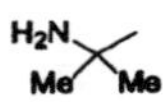	12.5	50	0.78	25	358	[48]
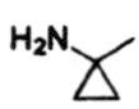	0.2	0.2	0.1	3.13	378	[48]
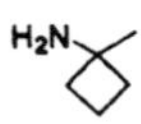	0.78	0.78	0.2	12.5	126	[48]
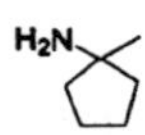	1.56	1.56	0.39	6.25	253	[48]
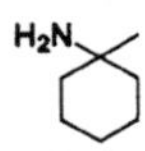	12.5	12.5	3.13	25	>800	[48]
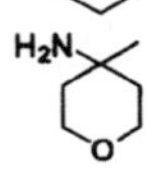	3.13	6.25	1.56	50	>800	[48]
Ciprofloxacin	0.1	12.5	<0.013	0.39	57	[48]

summarizes the data for another series of compounds with C-8 variations [51]. The rank order for potency is C–Cl = C–OMe > C–F = C–OEt > C–H > N. The C-8 methoxy analogue has been shown to have potent activity against Gram-positive bacteria and reduced phototoxicity as compared to the C-8 halogen analogues [52]. Table 15 contains another series of compounds differing in C-7 substituents [53–54]. Among these compounds, the C–F analogue is most active followed by the C–OMe and C–Cl analogues, and the C–H and N analogues are the weakest.

Table 16 shows that the C-8 methyl analogue of the 6-aminoquinolones is as active as the C-8 methoxy compound [55]. The ethyl analogue, however, is substantially weaker.

These findings have been rationalized as resulting from steric interactions between the C-8 and N-1 substituents causing a change in planarity of the ring system. This effect is particularly prominent in the 2-pyridone series covered in a section below.

Table 12. Comparison of *in vitro* MIC values for quinolones with a C–C linked C-7 substituent

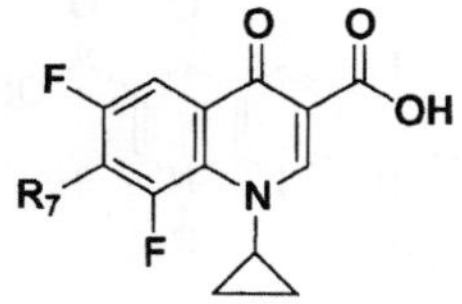

R7	MIC (μg/ml)			Ref.
	Sa 209P	Ec NIHJ	Pa 12	
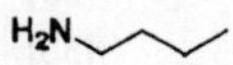	0.2	0.05	0.39	[49]
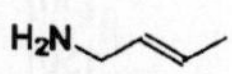	0.39	0.025	0.39	[49]
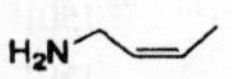	0.39	0.025	0.2	[49]
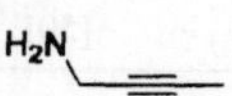	0.39	0.025	0.78	[49]
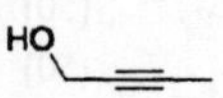	3.31	1.56	100	[49]
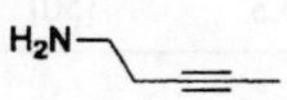	0.39	0.05	0.78	[49]
Sparfloxacin	0.05	0.0125	0.39	[49]

Novel structures targeting DNA gyrase and topoisomerase IV

Since the introduction of nalidixic acid in 1967, a substantial amount of work has been devoted to the replacement of the 4-naphthyridinone ring system. Over the years, the 4-quinolone ring system has emerged as the consentually optimal core for antibacterial activity. Recent chemical activity consequently has been centered upon providing incremental improvements of the 4-quinolone structure. However, development of novel core systems represents a very appealing strategy. Today this is more than ever attractive, despite the high risk involved with this kind of operation. This approach can effectively address the patentability issues associated with this presently very crowded research area and can provide compounds with higher potential to overcome the emergence of quinolone resistance. The most significant new core systems developed recently are the 2-pyridone and non-fluoroquinolone systems.

2-Pyridones

2-Pyridones are nitrogen translocation products of 4-oxo-1,4-dihydroquinolines or 4-oxo-1,4-dihydronaphthyridines so are double bioisosteres of the

Table 13. Comparison of *in vitro* MIC for quinolones with a various C-8 structure

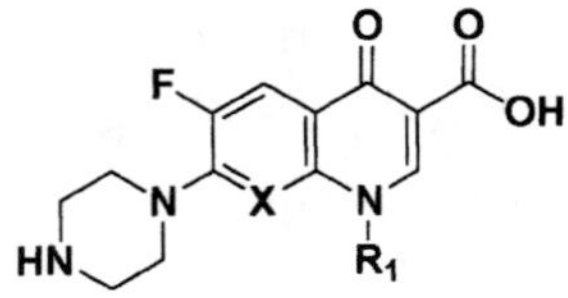

R1	X	MIC (μg/ml)				Ref.
		Sa H-228	Spy C203	Ec Vogel	Pa UI-18	
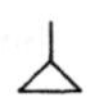	C—H	0.8	0.4	0.05	0.2	[50]
	N	1.6	1.6	0.05	0.2	[50]
	C—F	0.4	0.8	0.05	0.2	[50]
	C—Cl	0.1	0.4	0.05	0.2	[50]
	C—OMe	0.2	0.2	0.05	0.4	[50]
	C—OEt	0.4	0.8	0.1	1.6	[50]
	C—CF_3	0.4	0.8	0.1	1.6	[50]
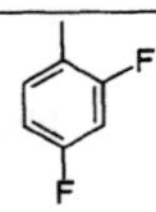	N	0.4	0.8	0.1	0.4	[50]
	C—F	3.1	0.16	0.2	1.6	[50]
	C—OMe	0.4	>3.1	0.2	0.8	[50]

Table 14. Comparison of *in vitro* MIC for quinolones with C-8 variation

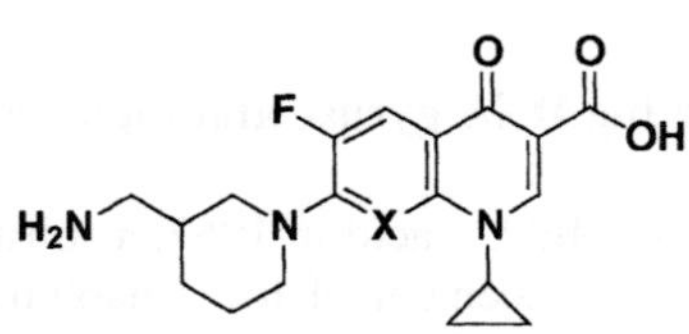

X	MIC (μg/ml)				Ref.
	Sa H228	Spy C203	Ec Vogel	Pa UI-18	
C—H	0.8	0.05	0.4	3.1	[51]
N	1.6	0.2	0.4	6.3	[51]
C—F	0.1	0.013	0.05	0.4	[51]
C—Cl	0.025	0.003	0.1	1.6	[51]
C—Ome	0.05	0.006	0.2	3.1	[51]
C—Oet	0.05	0.025	0.2	3.1	[51]
Ciprofloxacin	3.1	0.8	0.05	0.4	[51]

Table 15. Comparison of *in vitro* MIC for quinolones with C-8 variation

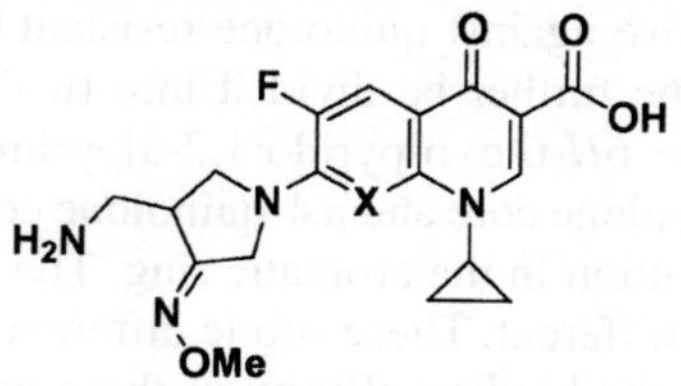

X	MIC (μg/ml)				Ref.
	Sa Cip-S	Sa Cip-R	Ec 10536	Pa 1012E	
C—H	0.008	4	<0.008	0.25	[53]
N	<0.008	4	<0.008	0.25	[53]
C—F	<0.008	0.5	<0.008	0.25	[53]
C—Cl	0.031	1	0.031	1	[53]
C—Ome	0.031	1	0.063	2	[53]
Ciprofloxacin	0.13	64	0.016	0.13	[53]

Table 16. Comparison of *in vitro* MIC values for quinolones with various C-8 substituents

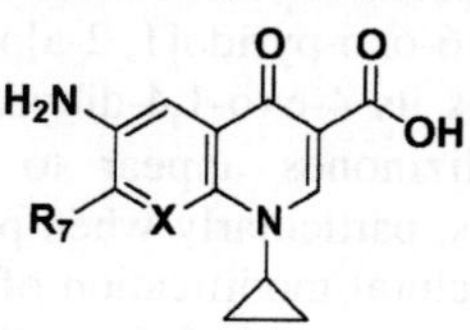

R7	X	MIC (μg/ml)				Ref.
		Sa Cip-S	Sa Cip-R	Ec 25922	Pa 9027	
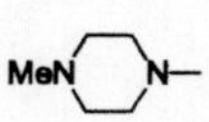	C—Me	1	>16	0.03	2	[55]
	C—Et	>16	>16	>16	>16	[55]
	C—OMe	2	>16	0.125	1	[55]
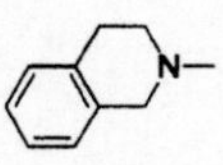	C—Me	<0.016	2	0.125	8	[55]
	C—Et	4	>16	16	>16	[55]
	C—OMe	<0.016	2	0.25	16	[55]
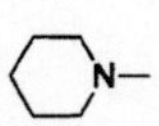	C—Me	0.06	8	0.125	4	[55]
	C—Et	8	>16	16	>16	[55]
	C—OMe	0.06	16	0.5	8	[55]
Ciprofloxacin		0.5	>16	<0.016	0.06	[55]

4-quinolones [56]. They were first reported in 1996 to be potent gyrase inhibitors and to be active against quinolone-resistant Gram-positive bacteria [57]. 2-Pyridones can be further be divided into two sub-classes, the *4H*-4-oxoquinolizines and the *6H*-6-oxo-pyrido[1,2-a]pyrimidines. The major difference between a 2-pyridone core and a 4-quinolone core is the apparent alteration in electron distribution in the aromatic ring. The geometries of the molecules are also slightly different. These subtle differences appear to be enough to impact favorably on the binding affinity of these molecules to their molecular targets and to make the 2-pyridones more active against mutationally resistant strains. The chemical formulae and numbering systems for these materials are illustrated in Figure 4. It is important to note that the alteration in the ring system changes the numbering system of the atoms from that used in the 4-pyridones.

2-Pyridones are potent inhibitors of bacterial type II DNA topoisomerases, which include two highly homologous enzymes – DNA gyrase and topoisomerase IV. In Gram-negative bacteria, DNA gyrase is the main target for 2-pyridones [58]; in Gram-positive bacteria, both DNA gyrase and topoisomerase IV are often equally important [59]. 2-Pyridones are significantly more active against resistant DNA gyrase and topoisomerase IV (Tab. 17) than are their quinolone counterparts.

Comparing the two 2-pyridone cores, the 4-oxoquinolizine ring system is clearly more active than the 6-oxo-pyrido[1, 2-a]pyrimidine system. The latter is about equally active as is its 4-oxo-1,4-dihydronaphthyridine bioisostere, however, the 4-oxoquinolizinones appear to be more active than the 4-oxo-1,4-dihydroquinolines, particularly when position 9 is substituted with a methyl group. So far structural modification of the 2-pyridone ring system has been performed only at positions 1, 6, 8 and 9. The structure-activity rela-

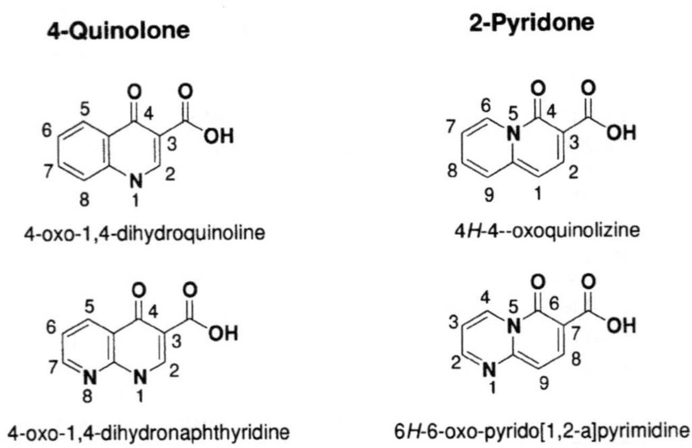

Figure 4. Comparison of the structural formulae and numbering systems of the 4-quinolone and 4-naphthyridinone systems with the corresponding 2-quinolone and 2-naphthyridinone systems.

Table 17. Comparison of DNA cleavage activity of ABT-719 and ciprofloxacin against purified type II DNA topoisomerases

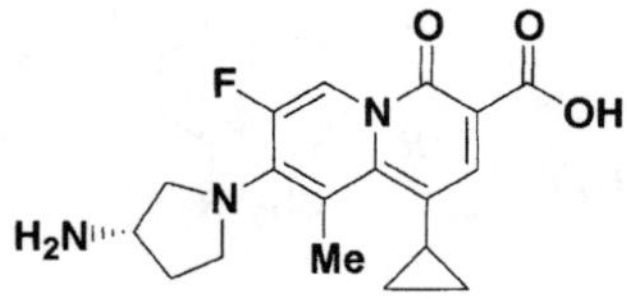

Compound	CC50 (μg/ml)					
	Sa gyrase	Sa Topo IV	Ec gyrase	Ec Topo IV	R-Ec gyrase	R-Ec Topo IV
ABT-719	0.05	0.024	0.02	2.2	1.2	3.4
Ciprofloxacin	3.5	0.18	0.1	9.6	300	190

tionships for the 2-pyridones are in general agreement with those of the classical 4-quinolones although with some subtle but important differences.

Position 1. Table 18 illustrates that the moiety at position 1 is critical for potent antibacterial activity. Among the various groups introduced, compounds with a small and lipophilic group at position 1 are most active. As with the quinolone series, 2-pyridones with a cyclopropyl or a 2,4-difluorophenyl group at position 1 appear to be optimal [57, 60]. Also, as with the quinolones, compounds without a substituent or with a polar group at position 1 are substantially less active.

Position 6. Modification at position 6 in this new series has not been extensively studied. The only substituent introduced at this position to date is a methyl group. The product compares unfavorably with the corresponding unsubstituted analogue (Tab. 19) [57].

Position 8. The substituents at the C-7 of traditional quinolones are believed to interact directly with DNA gyrase and topoisomerase IV. The moiety at this position is not only important for attaining potent antibacterial activities, but also is important for differentiating between bacterial and eukaryotic targets. In addition, modification of this position can be used for obtaining desirable physicochemical properties, enhancing pharmacokinetics, *in vivo* efficacy and safety/tolerability profiles. As in the quinolone system, the corresponding position 8 of 2-pyridones has been most thoroughly studied. Thus far several hundreds of 2-pyridone analogues with a variety of different types of amine substituents, constituting various steric and electronic situations have been prepared and evaluated [61]. The structure-activity relationships for this position are similar to that of the traditional fluoroquinolones in that aminopyrro-

Table 18. Comparison of *in vitro* MIC values for 2-pyridones with various C-1 substituents

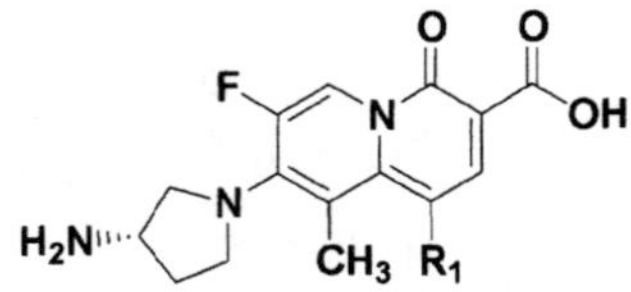

R1	MIC (μg/ml)							Ref.
	Sa Cip-S	Sa Cip-R	Ef	Sb	Spy	Ec	Pa	
—H	3.1	>100	25	50	12.5	0.39	3.1	[60]
—Me	0.05	>100	0.39	1.56	0.39	0.02	0.1	[60]
—Et	0.1	12.5	0.2	0.78	0.39	0.01	0.2	[57]
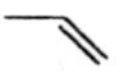	0.78	>100	1.56	6.2	3.1	0.2	0.78	[60]
—Pr^i	0.1	6.2	0.2	0.39	0.2	0.39	0.78	[60]
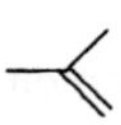	0.1	12.5	0.39	3.1	-	0.05	0.78	[60]
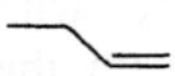	0.78	>100	1.56	6.2	6.2	1.56	0.78	[60]
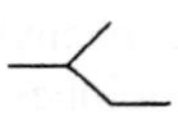	6.2	>100	12.5	>100	50	1.56	50	[60]
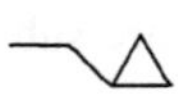	1.56	25	6.2	6.2	6.2	0.78	6.2	[60]
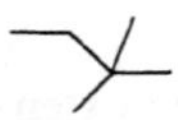	1.56	50	6.2	3.1	3.1	-	12.5	[60]
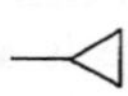	0.01	0.78	0.02	0.02	0.02	0.002	0.05	[60]
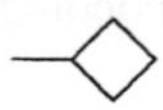	0.1	12.5	0.39	1.56	0.78	0.05	0.78	[60]
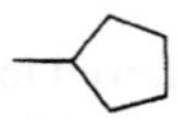	3.1	50	12.5	12.5	12.5	0.78	12.5	[60]
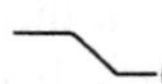 OMe	50	>100	>100	>100	-	12.5	50	[60]
Ciprofloxacin	0.39	>100	0.78	0.78	0.78	0.02	0.2	[60]

lidine substituents have provided the most potent antibacterial activity. The structure-activity relationships of this position have been comprehensively reviewed [56].

The effect of the stereochemistry at position 8 on bioactivity has also been studied in detail [61]. Table 20 illustrates that the potency difference between

Table 19. Comparison of *in vitro* MIC values for 2-pyridones with C-6 modifications

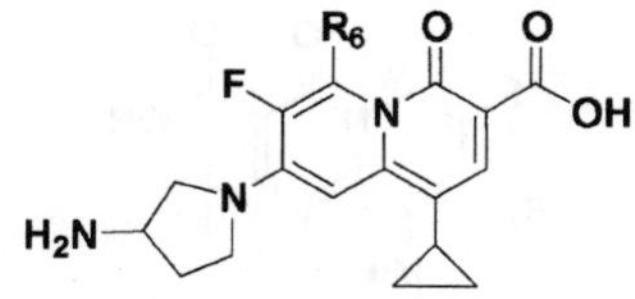

R6	MIC (µg/ml)							Ref.
	Sa Cip-S	Sa Cip-R	Ef	Sb	Spy	Ec	Pa	
—H	0.05	12.5	0.2	0.2	0.2	0.005	0.1	[15]
—Me	0.78	50	6.2	6.2	3.1	0.2	1.56	[14]
Ciprofloxacin	0.39	>100	0.78	0.78	0.78	0.02	0.2	[14]

the two enantiomers is unsubstantial lying within one-dilution difference in most cases. But, in some special cases, the differences appear to be significant. For example, the (*S*)-enantiomer of the 3-hydroxypyrrolidine substituted 2-pyridone is two to four fold more potent than the (*R*)-enantiomer and the (3*S*,4*R*)-enantiomer of the 3-methylamino-4-methylpyrollidine derivative is two to 15 fold more potent than the (3*R*,4*S*)-enantiomer. From the available data, it is very difficult to generalize what kind of group makes the activity of the compound sensitive to chirality.

Position 9. Groups at position 9 are critical for achieving potent antibacterial activity in the 2-pyridones. Table 5.1.5 summarizes the *in vitro* antibacterial activity of six 9-position analogues revealed to date. The structure-activity relationships for this position are somewhat different from those derived for the quinolone series. Unlike the quinolone series, introduction of a fluorine or chlorine group at this position does not improve the *in vitro* activity. However, introduction of a methyl group to this position provided compounds with significantly improved antibacterial activity. These analogs are not only highly potent against both Gram-positive and Gram-negative bacteria, but also are more potent against ciprofloxacin-resistant organisms.

Other modifications. Tricyclic 2-pyridones with a bridge between position 1 and 9 have also been prepared. These compounds are bioisosteres of levofloxacin. The chirality of the bridge is very important for the antibacterial activity of these analogs just as it was with the ofloxacin branch molecules. The (*R*)-isomer is substantially more potent than the (*S*)-enantiomer. However, these novel compounds are not more potent than the corresponding quinolone analogues [56].

Table 20. Comparison of *in vitro* MIC values for 2-pyridones with enantiomeric C-8 substituents

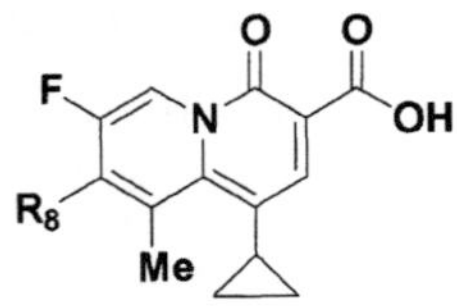

R8		MIC (μg/ml)						Ref.
		Sa Cip-S	Sa Cip-R	Ef	Sb	Spy	Ec	Pa	
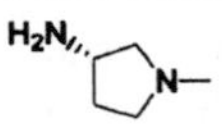	(S)	0.01	0.78	0.02	0.02	0.02	0.002	0.02	[57]
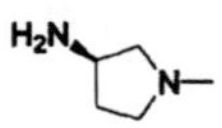	(R)	0.01	1.56	0.05	0.1	0.05	0.005	0.05	[57]
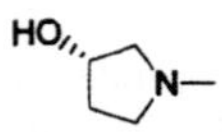	(S)	0.005	0.39	0.05	0.1	-	0.02	0.39	[57]
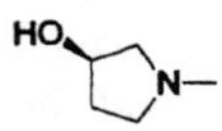	(R)	0.02	1.56	0.2	0.2	-	0.1	0.78	[57]
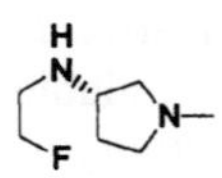	(S)	0.01	0.39	0.1	-	0.1	0.2	0.78	[61]
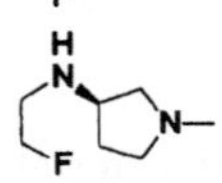	(R)	0.02	0.39	0.1	-	0.05	1.56	1.56	[61]
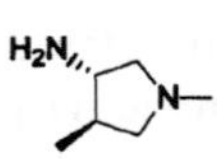	(SR)	0.02	0.78	0.05	-	0.05	0.05	0.2	[61]
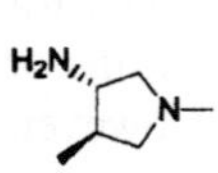	(RS)	0.05	0.78	0.2	-	0.1	0.1	0.39	[61]
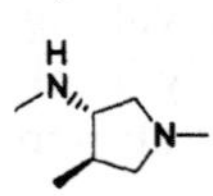	(SR)	0.01	0.39	0.1	-	0.02	0.05	0.2	[61]
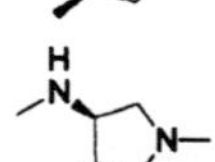	(RS)	0.05	0.78	0.2	-	0.1	0.2	3.1	[61]
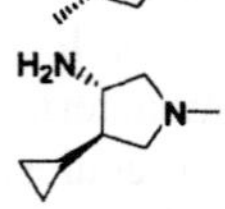	(SR)	0.05	0.78	0.1	-	0.05	0.2	0.39	[61]
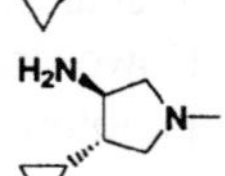	(RS)	0.02	0.78	0.1	-	0.1	0.2	0.39	[61]

(Continued on next page.)

Table 20. (Continued)

R8	MIC (μg/ml)							Ref.
	Sa Cip-S	Sa Cip-R	Ef	Sb	Spy	Ec	Pa	
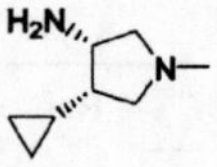 (SS)	0.005	0.39	0.05	-	0.02	0.1	0.39	[61]
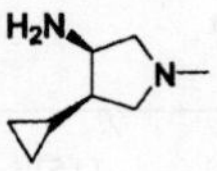 (RR)	0.02	0.78	0.1	-	0.1	0.2	0.39	[61]
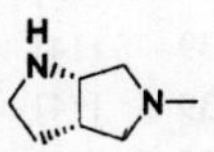 (SS)	0.05	3.1	0.1	0.1	-	0.02	0.2	[61]
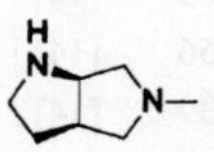 (RR)	0.1	6.2	0.2	0.39	-	0.05	0.39	[61]
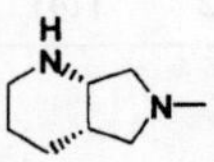 (SS)	0.01	0.39	0.1	0.05	0.05	0.005	0.2	[61]
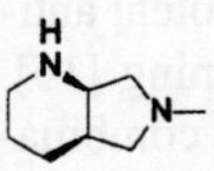 (RR)	0.05	0.78	0.1	0.05	0.05	0.05	0.78	[61]
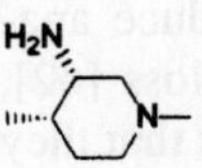 (SS)	0.05	1.56	0.2	-	0.1	0.2	0.78	[34]
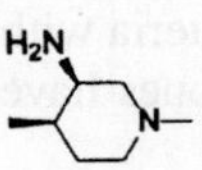 (RR)	0.1	3.1	0.39	-	0.39	0.78	1.56	[34]
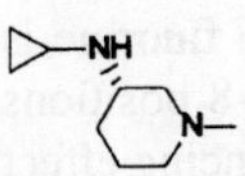 (S)	0.01	0.39	0.1	-	0.02	0.05	0.2	[34]
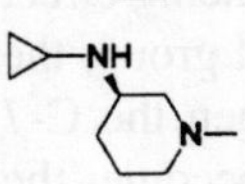 (R)	0.01	3.1	0.05	-	0.02	0.1	0.78	[34]
Ciprofloxacin	0.39	>100	0.78	0.78	0.78	0.02	0.2	[34]

Non-fluorinated quinolones

Since the introduction of the first clinically significant fluoroquinolone, norfloxacin, in 1983, a fluorine substituent at the C-6 position has become an integral part of all subsequently important quinolone molecules. It is widely

Table 21. Comparison of *in vitro* MIC values for 2-pyridones with position 9 modifications

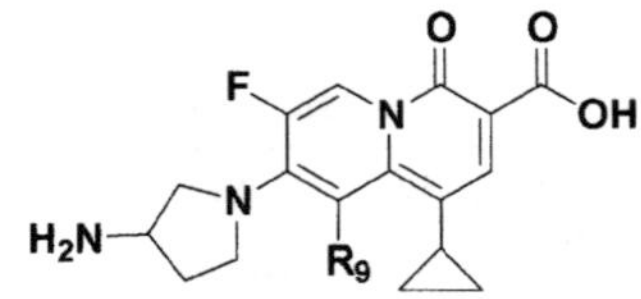

R9	MIC (μg/ml)							Ref.
	Sa Cip-S	Sa Cip-R	Ef	Sb	Spy	Ec	Pa	
—H	0.05	12.5	0.2	0.2	0.2	0.005	0.1	[15]
—F	0.1	6.2	0.78	0.78	0.78	0.01	0.39	[14]
—Cl	0.2	6.2	0.39	0.78	0.39	0.05	0.39	[14]
—Me	0.01	0.78	0.02	0.02	0.02	0.002	0.05	[14]
—Et	0.1	6.2	0.39	-	0.39	0.2	1.56	[14]
—OMe	0.05	3.1	0.2	0.39	0.2	0.02	0.39	[14]
Ciprofloxacin	0.39	>100	0.78	0.78	0.78	0.02	0.2	[14]

accepted that the fluorine at the C-6 position is essential for having potent antibacterial activity. The evidence to support this notion is overwhelming [15]. However, recent studies suggest that removal of the C-6 fluorine, in combination with certain other modifications at the C-8 position, can produce analogues with potent antibacterial activity that compensates for this loss [62]. One of the most significant features of these non-fluoroquinolones is that they tend to be more active against quinolone-resistant Gram-positive bacteria with both GyrA and ParC mutations [63]. In addition, non-fluoroquinolones have been reported to possess improved safety profiles [64, 65].

The data in Table 22 illustrates the fact that the role of the C-6 fluorine is dependent upon the specific substituents present at the C-7 and C-8 positions [62]. When the C-7 group is a N-methylpiperazinyl group, the enhancing effect of the fluorine is substantial. When the C-7 moiety is a piperidinyl group, the non-fluoroquinolone is as potent as the fluorinated analogue. When the C-7 group is a tetrahydroisoquinolinyl group, the C-6 amino analogue becomes the most potent compound. A very important lesson one can learn from this work is that it is dangerous and often misleading to single out a particular group for developing structure-activity relationships without taking other groups in the molecule into consideration. Another interesting observation from this work is the poor correlation between the gyrase inhibitory activity and the antibacterial MICs. Although not a surprising result, it suggests that DNA gyrase may not be the primary or sole target for these compounds, at least in some cases.

Several particular groups at the C-8 position have been demonstrated to enhance antibacterial activity in the absence of the C-6 fluorine. Table 23 summarizes the MICs for a series of nonfluoroquinolones with a methyl group at

Table 22. Comparison of *in vitro* MIC values for 6-desfluoroquinolones [62]

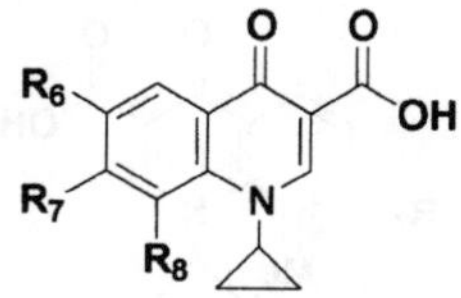

Compound			Mean MIC (μg/ml)		Ec Gyrase
R7	R6	R8	Gram-(+)	Gram-(–)	IC_{50} (μg/ml)
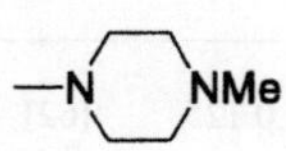	F	H	0.65	0.11	1.5
	F	Me	0.27	0.15	5.9
	H	Me	1.09	0.61	28.5
	NH2	Me	3.36	0.46	3.8
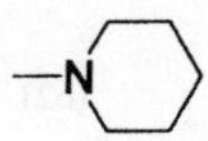	F	H	0.50	0.71	32.1
	F	Me	0.02	0.29	2.4
	H	Me	0.05	0.53	3.3
	NH2	Me	0.34	1.00	3.2
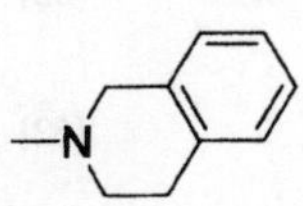	F	H	0.21	1.15	10.8
	F	Me	0.07	0.87	3.0
	H	Me	0.27	1.85	7.8
	NH2	Me	0.07	1.00	3.6

the C-8 position [63]. The compounds in this series are more potent than ciprofloxacin against Gram-positive organisms. The potency of this series depends upon the substituent at position 7. General speaking, a hydrophobic group at the C-7 position tends to give better activity against Gram-positive bacteria, while a hydrophilic group tends to give better activity against Gram-negative organisms.

The methoxy group has also been investigated as a potency enhancer for the nonfluoroquinolones. The antibacterial activity (MIC_{90}) of N-1-cyclopropyl-8-methoxy-4-oxo-1,4-dihydro-3-quinolinecarboxylic acids with three different C-7 amines against *E. coli*, PRSP, and MRSA were compared with that of ciprofloxacin, trovafloxacin, gatifloxacin and clinafloxacin (Tab. 24) [66, 67]. All three non-fluorinated quinolones are more potent than ciprofloxacin, trovafloxacin and gatifloxacin against penicillin-resistant *Streptococcus pneumoniae* (PRSP) and methicillin-resistant *Staphylococcus aureus* (MRSA). They are slightly less active than the reference agents against *E. coli*. These non-fluorinated quinolones are also less susceptible than the reference compounds to existing mechanisms of quinolone resistance [66, 67].

The specific nature of the C-7 group has a significant impact on the antibacterial activity of this 8-methoxy non-fluorinated quinolone system [68].

Table 23. Comparison of *in vitro* MIC for 8-methyl nonfluoroquinolones

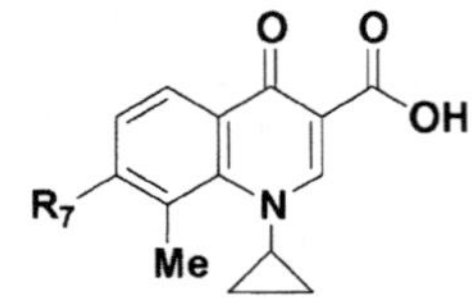

R7	MIC (μg/ml)							Ref.
	Sa ATCC Cip-S	Sa OBT687 Cip-R	Ef LEPBr	Spy OMNFI	Hf	Ec ATCC	Pa ATC1C	
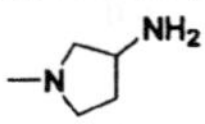	0.125	4	1	1	<0.016	<0.016	0.125	[62]
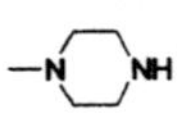	0.5	16	2	2	0.03	0.03	0.125	[62]
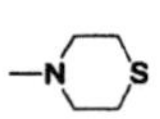	<0.016	2	1	0.5	<0.016	0.125	4	[62]
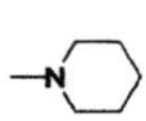	<0.016	1	1	0.03	<0.016	0.03	4	[62]
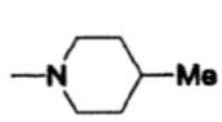	<0.016	1	0.5	0.125	<0.016	0.03	2	[62]
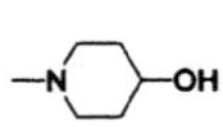	<0.016	0.5	0.5	2	0.25	0.06	2	[62]
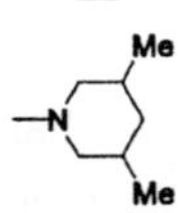	<0.016	2	1	0.5	0.25	1	8	[62]
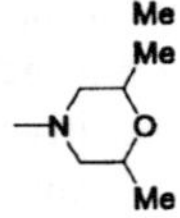	0.125	1	1	0.5	1	1	16	[62]
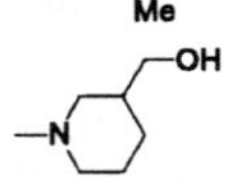	<0.016	1	0.5	0.5	<0.016	0.125	4	[62]
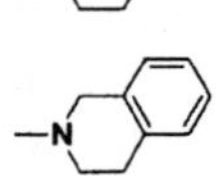	<0.016	2	1	0.25	0.06	1	>16	[62]
Ciprofloxacin	0.5	>16	1	0.5	<0.016	<0.016	0.06	[62]

The data in Table 23 indicates that introducing a small alkyl group in the vicinity of the terminal amino group can significantly improve the overall potency.

The C-8 difluoromethoxy group was demonstrated to be superior to a methoxy group as a potency enhancer for the non-fluorinated quinolones [69, 70]. So far, the study only involved a 2,3-dihydro-1H-5-isoindolyl group at the

Table 24. Comparison of MIC_{90} values for three 8-methoxy nonfluoroquinolones

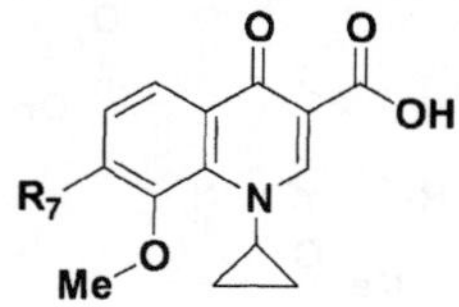

R7	MIC90 (µg/ml)			Ref.
	E. coli (n = 20)	PRSP (n = 23)	MRSA (n = 34)	
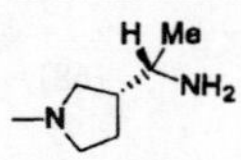	0.125	0.031	2.0	[66, 67]
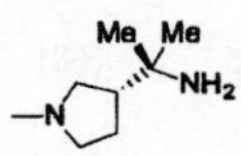	0.25	0.125	2.0	[66, 67]
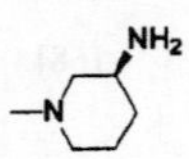	0.125	0.125	2.0	[66, 67]
Ciprofloxacin	0.031	2	>64	[66, 67]
Trovafloxacin	0.125	0.25	32	[66, 67]
Gatifloxacin	0.063	0.5	16	[66, 67]
Clinafloxacin	0.016	0.125	2.0	[66, 67]

position 7 [71]. How general this conclusion will be when there is a different C-7 substituent remains to be seen.

Table 26 compares the antibacterial activities for several different 8-difuoromethoxy analogues. The 8-difluoromethoxy analogues are significantly more active than both the 8-unsubstituted and 8-methoxy analogues against both wild type and quinolone-resistant bacteria.

Benzonaphthyridones

A series of benzo[b]naphthyridones has been shown to have potent antibacterial activity [72]. Although they are structurally related to quinolones, these benzonaphthyridones have been shown to be equally active against quinolone-susceptible and quinolone-resistant organisms (Tab. 27). Mutations in genes encoding DNA gyrase and topoisomerase IV that confer high level quinolone resistance have no effect on these compounds indicating that these compounds may have a different mode of action than the classical quinolones [73]. However, the mechanism of action of these compounds has not been elucidated as yet.

Table 25. Comparison of MIC_{90} values for three additional 8-methoxy nonfluoroquinolones

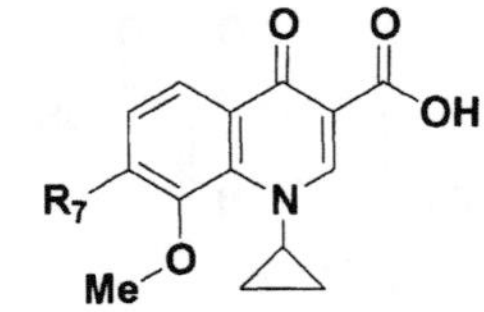

R7	MIC_{90} (μg/ml)					Ref.
	Sa Cip-S	Sa Cip-R	Sp	Ec	Pa	
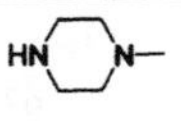	1	>32	8	0.5	4	[68]
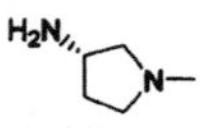	<0.06	4	1	<0.06	0.5	[68]
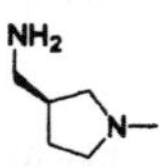	<0.06	1	0.12	0.12	2	[68]
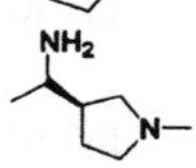	0.008	0.06	0.016	0.03	0.25	[68]
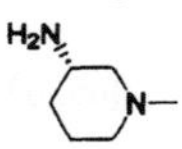	0.016	0.25	0.03	0.03	0.5	[68]
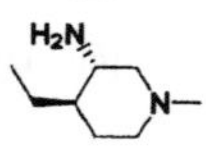	<0.008	0.06	<0.008	<0.008	0.5	[68]

Table 26. Comparison of *in vitro* MIC values for 8-difluoromethoxy des-fluoroquinolones

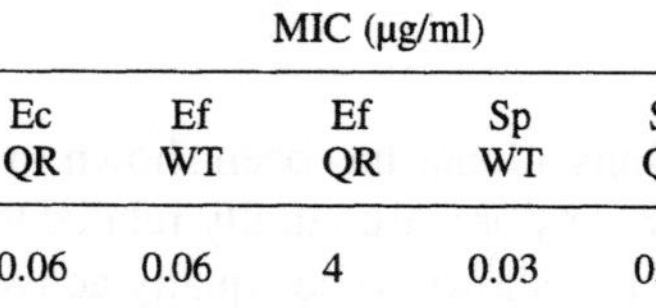

R8	MIC (μg/ml)								Ref.
	Ec WT	Ec QR	Ef WT	Ef QR	Sp WT	Sp QR	Sa WT	Sa QR	
—H	0.007	0.06	0.06	4	0.03	0.25	0.015	4	[71]
—OCH_3	0.015	0.25	0.25	2	0.125	2	0.03	4	[71]
—$OCHF_2$	0.015	0.06	0.06	1	0.015	0.125	0.007	0.5	[71]
Ciprofloxacin	0.007	0.125	0.5	32	1	16	0.125	64	[71]
Moxifloxacin	0.015	0.25	0.25	8	0.25	1	0.03	2	[71]
Levofloxacin	0.03	0.25	0.5	8	0.5	4	0.125	64	[71]

Table 27. Comparison of MIC values for benzo[b]naphthyridones

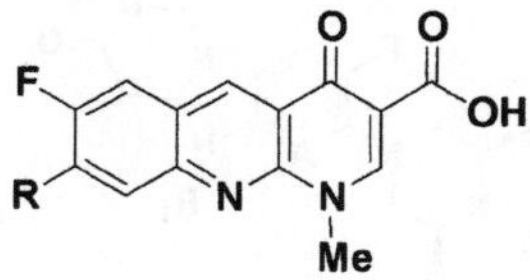

R	MIC (μg/ml)		Ref.
	Sa Cip-S	Sa Cip-R	
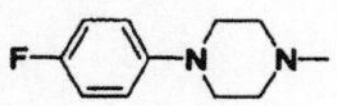	0.25	0.50	[72]
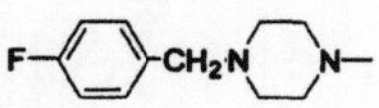	0.50	1	[72]
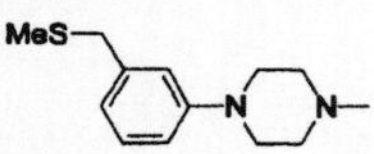	4	4	[72]
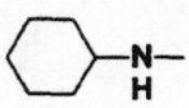	1	1	[72]
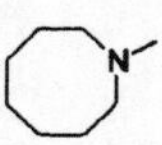	1	1	[72]
Pefloxacin	0.5	128	[72]

Other novel structures

In contrast to the successes achieved with the 2-pyridones and the non-fluorinated quinolones, there have been many failed attempts in altering the core structure of quinolones during the last decade. Those novel structures, which did not possess significant improvement over the traditional quinolones, will not be discussed in detail in this review. Instead, they are listed with references in Figure 5 so that the interested reader can easily find the original publications for details of these compounds.

Research emphasis in the next five years

From the chemical standpoint, the next 5 years will hopefully decide through evaluation of analogs what the clinical future of the 2-pyridones and the 6-desfluoro series will be. The advancement of additional novel structures exploiting topoisomerase targets would be desirable. Agents able to overcome the resistance problem would be highly desirable. The details of the molecular mode of action of the quinolones is as yet unsettled. A clearer picture of the

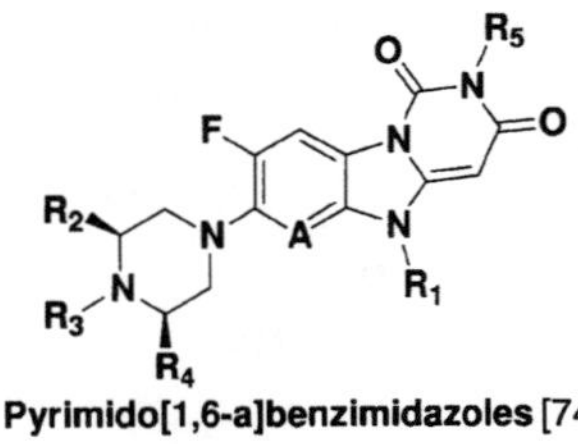

Pyrimido[1,6-a]benzimidazoles [74]

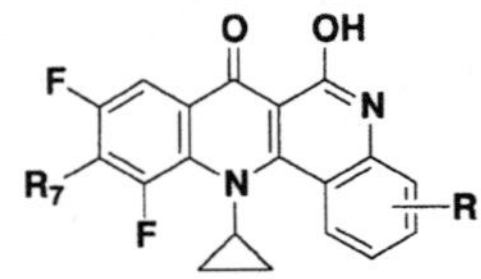

Dibenzo[1,6]naphthyridiones [75]

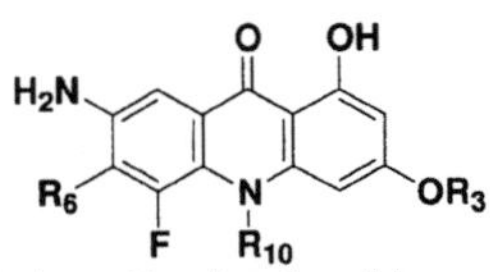

1-Hydroxy-7-amino-9-acridones [76]

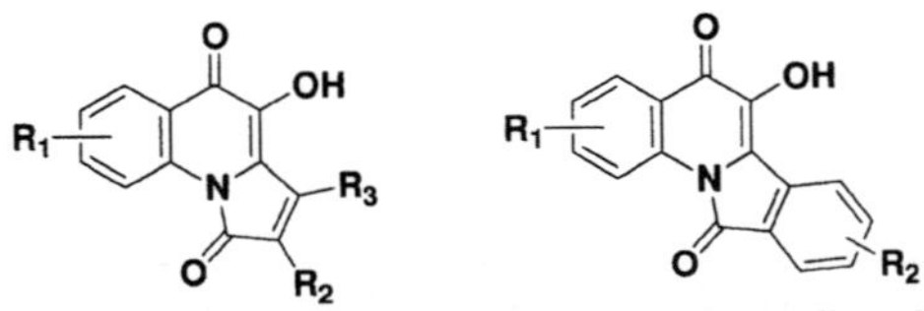

Pyrrolo[1,2-a]quinolines and Isoindolo[2,1-a]quinolines [77]

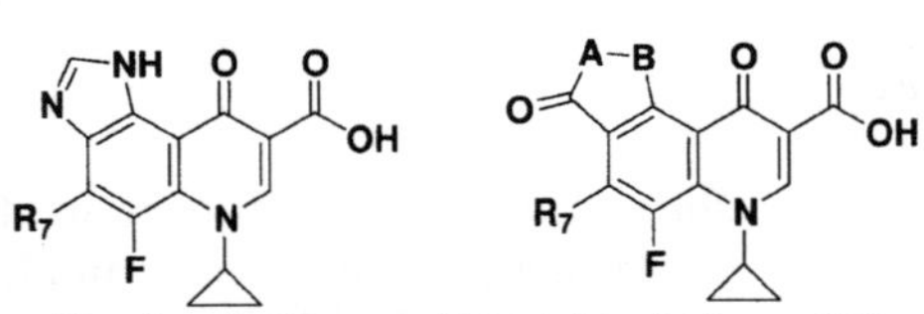

Pyrroloquinolones and Pyrazoloquinolones [78]

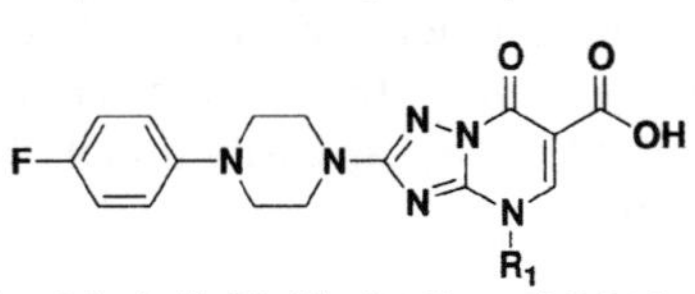

2-[4-(4-Fluorophenyl)piperizin-1-yl]-4,7-dihydro-7-oxo-1,2,4-triazolo[1,5-a]pyrimidine-6-carboxylic Acids [79]

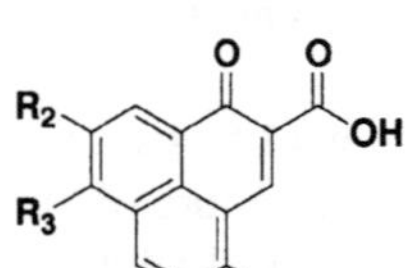

p-Quinone Methides [80]

Figure 5. Structures and references for quinolone analogs that have not achieved high activity.

relationship between structure and activity against DNA gyrase, bacterial topoisomerase IV, and human topoisomerase II is coming into focus and should be more settled by that time.

These are all comparatively safe projections based upon events currently in progress and their successful realization would materially enhance the desirability of these important antiinfective weapons.

References

1 Teoh-Chan CH, Cowlishaw A, Eley A, Slater G, Greenwood D (1985) Laboratory evaluation of enoxacin: comparison with norfloxacin and nalidixic acid. *J Antimicrob Chemother* 15: 45–52
2 Ohshita Y, Hayashi N, Amano H, Hirao Y, Niino Y, Yazaki A, Kobayashi Y (1998) WQ-3034, A novel acidic fluoroquinolone: *in vitro* and *in vivo* antimicrobial activities. 38th Interscience Conference on Antimicrobial Agents and Chemotherapy, San Diego. Poster F-084
3 Huczko E, Valera L, Conetta B, Stickle T, Macko A, Fung-Tomc J (1999) Susceptibility of bacterial isolates to gatifloxacin and ciprofloxacin from the clinical trails during the 1997–1998 Period. 39th Interscience Conference on Antimicrobial Agents and Chemotherapy, San Francisco. Poster F-0351
4 Fass RJ (1997) *In vitro* activity of Bay 12-8038, a new 8-methoxyquinolone. *Antimicrob Agts Chemother* 41: 1818–1824
5 Barry AL, Jones RN (1989) *In vitro* activities of temafloxacin, tosufloxacin (A-61827) and five other fluoroquinolone agents. *J Antimicrob Chemother* 23: 527–35
6 Wise R, Andrews JM (1999) Gemifloxacin: the *in vitro* activity and a tentative breakpoint of a new fluoroquinolone. 39th Interscience Conference on Antimicrobial Agents and Chemotherapy, San Francisco. Poster F-2309
7 Garey KW, Amsden GW (1999) Trovafloxacin: an overview. *Pharmacotherapy* 19: 21–34
8 Wise R, Andrews JM, Matthews R, Wolstenholme M (1992) The *in vitro* activity of two new quinolones: rufloxacin and MF-961. *J Antimicrob Chemother* 29: 649–660
9 Morita S, Otsubo K, Uchida M, Kawabata S, Tamaoka H, Shimizu (1990) A synthesis and antibacterial activity of the metabolites of 9-fluoro-6,7-dihydro-8-(4-hydroxy-1-piperidyl)-5-methyl-10-benzo[i.j]quinolizine-2-carboxylic acid (OPC-7251). *Chem Pharm Bull* 38: 2027–2029
10 Albrecht R (1977) Development of antibacterial agents of the nalidixic acid type. *Prog Drug Res* 21: 9–104
11 Domegala J, Heifetz C, Siporin (eds) (1990) *The new generation of quinolones*. Marcel Dekker, Inc., New York
12 Radl S (1990) Structure-activity relationships in DNA gyrase inhibitors. *Pharmac Ther* 48: 1–17
13 Rosen T (1990) The fluoroquinolone antibacterial agents. *Prog Med Chem* 27: 235–295
14 Wentland MP (1990) Structure-activity relationships of fluoroquinolones. *In*: J Domagala, C Heifetz, C Siporin (eds): *The new generation of quinolones*. Marcel Dekker, Inc., New York, 1–43
15 Mitscher LA, Devasthale P, Zavod R (1993) Structure-activity relationships. *In*: JS Wolfson, DC Hooper (eds): *Quinolone antibacterial agents, 2nd ed.* American Society for Microbiology, Washington, 3–52
16 Wolfson JS, Hooper DC (eds) (1993) *Quinolone antibacterial agents, 2nd ed.* American Society for Microbiology, Washington
17 Domagala JM (1994) Structure-activity and structure-side-effect relationships for the quinolone antibacterials. *J Antimicrob Chemother* 33: 685–706
18 Gootz TD, Brighty KE (1996) Fluoroquinolone antibacterials. *Med Res Reversus* 16: 433–86
19 Drlica K, Zhao X, (1997) DNA gyrase, topoisomerase IV, and the 4-quinolones, *Microbiol Mol Biol Rev* 61: 377–92
20 Brighty KE, Gootz TD (1997) The chemistry and biological profile of trovafloxacin. *J Antimicrob Chemother* 39 Suppl. B: 1–14
21 Andriole VT (ed) (1998) *The Quinolones, 2nd ed.* Academic Press, New York
22 Bonomo RA (1998) Fluoroquinolones. *Clinical Microbiology Newsletter* 20: 197–201
23 Blondeau JM (1999) Expanded activity and utility of the new fluoroquinolones: a review. *Clin Ther* 21: 3–40

24 Rubenstein E (2001) History of quinolones and their side-effects. *Chemotherapy* 47, Suppl. 3: 3–8
25 Takemura M, Hayakawa I (2001) Recent advances in the field of quinolones. *Farmaco* 56: 37–40
26 Peterson LR (2001) Quinolone molecular structure-activity relationships: what we have learned about improving antimicrobial activity. *Clin Infect Dis* 33 Suppl 3: S180–S186
27 Kim OK, Ohemeng K, Barrett JF (2001) Advances in DNA gyrase inhibitors. *Expert Opin Investig Drugs*, 10: 199–212
28 Berger JM, Gamblin SJ, Harrison SC, Wang JC (1996) Structure and mechanism of DNA topoisomerase II, *Nature* 379: 225–32
29 Kato J, Nishimura Y, Imamura R, Niki H, Hiraga S, Suzuki H (1990) New topoisomerase essential for chromosome segregation in *E. coli*. *Cell* 63: 393–404
30 Hanessian S, Saladino R, Nunez JC (1996) On the binding site of quinolone antibactrerials. An attempt to probe the Shen model. *Biorg Med Chem Lett* 6: 2333–8
31 Batori S, Timari G, Koczka I, Hermecz I (1996) Synthesis and biological evaluation of N-(1-aziridino)-6-fluoroquinolone-3-carboxylic acids. *Biorg Med Chem Lett* 6: 1507–1510
32 Al-Masoudi NA, Al-Soud YA, Eherman M, Clercq ED (1998) Quinolone nucleoside: 6,7-dihalo-N-beta- and alpha-glycosyl-1,4-dihydro-4-oxoquinoline-3-carboxylic acids and derivatives. Synthesis, antimicrobial and antiviral activity. *Nucleosides, Nucleotides* 17: 2255–66
33 Al-Masoudi NA, Al-Soud YA, Eherman M, Clercq ED (2000) Synthesis of acyclic 6,7-dihaloquinolone nucleoside analogues as potential antibacterial and antiviral agents. *Bioorg Med Chem* 8: 1407–13
34 Kawakami K, Takahashi H, Ohki H, Kimura K, Miyauchi S, Miyauchi R, Takemura M (2000) Studies on 8-methoxyquinolones: synthesis and antibacterial activity of 7-(3-amino-4-substituted)pyrrolidinyl derivatives. *Chem Pharm Bull* 48: 1667–72
35 Hayashi N, Amano H, Ohshita Y, Niino Y, Yoshida J, Yazaki A (1996) *In vitro* and *in vivo* activities, pharmacokinetics and toxicity of WQ-2756 and WQ-2765, two novel fluoroquinolones. 36th Interscience Conference on Antimicrobial Agents and Chemotherapy. New Orleans. Abstr. F051
36 Amano H, Hayashi N, Ohshita Y, Niino Y, Yazaki A (1997) WQ-2724 and WQ-2743, novel fluoroquinolones: *in vitro* and *in vivo* activities, pharmacokinetics and toxicity. 37th Interscience Conference on Antimicrobial Agents and Chemotherapy, Toronto. Abstr. F163
37 Hayashi N, Ohshita Y, Amano H, Hirao Y, Niino Y, Yazaki A (1999) WQ-3330 and WQ-2942, structure-activity relationships of novel 8-methyl quinolones containing an aminophenyl group at the N1-position. 39th Interscience Conference on Antimicrobial Agents and Chemotherapy. San Francisco. Abstr. F557
38 (38) Hayashi N, Hashimoto K, Yazaki A (2001) A novel substituent at the 1-position markedly decreases the phototoxicity of an 8-chloro fluoroquinolone, WQ-2756, *in vivo* and *in vitro*. 41st Interscience Conference on Antimicrobial Agents and Chemotherapy. Chicago. Abstr. F556
39 Jung J-C, Jung Y-J, Park O-S (2001) Synthesis of 4-hydroxyquinolone-2(1H)-one analogues and 2-substituted quinolone derivatives. *J Heterocyclic Chem* 38: 61–67
40 Matsuoka M, Segawa J, Amimoto I, Masui Y, Tomii Y, Kitano M, Kise M (1999) Synthesis and antibacterial activity of novel 7-substituted-6-fluoro-1-fluoromethyl-4-xox-4H-[1, 3]-thiazeto[3, 2-a]quinoline-3-carboxylic acid derivatives. *Chem Phar Bull* 47: 1765–1773
41 Matsuoka M, Segawa J, Amimoto I, Masui Y, Tomii Y, Kitano M, Kise M (1999) Synthesis and antibacterial activity of novel 7-substituted-6-fluoro-1-methylene-4-xox-4H-[1, 3]-thiazeto[3, 2-a]quinoline-3-carboxylic acid derivatives. *Heterocycl* 51: 2915–2930
42 Cecchetti V, Fravolini A, Lorenzini MC, Tabarrini O, Terni P, Xin T (1996) Studies on 6-aminoquinolones: synthesis and antibacterial evaluation of 6-amino-8-methylquinolones. *J Med Chem* 39: 436–445
43 Hong CY, Kim SH, Kim YK (1997) Novel 5-amino-6-methylquinolone antibacterials: a new class of non-6-fluoroquinolones. *Bioorg Med Chem Lett* 7: 1875–1878
44 Gootz TD, McGuirk PR, Moynihan MS, Haskell SL (1994) Placement of alkyl substituents on the c-7 piperizine ring of fluoroquinolones: dramatic differential effects on mammalian topoisomerase II and DNA gyrase. *Antimicrob Agents Chemother* 38: 130–133
45 Renau TE, Sanchez JP, Gage JW, Dever JA, Shapiro MA, Gracheck SJ, Domagala JM (1996) Structure-activity relationships of the quinolone antibacterial against mycobacteria: effect of structural changes at the N-1 and C-7. *J Med Chem* 39: 729–735
46 Hong CY, Kim YK, Chang JH, Kim SH, Choi H, Nam HKim YZ, Kwak JH (1997) Novel fluoroquinolone antibacterial agents containing oxime-substituted (aminomethyl)pyrrolidines: synthesis and antibacterial activity of 7-(4-(aminomethyl)-3-(methoxyimino)pyrrolidin-1-yl)-1-cyclo-

propyl-6-fluoro-4-oxo-1,4-dihydro[1, 8]naphthyridine-3-carboxylic acid (LB20304). *J Med Chem* 40: 3584–3593
47 Fujita M, Chiba K, Tominaga Y, Hino K (1998) 7-(2-Aminomethyl-1-azetidinyl)-4-oxoquinoline-3-carboxylic acids as potent antibacterial agents: design, synthesis, and antibacterial activity. *Chem Pharm Bull* 46: 787–796
48 Haramura M, Okamachi A, Makino T, Kohda A, Katoh Y, Munemura K, Ito T, Matsumoto M, Kojima K, Yokota T (1994) Synthesis and biological activity of new 8-methoxyquinolones possessing 7-aminoalkyl group. 34th Interscience Conference on Antimicrobial Agents and Chemotherapy, Orlando. Abstr. F36
49 Fujita M, Chiba K, Nakano J, Tominaga Y, Matsumoto J (1998) Synthesis and structure-antibacterial activity relationships of 7-(3-amino-1-propyl and 3-amino-1-propyl)quinolones. *Chem Pharm Bull* 46: 631–638
50 Renau TE, Gage JW, Dever JA, Roland GE, Joannides ET, Shapira MA, Sanchez JP, Gracheck SJ, Domagala JM, Jacobs MR, Reynolds RC (1996) Structure-activity relationships of quinolone agents against mycobacteria: effect of structural modification at the 8 position. *Antimicrob Agents Chemother* 40: 2363–2368
51 Sanchez JP, Gogliotti RD, Domagala JM, Gracheck SJ, Huband MD, Sesnie JA, Cohen MA, Shapiro MA (1995) The synthesis, structure-activity, and structure-side effect relationships of a series of 8-alkoxy- and 5-amino-8-alkoxyquinolone antibacterial agents. *J Med Chem* 38: 4478–4487
52 Kitani H, Kurada T, Moriguchi A, Ao H, Hirayama F, Ikeda Y, Kawakita T (1997) Synthesis and structural optimization of 7-(3,3-disubstituted-1-pyrrolidinyl)-1-cyclopropyl-6-fluoro-1,4-dihydro-8-methoxy-4-oxo-3-quinolinecarboxylic acids as antibacterial agents. *Bioorg Med Chem Lett* 7: 515–520
53 Hong CY, Kim YK, Chang JH, Kim SH, Choi H, Nam H, Kim YZ, Kwak H (1997) Novel fluoroquinolone antibacterial agents containing oxime-substituted (aminomethyl)pyrrolidines: synthesis and antibacterial activity of 7-(4-(aminomethyl)-3-(methoxyimino)pyrrolidine-1-yl)-1-cyclopropyl-6-fluoro-4-oxo-1,4-dihydro[1, 8]naphthyridine-3-carboxylic acid (LB20304). *J Med Chem* 40: 3584–3593
54 Hong CY, Kim YK, Lee YH, Kwak JH (1998) Methyloxime-substituted aminopyrrolidine: a new surrogate for 7-basic group of quinolone. *Bioorg Med Chem Lett* 8: 221–226
55 Cecchetti V, Tabarrini O, Sabatini S, Miao H, Filipponi E, Fravolini A (1999) Studies on 6-aminoquinolones: synthesis and antibacterial evaluation of 6-amino-8-ethyl- and 6-amino-8-methoxyquinolones. *Bioorg Med Chem Lett* 7: 2465–2471
56 Li Q, Mitscher LA, Shen LL (2000) The 2-pyridone antibacterial agents. *Med Res Rev* 20: 231–293
57 Li Q, Chu DTW, Claiborne A, Cooper CS, Lee CM, Raye K, Berst KB, Donner P et al (1996) Synthesis and structure-activity relationships of 2-pyridones: A novel series of potent DNA gyrase inhibitors as antibacterial agents. *J Med Chem* 39: 3070–3088
58 Shen LL, Tanaka SK, Chu DTW (1997) Quinolones, 2-pyridones and resistant type II DNA topoisomerases. *Current Pharmaceutical Design* 3: 169–176
59 Saiki AYC, Shen LL, Chen CM, Baranowski J, Lerner CG (1999) DNA Cleavage activities of *Staphlococcus aureus* gyrase and topoisomerase IV stimulated by quinolones and 2-pyridones. *Antimicrob Agents Chemother* 43: 1574–1577
60 Klein LL, DeGoey DA, Thomas SA, Yeung CM, Leone CL, Grampovnik DJ, Chu DT, Lartey PA (1997) Preparation and antibacterial activity of pyridopyridone analogs: C-1 modifications. *Bioorg Med Chem Lett* 7: 1167–1170
61 Ma Z, Chu DTW, Cooper CS, Li Q, Fung AKL, Wang S, Shen LL, Flamm RK, Nilius AM, Alder JD, Meulbroek JA, Or YS (1999) Synthesis and antimicrobial activity of 4H-4-oxoquinolizine derivatives: Consequences of structural modification at the C-8 position. *J Med Chem* 42: 4202–4213
62 Cecchetti V, Fravolini A, Palumbo M, Sissi C, Tabarrini O (1996) Potent 6-desfluoro-8-methylquinolones as new lead compounds in antibacterial chemotherapy. *J Med Chem* 39: 4952–4957
63 Takahata M, Mitsuyama J, Yamashiro Y, Yonezawa M, Araki H, Todo Y, Minami S, Watanabe Y, Narita H (1999) *In vitro* and *in vivo* antimicrobial activities of t-3811me, a novel des-f(6)-quinolone. *Antimicrob Agents Chemother* 43: 1077–1084
64 Nagai A, Takahata M, Miyazaki M, Kawamura Y, Kodama T, Todo Y, Watanabe Y, Narita H (1997)

T-3811, a novel des-f(6)-quinolone: toxicological evaluation. *In*: Abstracts of the 37th ICAAC, Toronto Abstract F-162, p.173. American Society for Microbiology, Washington, DC
65 Murphy VA, Ledoussal B, Renick PJ, Twinem TL, Morris TW (2001) Clastogenicity and human topoisomerase II inhibition profiles of non-fluorinated quinolones (NFQs). 41st Interscience Conference on Antimicrobial Agents and Chemotherapy, Chicago. Abstr. F563
66 Roychoudhury S, Twinem TL, Makin KM, McIntosh EJ, Ledoussal B, Catrenich CE (2001) Activity of non-fluorinated quinolones (NFQs) against quinolone-resistant *Escherichia coli* and *Streptococcus pneumoniae*. *J Antimicrob Chemother* 48: 29–36
67 Roychoudhury S, Catrenich CE, McIntosh EJ, McKeever HD, Makin KM, Koenigs PM, Ledoussal B (2001) Quinolone resistance in staphylococci: activities of new nonfluorinated quinolones against molecular targets in whole cells and clinical isolates. *Antimicrob Agents Chemother* 45: 1115–1120
68 Ledoussal B, Almstead JK, Gallagher CP, Gray JL, Hu XE, Kim NK, Mckeever HD, Taylor CJ, Twinem TL (2001) New 7-piperidinyl non-fluorinated quinolones (NFQs), synthesis and structure-activity relationships. 41st Interscience Conference on Antimicrobial Agents and Chemotherapy, Chicago. Abstr. F564
69 Takahata M, Mitsuyama J, Yamashiro Y, Yonezawa M, Araki H, Todo Y, Minami S, Watanabe Y, Narita H (1999) *In vitro* and *in vivo* antimicrobial activities of T-3811ME, a novel des-F(6)-quinolone. *Antimicrob Agents Chemother* 43: 1077–1084
70 Lawrence LE, Wu P, Fan L, Gouveia KE, Card A, Casperson M, Denbleyker K, Barrett JF (2001) The inhibition and selectivity of bacterial topoisomerases by BMS-284756 and its analogues. *J Antimicrob Chemother* 48: 195–201
71 Hayashi K, Todo Y, Hamamoto S, Ojima K, Yamada M, Kito T, Takahata M, Watanabe Y, Narita H (1997) T-3811, a novel des-F(6)-quinolones: synthesis and *in vitro* activity of 7-(isoindolin-5-yl) derivatives. 37th Interscience Conference on Antimicrobial Agents and Chemotherapy, Toronto. Abstr. F158
72 Tabart M, Picaut G, Berthaud N, Desconclois J-F (2000) Synthesis and biological evaluation of RP60556A, a new tropical antibacterial agent. 40th Interscience Conference on Antimicrobial Agents and Chemotherapy, Toronto. Abstr. 1512
73 Berthaud N, Dutka-Malen S, Boisrobert V, Efremenko F, Gouin A-M, Martin J, Rousseau J, Desnottes J-F (2000) RP60556A, a new tropical benzonaphthyridone derivative: *in vitro* bacteriostatic activity against Gram-positive cocci resistant to quinolones. 40th Interscience Conference on Antimicrobial Agents and Chemotherapy, Toronto, Abstr. 1514
74 Sraga J, Guerry P, Kompis I (1994) Synthesis and biological activity of tetrahydropyrido[2', 3': 4, 5]imidazo[1, 2-c]pyrimidine-6,8-diones. *Helv Chim Acta* 77: 1057–1064
75 Cecchetti V, Fravolini A, Sabatini S, Tabarrini O, Xin T (1998) Dibenzo[1, 6]naphthyridiones as modified quinolone antibacterials. *Eur J Med Chem* 33: 899–903
76 Tabarrini O, Cecchetti V, Fravolini A, Nocentini G, Barzi A, Sabatini S, Miao H, Sissi C (1999) Design and synthesis of modified quinolones as antitumoral acridones. *J Med Chem* 42: 2136–2144
77 Sui Z, Altom J, Nguyen VN, Fernandez J, Bernstein JI, Hiliard JJ, Barrett JF, Podlogar BL, Ohemeng KA (1998) Synthesis and inhibitory activity of novel tri- and tetracyclic quinolines against topoisomerases. *Bioorg Med Chem* 6: 735–742
78 Fujita M, Egawa H, Miyamoto T, Nakano J, Matsumoto J (1996) Pyrroloquinolones and pyrrazoloquinolones as potential antibacterial agents. synthesis and antibacterial activity. *Eur J Med Chem* 31: 981–988
79 Abdelal AM, Gineinah MM, Kheira MM (1999) Synthesis and antibacterial activity of 2-[4-(4-fluorophenyl)piperizin-1-yl]-4-substituted-4,7-dihydro-7-oxo-1,2,4-triazolo[1, 5-a]pyrimidine-6-carboxylic acids and its analogs. *Med Chem Res* 9: 277–290
80 Chung S-K, Lee JW, Shim NY, Kwon TW (1996) p-Quinone methides as geometric analogues of quinolone carboxylate antibacterials. *Bioorg Med Chem Lett* 6: 1309–1312

Fluoroquinolone Antibiotics
ed. by A.R. Ronald and D.E. Low

Epidemiology and mechanisms of resistance

Pak-Leung Ho and Vincent C.C. Cheng

Division of Infectious Diseases, Department of Microbiology, Queen Mary Hospital, The University of Hong Kong, Pokfulam Road, Pokfulam, Hong Kong SAR, China

Introduction

The fluoroquinolones is the first group of synthetic antibacterial agents available for clinical use. Since their introduction in the late 1980s, there has been a great expansion in the usage of fluoroquinolones as antimicrobial agents. Initially, these agents were primarily indicated in therapy of infections due to Gram negative bacteria and for prophylaxis in neutropenia or liver cirrhosis. With the introduction of agents with enhanced anti-Gram positive activities such as gatifloxacin and moxifloxacin, their indications have expanded to include acute bacterial infections of the respiratory tract and skin and soft tissue infections. Expectedly, resistance has become more prevalent among some organisms as the usage of this group of agents increased [1, 2]. The first resistant strains were found in microorganisms that are inherently less susceptible such as staphylococci and *Pseudomonas aeruginosa*. However, reduced susceptibility or resistance has been recently broadened to *Escherichia coli*, *Salmonella* spp., *Campylobacter* spp., *Neisseria gonorrhoeae* and *Streptococcus pneumoniae*. Wide variations in the rates of resistance have been reported depending on the bacterial species, clinical settings, origins of strains, geographic locations and pattern of usage. Generally speaking, resistance is more prevalent in developing countries than in developed parts of the world. In areas where there has been extensive veterinary use, particularly among food animals, resistance rates were also higher.

Nonetheless, concerns about resistance and technological advances have provided the impetus for better understanding of the mode of fluoroquinolone actions and the ways that microorganisms develop resistance. Important achievement in recent years include identification of quinolone-induced DNA strand breaks as a critical step in bacterial killing [3], modeling of the DNA-gyrase interaction at the breakage-reunion domain by crystallography [4], and characterization of fluoroquinolone efflux pumps such as PmrA in *S. pneumoniae* [5] and MexAB-OprM in *P. aeruginosa* [6]. In the following text, the latest epidemiology of fluoroquinolone resistance in medically important bacteria and their mechanisms of resistance will be reviewed.

Current situation of quinolone resistance in specific bacteria

Gram positive bacteria

Staphylococci

Within a few years after the introduction of fluoroquinolones for clinical use, fluoroquinolone resistance had developed in clinical isolates of staphylococci. Interestingly, fluoroquinolone-resistant isolates were mostly distributed among the oxacillin-resistant staphylococci. Since mid-1990s, these strains have been reported from virtually all countries. In the past few years, fluoroquinolone resistance rates remain high (>50% to 99%) among oxacillin-resistant staphylococci. Among the oxacillin-susceptible strains, fluoroquinolone resistance rates were generally perceived to be <5% (Tab. 1).

Table 1. Fluoroquinolone susceptibility of staphylococci in SENTRY and SCOPE programs

Source (ref)	No. tested	Year(s) of study	Geographical area (% isolates susceptible to ciprofloxacin)
Oxacillin susceptible *S. aureus*			
[93]	1072	1997	USA (94.1%), Canada (98.5%) and Latin America (86.6%)
[94]	50	1995–1996	USA (96%)
Oxacillin susceptible CoNS			
[93]	222	1997	USA (91.9%), Canada (94.9%), Latin America (97.5%)
[94]	127	1995–1996	USA (84%)
Oxacillin resistant *S. aureus*			
[93]	395	1997	USA (10.6%), Canada (50%) and Latin America (13.3%)
[94]	100	1995–1996	USA (8%)
Oxacillin resistant CoNS			
[93]	557	1997	USA (42.2%), Canada (55.0%), Latin America (42.9%)
[94]	173	1995–1996	USA (39%)

CA, community-acquired; HA, hospital-acquired; CoNS, coagulase-negative staphylococcus.

Streptococcus pneumoniae

National and international surveillance has established that quinolone-resistant *S. pneumoniae* (QRSP) remains a rare occurrence (Tab. 2). However, more focused studies suggested that fluoroquinolone resistance in *S. pneumoniae* might begin to emerge in some areas. In Canada, a study of 7551 isolates found an increase in ciprofloxacin resistance (MIC $\geq$ 4 μg/ml) from 0% in 1993 to 1.7% in 1997–1998 [7]. In the United States, a study involving 12,045 isolates found the proportion of isolates that were resistant to ofloxacin

Table 2. Susceptibility of *Streptococcus pneumoniae* to fluoroquinolones

Source (ref)	Specimen source	Year(s) of study	Geographical area(s)	% Levofloxacin nonsusceptible (n)
TRUST [20]	Multiple sources	1997–2000	USA	0.5% (n = 15,123)
Sahm et al. [14]	Multiple sources	1997–1998	USA	0.3%[a] (n = 5640)
SENTRY [91]	Respiratory and blood	1997–1998	Europe	0.4% (n = 698)
SENTRY [93]	Blood	1997	USA Canada Latin America	0.3% (n = 341) 2% (n = 102) 0% (n = 32)
SENTRY [24]	Pneumonia	1998	USA	0% (n = 195)
SENTRY [88]	Respiratory	1999	North America	1.1% (n = 1201)
SENTRY [89]	Respiratory and blood	1997–1998	USA	0.5% (n = 3049)
SENTRY [87]	Respiratory	1997	USA and Canada	0.8% (n = 1100)
SENTRY [90]	Respiratory and blood	1997	USA, Canada, Latin America and Europe	0.6% (n = 2284)
Chen et al.	Multiple sources	1997–1998	Canada	1.7%[a], 0.6% (n = 1844)

[a] Figure for ciprofloxacin given. The breakpoints for nonsusceptibility were ≥ 4 μg/ml for both ciprofloxacin and levofloxacin.

increased significantly from 2.6% in 1995 to 3.8% in 1997 [8]. In another study of 7,246 isolates from the United States, there has been a small but statistically significant increase in the prevalence of levofloxacin resistance from 0.1% in 1997–1998 to 0.6% in 1998–1999 [9]. Similarly, the SENTRY program has demonstrated an increase in levofloxacin-resistant isolates from 0.2 to 0.8%, between the respiratory disease seasons of 1997–1998 and 1998–1999 [10]. In southeast Asia, levofloxacin-resistant strains remain rare except in Hong Kong. In Hong Kong, two consecutive studies involving 361 pneumococci from hospitals have demonstrated an increase in the proportion of levofloxacin nonsusceptible (MIC ≥ 4 μg/ml) isolates from 5.5% in 1998 to 13.3% in 2000 [11, 12]. In a case-control study, presence of chronic obstructive pulmonary disease, nosocomial acquisition, nursing home residence and exposure to fluoroquinolones were independently associated with QRSP in the logistic regression model [13]. The isolates from Hong Kong were clonal while those from Canada and the United States [7, 8, 14] were not clonally related. Importantly, QRSP isolates in Hong Kong were multiply resistant and were related to the prevalent Spanish 23F clone [15]. This raises concern that the QRSP clone might spread to other countries, particularly when other Asian countries like Taiwan and Singapore have also reported the appearance of levofloxacin-resistant isolates [16, 17]. In Spain, 30% of the ciprofloxacin-resistant pneumococci belonged to two internationally spread epidemic clones (France^{9V}-3 and Spain^{23F}-1), further highlighting the potential role of clonal dissemination in the emergence of fluoroquinolone resistance [18].

Several studies from Hong Kong, Ireland and Canada have demonstrated a statistically significant association between reduced quinolone susceptibility and penicillin resistance [7, 11, 19]. At present, fluoroquinolone resistance was absent among isolates from the paediatric populations. Among the adult populations, FQ resistance was more frequent among isolates from the elderly and among respiratory isolates. Using the phenotype of a ciprofloxacin MIC of ≥ 4 μg/ml to mark reduced susceptibility, Chen et al. found a prevalence of 2.6% among isolates from those ≥ 65 years comparing to 1.0% among those 15–64 years of age [7]. In a study of 5,640 isolates collected from the United States during the 1997 to 1998 respiratory season, similarities with the findings of Chen et al. were noted when the same phenotype was used to analyze the results [14]. Reduced susceptibility among isolates from those ≥ 65 years of age (0.6%) was significantly higher than those among persons aged <15 years of age (0%). The prevalence of the phenotype was 0.5% among the respiratory isolates comparing to 0.1% among blood isolates [14]. In the SENTRY study, levofloxacin resistance was significantly higher among penicillin intermediate (2.3%) or resistant (2.8%) isolates, than in penicillin sensitive (0.1%) isolates [10]. Similarly, the Active Bacterial Core Surveillance program has found a link between levofloxacin resistance and penicillin resistance among the invasive pneumococci [8]. Nonetheless, one large study involving 15,123 isolates from the US concluded that levofloxacin resistance was not statistically associated with advanced patient age or penicillin resistance [20].

Gram negative bacteria

Enterobacteriaceae

Among the Gram-negative bacteria, the risk of development of resistance among members of the family *Enterobacteriaceae* was considered to be extremely low [21]. In one center, there was no increase in quinolone resistance among the Enterobacteriaceae 6 years after introduction of ciprofloxacin [22]. Table 3 showed the ciprofloxacin susceptibility of members in the family *Enterobacteriaceae* in recent studies. Generally speaking, the fluoroquinolones continue to be active against most (>90–97%) *E. coli*, *Klebsiella*, *Citrobacter*, *Enterobacter* and *Serratia* species isolated from Canada and the United States [23, 24]. In contrast, fluoroquinolone resistance has been detected in 10–25% of these isolates from Latin America [23, 25, 26]. In Europe, variations in quinolone resistance rates existed, with the highest rates reported in southern Europe (namely Greece, Italy, Portugal and Spain). In some regions, quinolone resistance has also become an important issue among the *Enterobacteriaceae* that caused nosocomial bacteremia. In a study of nosocomial bacteremia in 61 hospitals within the United Kingdom between 1997 to 1999, ciprofloxacin resistance was found in 8% and 14% of the *E. coli* and *Klebsiella* spp. isolates respectively [27]. Another study from South Korea

Table 3. Ciprofloxacin susceptibility of *Enterobacteriaceae* in 1997–1998

Geographic area	% susceptible			
	E. coli	*Klebsiella* spp.	*Enterobacter* spp.	*Citrobacter* spp.
Canada	97–98.9 (100)	93.8–94.7 (92.3)	91.7–97.2	93.8
United States	97.4–97.8	93.2–98.1 (96.4)	91.3–94.2 (95.4)	96
Latin America	86.8–93.9 (77.5)	81.9–84 (89.6)	77.5–91.7 (64.3)	80
Austria	100	100	–	–
Belgium	94.7	91.7	–	–
France	94.6–96.0	96.8–100	–	–
Germany	91.8–98.0	96.2–100	–	–
Greece	93.5	84.8	–	–
Italy	93.4–90.5	77.3–88.9	–	–
The Netherlands	94.9	100	–	–
Poland	82.9–100	54.6–86.7	–	–
Portugal	77.8	100	–	–
Spain	76.7–88.0	88.9–100	–	–
Switzerland	100	100	–	–
United Kingdom	92	92.6	–	–

Figures extracted from the SENTRY antimicrobial surveillance program data. Data for countries in Europe were derived from testing isolates obtained between 1997–1998 [95]. Data for other countries were obtained from surveillance in 1997 or in 1998 [23–26, 58, 59]. Range indicates variations in isolates from different specimen sites or centers.

reported a quinolone resistance rate of 16% among *E. coli* isolates causing bloodstream infection in a hospital [28].

Except among isolates from patients with cancer or cirrhosis that were given fluoroquinolone prophylaxis, development of quinolone resistance in *E. coli* has been rare until the past several years. Of note were several reports [29–31] that associated increasing use of quinolones with resistance in community urinary isolates of *E. coli*. In The Netherlands, a surveillance of >90,000 *E. coli* urinary isolates demonstrated an increase in resistance to norfloxacin from 1.3% in 1989 to 5.8% in 1998. Resistance among community isolates was associated with previous fluoroquinolones use but was independent of age, gender and origin of the isolate [31]. At one institute in Spain, as fluoroquinolone consumption increase from 1392 g in 1990 to 3203 g in 1996, a drastic increase in ciprofloxacin resistance from 3% to 20% was observed in *E. coli* isolated from urine samples [30]. Interestingly, quinolone resistance in *E. coli* isolated from blood or other sample cultures was not increased [30]. In a case control study by Ena et al., risk factors independently associated with urinary tract infection by quinolone-resistant *E. coli* include prior treatment with fluoroquinolones, urinary tract abnormalities, age 65 years or above and urinary catheterization [32]. In regions with greater consumption of fluoroquinolones, there has been a significant increase not only in quinolone-resistant *E. coli* isolated from urine samples, but also bloodstream infections [28, 35]. In contrast, a survey of >100,000 urinary isolates from the United States demonstrated that >98% of *E. coli* in community-acquired urinary tract infection remain susceptible to the fluoroquinolones [33].

Quinolone-resistant *E. coli* [19, 28, 34, 35] as well as *Klebsiella* spp. [36] isolates were often also resistant to multiple antibiotics of unrelated classes. An association with production of extended-spectrum β-lactamase has been repeatedly observed [36, 37]. In instances that involve ESBL-producing strains, Paterson et al. reported this to be due to the dissemination of a limited number of resistant clones [36]. Among isolates that were not producing ESBL, studies from Europe and South Korea have found little evidence of clonal spread [28, 34].

Campylobacter and Salmonella

Quinolone resistance among the campylobacters in both humans and food animals is rapidly emerging worldwide since the early 1990s [38]. This was widely believed to be the result of using quinolones, such as enrofloxacin and sarafloxacin as growth promoter in animal husbandry. In Denmark, 24% of *Campylobacter coli* isolates from pigs were resistant to enrofloxacin, whereas 29% isolates from humans were resistant when 123 isolates were tested in 1997 [39]. In the same year, *C. jejuni* with ciprofloxacin MIC of >256 µg/ml occurred in 12% of strains isolated from humans with acute gastrointestinal infections in North-West England and Wales [40]. In Spain, an extremely high frequency of ciprofloxacin resistance was detected among *Campylobacter* strains in 1997–1998, particularly those isolated from boilers and pigs (99%), with a slightly lower result for humans (72%) [41]. A similar trend has also been observed in North America. In Quebec, ciprofloxacin-resistant *C. jejuni* increased from 3.5% in 1992–1993 to 12.7% in 1995–1997 [42]. In Minnesota, the proportion of ciprofloxacin-resistant *C. jejuni* isolates in humans increased from 1.3% in 1992 to 10.2% in 1998 after the licensure of sarafloxacin and enrofloxacin in 1995 and 1996 respectively for animal use [43].

Since quinolone became the major alternative therapy for patients suffering from typhoid fever in the Indian sub-continent and Southeast Asian countries in the early 1990s, strains of *Salmonella enterica* serotype Typhi with reduced susceptibility to ciprofloxacin were increasingly recognized in these areas [44]. In Vietnam, the proportion of *S. enterica* serotype Typhi with reduced susceptibility to ciprofloxacin increased slowly from 4% in 1993 to 12% in 1997 [45]. An epidemic of *S. enterica* serotype Typhi with reduced susceptibility to ciprofloxacin was first reported in Tajikistan (which is located to the north of Afganistan), where more than 6000 cases were identified within the first 3 months of 1997 in the capital [46]. Transcontinental spread of *S. enterica* serotype Typhi with reduced susceptibility to ciprofloxacin has also been reported [47]. In the UK, isolates obtained from travelers returning from Sri Lanka, Nepal, Bangladesh and Thailand demonstrated an increasing trend of

S. enterica serotype Typhi with reduced susceptibility to ciprofloxacin (MIC ≥ 0.25 μg/ml), from 3% in 1995 to 23% in 1999. Furthermore, more than 50% of these isolates were also resistant to chloramphenicol, ampicillin, and trimethroprim [47].

Strains of *S. enterica* serotype Typhi with high level resistance to fluoroquinolones have not been reported if the accepted British Society for Antimicrobial Chemotherapy and National Committee for Clinical Laboratory Standard breakpoints for ciprofloxacin (MIC of 2 μg/ml and 4 μg/ml respectively) for *Enterobacteriaceae* are used [48, 49]. In some instances, reduced susceptibility to ciprofloxacin has been associated with fluoroquinolone treatment failure in typhoid fever [50]. Fully quinolone-resistant strains will likely appear, perhaps in the near future. These strains would pose a major health problem particularly in areas where typhoid fever is endemic and public health measures inadequate. If high level resistance to quinolones emerge in *S. enterica* serotype Typhi, the remaining therapeutic options will be limited.

Salmonella enterica serotypte Typhimurium phage type DT 104 with multiresistant profile (ampicillin, chloramphenicol, streptomycin, sulphonamide, tetracycline) has emerged as an important food-borne salmonella infection in industrialized countries since 1997. Currently, it accounts for 8–9% of *Salmonella* isolates in the US [51]. In the UK, 12% of multi-resistant DT 104 had reduced sensitivity to the fluoroquinolones (ciprofloxacin MIC ≥ 0.5 μg/ml) [52]. A study from Denmark in 1998 demonstrated the first community outbreak of quinolone less susceptible and multi-resistant DT 104 infection, in which 11 of 25 patients were hospitalized and two of them died. Epidemiological analysis suggested the resistant strains were spread from food animals to human [53]. In *S. enterica* serotype choleraesuis, a recent study from Taiwan suggested that fluoroquinolone resistance might be also emerging [54]. Among isolates obtained in two medical centers, ciprofloxacin resistance increased from 0% between 1987 through 1999 to 60% in the third quarter of 2001. By molecular typing, most patient isolates had an identical profile to isolates recovered from pigs, suggesting that fluoroquinolone-resistant *S. enterica* serotype choleraesuis can spread from swine to human [54]. The link between animal use of quinolones and resistance in campylobacters and the salmonellae will be further discussed later.

Pseudomonas aeruginosa

A wide range of quinolone resistance rates continued to exist among recent isolates of *P. aeruginosa.* At present, the fluoroquinolones is the only class of agents that can be given orally to treat infections due to *P. aeruginosa*. Hence, they were used more often in outpatient than in inpatient settings. In the ICARE Project, quinolone-resistant *P. aeruginosa* is the only organism, for which resistance rates in the outpatient areas (20%) were higher than those in inpatients (16.4–17.6%) [55]. In inpatients, quinolone resistance were particular common in the settings of cystic fibrosis, ventilator-associated pneumonia and nosocomial urinary tract infection. In North America, the overall rates of ciprofloxacin-resistant *P. aeruginosa* have increased from 5–10% in early 1990s [21, 56, 57] to >10% and up to 28% in 1997 [23, 25, 58, 59]. In Latin America, much higher ciprofloxacin resistance rates have been found, ranging from 26% in blood isolates [23], 32% in pneumonia isolates [26] to 69% in urinary isolates [25]. In the UK, 15% of *P. aeruginosa* isolates causing nosocomial bacteremia were ciprofloxacin resistant [27].

Haemophilus influenzae and Moraxella catarrhalis
Fluoroquinolone resistance in both *H. influenzae* and *M. catarrhalis* remains extremely rare. Identification of such isolates has been limited to isolated reports from diverse geographic locations. A recent update of the Alexander Project indicated that in 1995 and 1996, 0.37 and 0.14% of 4,663 *H. influenzae* strains were ofloxacin-resistant, respectively [60].

Gonococci
Among the gonococci, quinolone resistance (ciprofloxacin MIC ≥ 1 μg/ml) has increasingly been reported to correlate with treatment failure [61, 62]. Quinolone-resistant *Neisseria gonorrheae* (QRNG) is prevalent in Australia and most Southeast Asian countries. In these areas, studies such as those from the WHO Gonococcal antimicrobial susceptibility program (GAST) have revealed substantial increase in the incidence of resistance since the mid-1990s. In Australia and Singapore, the increase has been relatively modest, from 0.1% to 2.6% between 1992–96 and from 0.3% to 4% between 1993–96 respectively [63]. In Japan, one center reported an increase from 7% in 1993 to 24% in 1998 [64]. In Hong Kong, China, Korea, Cambodia and The Philippines, intermediate resistance to ciprofloxacin is now exhibited by >50% of the current isolates [63]. As a result, the fluoroquinolones have been discontinued as first line of treatment for gonorrhea in Hong Kong and Japan. In Canada and the US, the overall rates of fluoroquinolone resistance remain low, but sporadic QRNG isolates and endemic spread have been increasingly reported [65, 66]. The Gonorrhea Isolate Surveillance Project (GISP) has indicated that QRNG may be imported into and may spread in the US [65]. In Ohio, one study has documented the endemic spread of a single genotype within a few years [67]. These findings are important since the history of QRNG in the Far East indicated that rise in resistance can be rapid. Interestingly, most of the QRNG isolates in Japan and the US had chromosomally mediated penicillin resistance and were of Pro auxotype [66, 67]. Therefore, Pro gonococcal isolates may more easily acquire chromosomally mediated resistance not only to penicillin but also to the fluoroquinolones.

Animal use, suboptimal human use and bacterial resistance

In humans, there is evidence to link suboptimal use of quinolone such as using less active agents or giving recommended agents at sub-therapeutic dose with development of quinolone resistance in certain microorganisms. In tropical countries such as the Indian subcontinent and Vietnam where typhoid fever is endemic, emergence of strains with reduced susceptibility has been attributed to the widespread and indiscriminate use of fluoroquinolones. In the Philippines, the emergence of quinolone-resistant gonococci has also been attributed to the widespread use of less active fluoroquinolone such as rosoxacin and norfloxacin in the 1980s for therapy of gonococcal infections. Subsequently, when ciprofloxacin became the primary therapy for gonorrhea the drug was often given at subtherapeutic dose, and as many as 30% of commercial sex workers in the Philippines have reported using prophylactic quinolone in a low dosage, before scheduled routine examination [68]. Concerning the pneumococci, one case-control study showed that a history of previous fluoroquinolone use, mostly with less active agents such as ciprofloxacin and ofloxacin was common among patients with respiratory colonization or infection by quinolone-resistant strains [13].

According to the reports from the World Health Organization, it was estimated that about 50% of antibiotic production were used in the animal industry [69]. Quinolones are one of the commonly used groups of antimicrobial agents in food animals. There were 11 quinolones licensed for use in animals in different regions of the world in 1998. The annual consumption in areas such as the US, European countries, Japan, and South Korea has been estimated to be around 50 tons for proprietary quinolones and 70 tons for generic products [70]. In such a huge amount of antibiotic consumption, only a few were used as treatment or prophylaxis of infectious diseases in the animal. The majority of antibiotics were applied as growth promoters. Indiscriminate use of antibiotics including quinolones in animals might adversely affect human health in one of the following ways (Fig. 1).

Selection of quinolone resistance in enteric pathogens

There is evidence that quinolone use in food animals leads to the emergence of quinolone-resistant bacteria in animals. These resistant organisms are transmitted to humans *via* direct contact with the animal or through the consumption of contaminated food and water. Quinolone-resistant campylobacter is one such example of animal-to-human transmission, as has been observed in many European countries since the early 1990s [71, 72]. *Campylobacter* spp. develop resistance readily because it is intrinsically less susceptible to the quinolones. A single point mutation may be enough to increase the MIC to a level above the breakpoint. Recently, incidence of quinolone-resistant *Campylobacter* spp. in the UK has increased from 11% in 1995 to 18% in 1998, following the introduction of enrofloxacin for animal use in 1993 [73]. Similarly, one report from the UK found that 12% of *Salmonella typhimurium* DT 104 had reduced susceptibility to ciprofloxacin (MIC 0.1–1 μg/ml) [52]. Furthermore, one study in the US has found similar rates ciprofloxacin-resistant *C. jejuni* from human

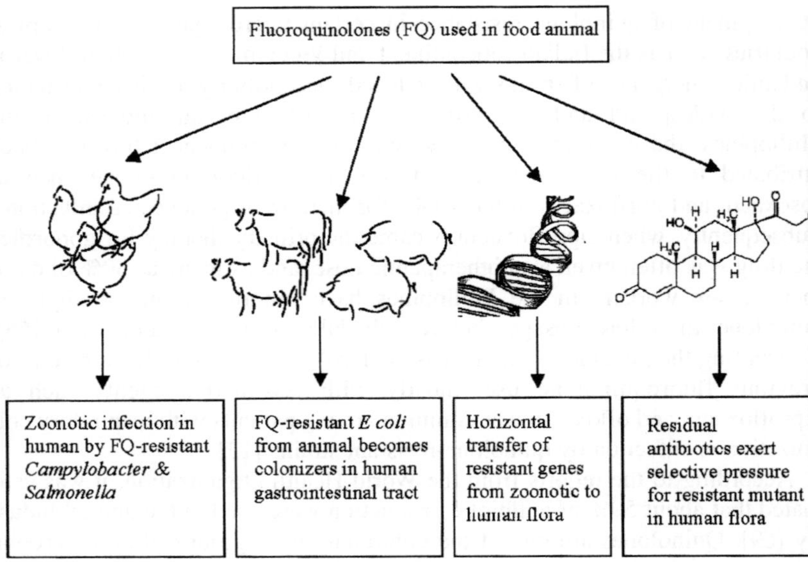

Figure 1. Ecological consequences of quinolone use in food animal

(10%) and domestic chicken (14%), and that the chicken isolates were identical to human isolates in the PCR-RFLP analysis [43].

Selection of quinolone resistance in colonizing flora

Quinolone-resistant *E. coli* has been isolated from poultry samples soon after the introduction of quinolone for animal use [74]. An increasing trend of quinolone-resistant *E. coli* isolation in poultry and pork has been observed in another study, in which up to 90% of chicken harbored quinolone-resistant *E. coli* [75]. The high level of resistance among animal isolates was not only linked to the asymptomatic carriage of quinolone-resistant *E. coli* in the feces of healthy adults (24%) and children (26%), but also related to quinolone-resistant *E. coli* bacteremia in the hospital [75]. The concomitant use of antibiotic in humans may increase the risk of infection with a quinolone-resistant *E. coli* once colonized the gut of human.

Acquisition of antimicrobial resistant gene via horizontal transfer

Acquisition of antimicrobial resistant genes from bacteria in food animals to the commensal strains of the gut flora *via* horizontal transmission is another concern. Excessive spread of resistant genes among Gram negative enteric bacilli, anaerobes, and Gram positive bacteria was previously demonstrated in the colon [76]. Transfer of the plasmid mediated resistant gene, CMY-2 from the food animal to human has recently been demonstrated in *Salmonella* and *E coli* [77]. While quinolone resistance determinants are encoded on the chromosome, the possibility that some of the resistant traits such as the efflux pumps becoming plasmid- or transposon-mediated cannot be completely ruled out. In fact, there has been one instance of a plasmid mediated quinolone resistance in a clinical isolate of *Klebsiella pneumoniae* although the mechanism of resistance remains undefined [78].

Direct absorption of residue antibiotic in animal food

Residual antibiotics in meat can pass from animal to human as a result of dietary intake. At permitted minimum residue levels, their impact on bacterial resistance in human is estimated to be small, according to one investigation [69]. However, the available evidence is only limited and in fact this has been identified as a priority for future studies in a recent World Health Organization meeting [69].

Mechanism of bacterial resistance

Fluoroquinolone mechanism of action

DNA topoisomerases are classified as type I or type II according to whether transient single-strand breaks (type I) or double strand breaks (type II) are made in the DNA when the double helical strands unwind during DNA processes. Bacteria contain two distinct type II enzymes, DNA gyrase and topoisomerase IV. Both enzymes are essential in the regulation of DNA topology. DNA gyrase is essential for maintaining the degree of supercoiling in the bacterial chromosome. By catalyzing negative DNA supercoiling, it relieves torsional stress that accumulates in front of the replication forks. The physiological function of topoisomerase IV is different from that of DNA gyrase. It is the enzyme that partitions the daughter chromosomes following DNA replication. Each of these enzymes comprises two subunits. DNA gyrase exists as an A_2B_2 heterotetramer, encoded by the *gyrA* and *gyrB* genes. Topoisomerase IV exists as a C_2E_2 heterotetramer, encoded by the *parC* and *parE* genes (sometimes referred to as *grlA* and *grlB* respectively in Gram-positive bacteria).

The fluoroquinolones are bactericidal. This group of agents acts by interacting with DNA gyrase and/or topoisomerase IV (Fig. 2). Depending on the bacterial species and quinolone used either DNA gyrase or topoisomerase IV serves as the primary intracellular target of drug action. The latest model on

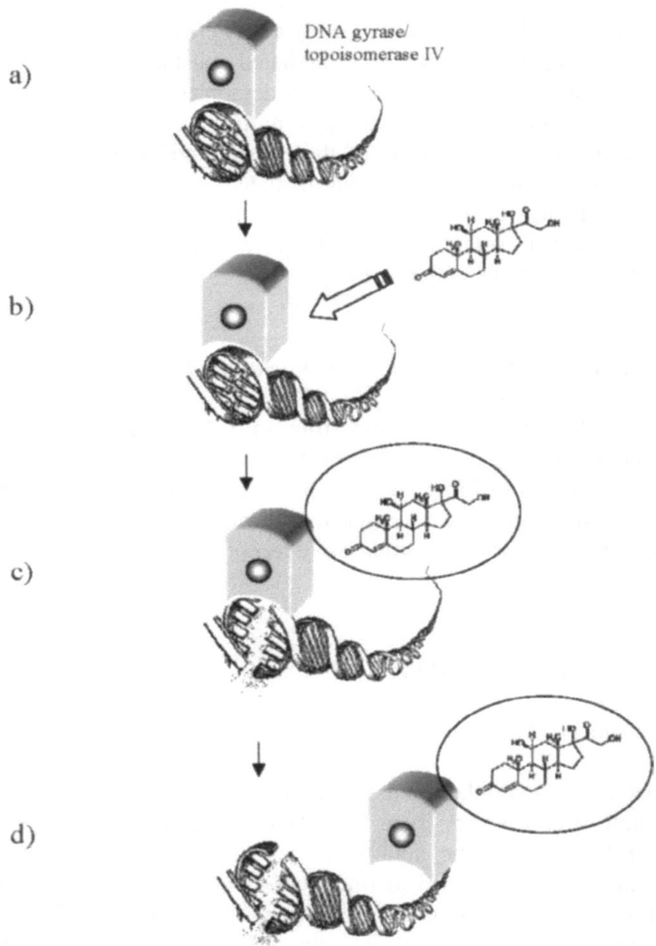

Figure 2. Diagrammatic representation of intracellular events involved in quinolone-mediated cell death. a) DNA bind to DNA gyrase or DNA topoisomerase IV in the "DNA accomodation groove" (represented by the concave surface). b) and c) Quinolone interact with the complexes of DNA–DNA gyrase or topoisomerase IV, converting it to a cleavage complex with double-stranded DNA break. d) By as yet undefined mechanisms including possiby collision between DNA tracking enzymes and the cleavage complex, transient enzyme-associated breaks are converted to permanent double-stranded breaks. As DNA breaks accumulate, the SOS response is activated which eventually induce cell death.

the intracellular actions of the quinolones is as follows [3, 4, 79]. The quinolones bind to the DNA gyrase/topoisomerase IV-DNA complex and inhibit the physiological functions of the enzymes. Inhibition of the enzymatic functions itself is not lethal. Rather, by enhancement of DNA cleavage or by blocking DNA relegation after double-stranded cleavage by the enzymes, the quinolones increase the intracellular concentrations of the cleavage complexes that are intermediates in the DNA gyrase/topoisomerase IV-mediated reactions. When DNA tracking enzymes such as polymerases or helicases collide with these cleavage complexes, transient enzyme-mediated DNA breaks become permanent. It is the release and accumulation of permanent double-strand DNA breaks that leads to bacterial cell death.

Mechanism of resistance

Fluoroquinolone resistance is mediated by target modifications and/or decreased intracellular accumulation. So far, there have been no reports of enzyme-mediated destruction or modification of the antibiotic. This could be due to the fact that the fluoroquinolones are synthetic compounds and thus have not been previously involved in physiological processes.

Target site modifications

Resistance to fluoroquinolones due to target site alteration tends to develop in a stepwise manner. The MIC of mutants increases with each additional mutation in the topoisomerases. In most organisms, particularly the Gram-positive bacteria high-level resistance to the fluoroquinolones generally only occurs in the presence of mutations involving both DNA gyrase and topoisomerase IV. Depending upon the bacterial species and the fluoroquinolone concerned, first step mutants occur reproducibly in either the DNA gyrase or the topoisomerase IV. In Gram-negative bacteria, DNA gyrase appears to be the primary cellular target for fluoroquinolones, whilst in Gram-positive bacteria topoisomerase IV is generally the primary target. However, variations from the aforementioned rule have been found. In *S. pneumoniae*, first-step mutants selected with the newer fluoroquinolones such as moxifloxacin and gatifloxacin, unlike older fluoroquinolones, bore mutations in DNA gyrase first.

Mutations in DNA gyrase and topoisomerase IV occur most commonly in the GyrA and ParC subunits respectively. The frequency of GyrB or ParE mutations, compared to GyrA and ParC respectively, has been relatively low. The deduced amino acid sequences of GyrA and ParC, and GyrB and ParE, respectively, show homology. However, many studies have failed to assign significance to mutations in GyrB and ParE. For instance, mutations in gyrB and parE among pneumococci had no apparent effect on the extent of quinolone susceptibility [80].

In GyrA, the most prevalent and resistant mutations occur over some hotspots within a small region near the N-terminus of the polypeptide. These mutations were closed to Tyr122, which is the site covalently bound to the DNA. Concerning GyrA, the enzyme from *E. coli* has been studied most intensively. Based on the amino acid sequence of the *E. coli* enzyme, the most com-

(A) GyrA

```
                     67                   83                                                122
E. coli              ARVV GDVIGKYHPH GDSAVYDTIV RMAQPFSLRY MLVDGQGNFG SIDGDSAAAM RYTEIR
S. typhi             ARVV GDVIGKYHPH GDSAVYDTIV RMAQPFSLRY MLVDGQGNFG SIDGDSAAAM RYTEIR
P. aeruginosa        ARVV GDVIGKYHPH GDTAVYDTIV RMAQPFSLRY MLVDGQGNFG SVDGDNAAAM RYTEVR
H. influenzae        ARVV GDVIGKYHPH GDSAVYDTIV RMAQPFSLRY MLVDGQGNFG SIDGDAPAAM RYTEVR
N. gonorrhoeae       ARIV GDVIGKYHPH GDSAVYDTIV RMAQNFAMRY VLIDGQGNFG SVDGLAAAAM RYTEIR
S. aureus            ARIV GDVMGKYHPH GDSSIYEAMV RMAQDFSYRY PLVDGQGNFG SMDGDGAAAM RYTEAR
S. pneumoniae        ARIT GDVMGKYHPH GDSSIYEAMV RMAQWWSYRY MLVDGHGNFG SMDGDSAAAQ RYTEAR
```

(B) ParC

```
                     64                   80                                                120
E. coli              ARTV GDVLGKYHPH GDSACYEAMV LMAQPFSYRY PLVDGQGNWG APDDPKSFAA MRYTES
S. typhi             ARTV GDVLGKYHPH GDSACYEAMV LMAQPFSYRY PLVDGQGNWG APDDPKSFAA MRYTES
P. aeruginosa        ARTV GDVLGKFHPH GDSACYEAMV LMAQPFSYRY PLVDGQGNWG APDDPKSFAA MRYTEA
H. influenzae        ARTV GDVLGKFHPH GDSACYEAMV LMAQPFSYRY PLVDGQGNWG APDDPKSFAA MRYTES
N. gonorrhoeae       ARVV GEILGKYHPH GDSSAYEAMV RMAQDFTLRY PLIDGIGNFG SRDGDGA.AA MRYTEA
S. aureus            AKTV GDVIGQYHPH GDSSVYEAMV RLSQDWKLRH VLIEMHGNNG SIDNDPP.AA MRYTEA
S. pneumoniae        AESV GNIMGNFHPH GDSSIYDAMV RMSQNWKNRE ILVEMHGNNG SMDGDPP.AA MRYTEA
```

Figure 3. Quinolone resistance determining regions (QRDR) of (A) GyrA and (B) ParC/GrlA from different bacteria. Amino acid substitutions known to associate with fluoroquinolone resistance are shaded. Numbering is based on those reported for *E. coli*. Underlined, the usual range of QRDR; boldface, tyrosine residue at the active site; and shaded, common substitution sites associated with resistance to quinolones. (Sequences were obtained from GenBank under the following accessions: NP_416734, CAD07504, NP_251858, NP_438419, AAA82128, BAA01370 and NP_358692 for GyrA; NP_417491, CAD03006, BAA37152, P43702, AAA82151, P50073 and NP_358351 for ParC/GrlA)

mon mutations that lead to drug resistance occur at Ser83 and Asp87 of the GyrA subunit. Other less frequent mutations occur at Ala67, Gly81, Ala84 and Gln106 (Fig. 3). Because of the consistent occurrence of mutations within the same region from amino acid position 67 to 106, this region is commonly referred to as the quinolones resistance-determining region (QRDR). Recently, the three-dimensional crystal structure of the "breakage-reunion" domain of *E. coli* GyrA dimer has been published and a model proposed to explain the interaction of the active site Tyr122 with the DNA helix [4]. According to the model, amino acid residues in the QRDR lie in close spatial proximity to the active tyrosine site in the "DNA accommodation groove." The current working hypothesis is that mutations in the QRDR distort the positioning of DNA in the "groove." As a result, binding of quinolone to the gyrase-DNA complex is reduced.

For many Gram-positive bacteria, as for *S. aureus* and *S. pneumoniae*, first-step quinolone resistance mutations occur in parC or, less commonly, parE. Based on the *S. pneumoniae* coordinates of parC, the hotspots most favoured for giving rise to quinolone resistance occur at Ser79 and Asp83. Other less frequent mutations occur at Asp78, Asp84, Arg95, Ala115 and Lys129 (Fig. 3). Accordingly, the corresponding active tyrosine site occurs at position 118.

Decrease cellular accumulation of quinolones

Reduced cellular accumulation of quinolones can occur as a result of decreased cellular entry and/or active drug efflux. In Gram-positive bacteria, active drug efflux was commonly inferred by MIC testing in the presence or absence of a efflux pump inhibitor such as reserpine or carbonyl cyanide m-chlorophenylhydrazone (CCCP). Susceptibility to quinolones typically increases by two- to eight-fold in the presence of an inhibitor. A number of efflux pumps, such as NorA in *S. aureus* and PmrA in *S. pneumoniae* have been identified in Gram-positive bacteria. NorA is expressed weakly in wild-type cells of all *S. aureus* isolates examined so far. In *S. aureus*, promoter mutation and the resultant upregulation of NorA lead to resistance to norfloxacin. In fluoroquinolone-resistant mutant *S. aureus*, it has been shown that enhanced efflux commonly precedes target site alteration. In *S. pneumoniae*, PmrA also appear to express at low level in wild-type cells. Studies with reserpine suggest that at least half of resistant pneumococcal clinical isolates had evidence of enhanced efflux expression. Generally speaking, quinolone efflux drug alone does not lead to high level resistance in the Gram-positive bacteria. This mechanism has only a trivial effect on the antimicrobial activities of the newer fluoroquinolones such as gatifloxacin and moxifloxacin. There is no cross-resistance to other structurally unrelated classes of antibiotics.

In contrast, drug efflux in Gram-negative bacteria such as *P. aeruginosa* can be the major mechanism of high-level quinolone resistance. Furthermore, drug efflux in the Gram-negative organisms tends to have broad substrate specificity, including fluoroquinolones and other structurally unrelated compounds such as the aminoglycosides and β-lactams. In Gram-negative bacteria, multi-drug transporters most commonly belong to the resistance-nodulation-division (RND) family. Each efflux transporter contains at least three subunits: a transporter protein, an outer membrane efflux protein (OEP) and a periplasmic membrane fusion protein (MFP) that links the two. A number of RND efflux transporters such as MexAB-OprM in *P. aerugionsa* and AcrAB-TolC in *E. coli* have been reported and characterized. These systems are an integral part of the normal genetic complement of the bacteria and appear to have roles in bacterial adaptation in different ecological niches. Expression of these transporters is highly regulated. The level of expression of these pumps affects the extent of efflux-mediated fluoroquinolone resistance. Mutations in global regulator loci such as marA, as well as in the specific pump regulator loci such as acrR have been associated with hyper-expression.

There are exceptions to the rule of stepwise development of quinolone resistance. Quinolone-resistant *S. aureus* obtained *in vitro* can harbor most of the mechanisms of resistance known, individually or in combination, and that mutations resulting in topoisomerase- and NorA-mediated FQ resistance can arise, alone or in combination, in a single step [81]. On the other hand, non-target gene mutations in the efflux regulatory loci can interact with target alterations in the development of fluoroquinolone resistance. For example, it has been shown that in *E. coli* non-target gene mutations regularly accumulate in second- and third-step mutants with topoisomerases alterations upon exposure to a fluoroquinolone. Therefore, it is likely that in most bacteria, mutations affecting fluoroquinolone efflux and drug binding to the target sites both contribute to resistance development *in vivo*.

Prevention of resistance

Fluoroquinolone resistance has important clinical implications. Surveillance and a better understanding of the mechanism of resistance are incomplete in the absence of efforts directed to reduce the scope of the problem. In some bacteria, it appears that a single occult mutation in one of the topoisomerase targets, such as single *parC* mutation in the pneumococci [82] or single *gyrA* mutation in *S. enterica* serotype cholerasuis [54] is a precursor to development of full resistance. To reduce the likelihood of selecting higher resistance, it may be important to be able to detect isolates with first-step mutations. Unfortunately, isolates with these resistance mechanisms will appear susceptible and could not be detected reliably using conventional susceptibility methods [54, 82]. This is an area that needs to be addressed in future studies.

Our knowledge in the pharmacodynamics of the fluoroquinolones has expanded. Many *in vitro* studies have been conducted to compare the pharmacodynamics of the fluoroquinolones and their correlation with the likelihood of selecting for resistance [83]. Different views exist regarding the importance of one or the other parameter, a C_{max}:MIC of ≥ 10 and an AUC_{0-24}:MIC of ≥ 100 to 125 have been associated with a lower risk of resistance development. Nonetheless, available clinical data were limited and were mainly of a retrospective nature [84, 85]. In a study of 107 acutely ill patients treated in four clinical trials treated with ciprofloxacin or a β-lactam, AUC_{0-24}:MIC ratio of <100 was a significant predictor of development of resistance [85]. Similarly, in a study of 635 patients with *Pseudomonas aeruginosa* infections, AUC_{0-24}:MIC ratio of <110 was also found to correlate with a higher risk of development of resistance to ciprofloxacin [84].

Concluding remarks

In conclusion, resistance to fluoroquinolones has become increasingly important in the past several years. In some areas, the current level of resistance has made this class of agents no longer appropriate as first-line agents for therapy of gonorrhoeae and campylobacter gastroenteritis. The emergence of resistance among *S. pneumoniae* and urinary isolates of *E. coli* in the community is of particular concern. The epidemiology of quinolone-resistant *S. pneumoniae* is being closely monitored, at least in the developed countries. However, there is little information on the molecular epidemiology of the quinolone-resistant

Table 4. International and national antimicrobial resistance surveillance data available at the Internet

Program	Countries	Internet address
Alexander Project	International	http://www.alexander-network.com
Gonococcal Isolate Surveillance Project	United States	http://www.cdc.gov/ncidod/dastlr/gcdir/gono.html
National Nosocomial Infection Surveillance	United States	http://www.cdc.gov/ncidod/hip/NNIS/members/members.htm#nnisreports
Public Health Laboratory Service	United Kingdom	http://www.phls.co.uk/publications/index.htm

E. coli from the community. One recent study demonstrated that increase in cotrimoxazole resistance among community uropathogenic *E. coli* in the US could be related to outbreak of a few successful clones [86]. Further study to determine whether the recent increase in quinolone resistance among *E. coli* could be due to the same mechanism would be a priority, as it presents a potential point for intervention to curtail resistance.

The fluoroquinolones are increasingly use for therapy of presumed or documented respiratory tract infections due to the atypical organisms. For the atypical pathogen such as *Legionella*, mycoplasma and chlamydia, there is a lack of resistance knowledge. Susceptibility testing of these organisms is more complicated and is not standardized. In the near future, centralized testing in few reference centers longitudinally would be preferred.

The main focus of most on-going surveillance is the susceptibility of the monitored organisms to a panel of antibiotics. Few have incorporated the usage of the fluoroquinolones from the areas where the organisms were obtained, as part of the monitoring program. Resistance often emerges after extensive and particularly suboptimal use. Hence, efforts to incorporate antibiotic usage data to existing surveillance should be intensified. The data should include not only the total usage but also the indications and dosage regimens.

International and national surveillance data is available on the internet (Tab. 4), facilitating accessibility and dissemination. However, only the Alexander Project homepage allow access to the database, user-specified search and analysis. The results of some major international initiatives such as the SENTRY project were not available on their website and the format of publications (e.g., year period, geographical regions and source of isolates) can be variable [24, 87–91]. Further research and development on this issue is important, as it is unlikely that a single published format can suit the needs of different persons who might range from clinicians to microbiologists, epidemiologists and health care administrators.

It is clear that there is a link between animal quinolone use and the emergence of resistance among some of the zoonotic pathogens. The sub-therapeutic use of antibiotics including the quinolones as growth promoters in food animals should be banned [92]. Antibiotic usage in food animals should be monitored and prescribed by a veterinarian only when there is a clear indication. Surveillance of resistant microorganisms in animals is less precisely coordinated as the ongoing program targeted at human pathogens. Because of the link between resistance in animal and human pathogens, programs that target the resistance in the zoonotic pathogens such as campylobacters and nontyphoidal salmonellae should try to standardize the methods and the panel of agents tested. It is only through a coordinated effort that one can make a meaningful comparison of data from animals and humans.

References

1 Kohler T, Pechere JC (2000) Bacterial resistance to quinolones: mechanisms and clinical implications., p. 139–167. *In:* VT Andriole (ed.): *The quinolones.* Academic Press, San Diego. *(This review summarizes the literature on quinolone resistance epidemiology in late 1980s to early 1990s in two large tables.)*
2 Turnidge J (1995) Epidemiology of quinolone resistance. Eastern hemisphere. *Drugs* 49 Suppl 2: 43–47 *(Describes the quinolone resistance epidemiology of a WHO study in 13 countries of the Western Pacific region between 1992–1993. Mainly of historic interests.)*
3 Chen CR, Malik M, Snyder M, Drlica K (1996) DNA gyrase and topoisomerase IV on the bacterial chromosome: quinolone-induced DNA cleavage. *J Mol Biol* 258: 627–637 *(This paper provides evidence that DNA breaks is a key mechanism in quinolone-mediated cell death.)*
4 Morais-Cabral JH, Jackson AP, Smith CV, Shikotra N, Maxwell A, Liddington RC (1997) Crystal structure of the breakage-reunion domain of DNA gyrase. *Nature* 388: 903–906
5 Gill MJ, Brenwald NP, Wise R (1999) Identification of an efflux pump gene, pmrA, associated with fluoroquinolone resistance in *Streptococcus pneumoniae. Antimicrob Agents Chemother* 43: 187–189
6 Li XZ, Nikaido H, Poole K (1995) Role of mexA-mexB-oprM in antibiotic efflux in *Pseudomonas aeruginosa. Antimicrob Agents Chemother* 39: 1948–1953
7 Chen DK, McGeer A, de Azavedo JC, Low DE (1999) Decreased susceptibility of *Streptococcus pneumoniae* to fluoroquinolones in Canada. Canadian Bacterial Surveillance Network. *N Engl J Med* 341: 233–239 *(A widely cited paper. It proved the emergence of* S. pneumoniae *with reduced susceptibility to quinolones.)*
8 Whitney CG, Farley MM, Hadler J, Harrison LH, Lexau C, Reingold A, Lefkowitz L, Cieslak PR, Cetron M, Zell ER, Jorgensen LH, Schuchat A (2000) Increasing prevalence of multidrug-resistant *Streptococcus pneumoniae* in the United States. *N Engl J Med* 343: 1917–1924
9 Sahm DF, Karlowsky JA, Kelly LJ, Critchley IA, Jones ME, Thornsberry C, Mauriz Y, Kahn J (2001) Need for annual surveillance of antimicrobial resistance in *Streptococcus pneumoniae* in the United States: 2-year longitudinal analysis. *Antimicrob Agents Chemother* 45: 1037–1042
10 Jones RN, Pfaller MA (2000) Macrolide and fluoroquinolone (levofloxacin) resistances among *Streptococcus pneumoniae* strains: significant trends from the SENTRY Antimicrobial Surveillance Program (North America, 1997–1999). *J Clin Microbiol* 38: 4298–4299
11 Ho PL, Que TL, Tsang DN, Ng TK, Chow KH, Seto WH (1999) Emergence of fluoroquinolone resistance among multiply resistant strains of *Streptococcus pneumoniae* in Hong Kong. *Antimicrob Agents Chemother* 43: 1310–1313
12 Ho PL, Yung RW, Tsang DN, Que TL, Ho M, Seto WH, Ng TK, Yam WC, Ng WW (2001) Increasing resistance of *Streptococcus pneumoniae* to fluoroquinolones: results of a Hong Kong multicentre study in 2000. *J Antimicrob Chemother* 48: 659–665
13 Ho PL, Tse WS, Tsang KW, Kwok TK, Ng TK, Cheng VC, Chan RM (2001) Risk factors for acquisition of levofloxacin-resistant *Streptococcus pneumoniae*: a case-control study. *Clin Infect Dis* 32: 701–707
14 Sahm DF, Peterson DE, Critchley IA, Thornsberry C (2000) Analysis of ciprofloxacin activity

against *Streptococcus pneumoniae* after 10 years of use in the United States. *Antimicrob Agents Chemother* 44: 2521–2524

15 Ho PL, Yam WC, Cheung TKM, Ng WWS, Que TL, Tsang DNC, Ng TK, Seto WH (2001) Fluoroquinolone resistance among *Streptococcus pneumoniae* in Hong Kong linked to the Spanish 23F clone. *Emerg Infect Dis* 7: 906–908

16 Hsueh PR, Teng LJ, Wu TL, Ho SW, Luh KT (2001) First clinical isolate of *Streptococcus pneumoniae* exhibiting high-level resistance to fluoroquinolones in Taiwan. *J Antimicrob Chemother* 48: 316–317

17 Kumarasinghe G, Chow C, Tambyah PA (2000) The emergence of resistance to levofloxacin before clinical use in a university hospital in Singapore. *J Antimicrob Chemother* 46: 862–863

18 Alou L, Ramirez M, Garcia-Rey C, Prieto J, de Lencastre H (2001) *Streptococcus pneumoniae* isolates with reduced susceptibility to ciprofloxacin in Spain: clonal diversity and appearance of ciprofloxacin-resistant epidemic clones. *Antimicrob Agents Chemother* 45: 2955–2957

19 Goldsmith CE, Moore JE, Murphy PG, Ambler JE (1998) Increased incidence of ciprofloxacin resistance in penicillin-resistant pneumococci in Northern Ireland. *J Antimicrob Chemother* 41: 420–421

20 Selman LJ, Mayfield DC, Thornsberry C, Mauriz YR, Sahm DF (2000) Risk factors associated with antimicrobial resistance among *Streptococcus pneumoniae* in the United States. Abstracts of the 40th Interscience Conference on Antimicrobial Agents and Chemotherapy, Toronto, Canada, 2000. Abstract 1800, p. 111. 2000. Washington, DC, American Society for Microbiology

21 Peterson LR (1993) Quinolone resistance in clinical practice: occurrence and importance., p. 119–137. *In:* DC Hooper, JS Wolfson (eds): *Quinolones antimicrobial agents*. American Society for Microbiology, Washington

22 Pieroni P, Goodfellow J, Reesor L, Louie M, Simor AE (1997) Antimicrobial susceptibilities of blood culture isolates obtained before and after the introduction of ciprofloxacin. *J Antimicrob Chemother* 39: 419–422

23 Diekema DJ, Pfaller MA, Jones RN, Doern GV, Winokur PL, Gales AC, Sader HS, Kugler K, Beach M (1999) Survey of bloodstream infections due to Gram-negative bacilli: frequency of occurrence and antimicrobial susceptibility of isolates collected in the United States, Canada, and Latin America for the SENTRY Antimicrobial Surveillance Program, 1997. *Clin Infect Dis* 29: 595–607

24 Mathai D, Lewis MT, Kugler KC, Pfaller MA, Jones RN (2001) Antibacterial activity of 41 antimicrobials tested against over 2773 bacterial isolates from hospitalized patients with pneumonia: I – results from the SENTRY Antimicrobial Surveillance Program (North America, 1998). *Diagn Microbiol Infect Dis* 39: 105–116

25 Gales AC, Jones RN, Gordon KA, Sader HS, Wilke WW, Beach ML, Pfaller MA, Doern GV (2000) Activity, spectrum of 22 antimicrobial agents tested against urinary tract infection pathogens in hospitalized patients in Latin America: report from the second year of the SENTRY antimicrobial surveillance program (1998). *J Antimicrob Chemother* 45: 295–303

26 Sader HS, Jones RN, Gales AC, Winokur P, Kugler KC, Pfaller MA, Doern GV (1998) Antimicrobial susceptibility patterns for pathogens isolated from patients in Latin American medical centers with a diagnosis of pneumonia: analysis of results from the SENTRY Antimicrobial Surveillance Program (1997) SENTRY Latin America Study Group. *Diagn Microbiol Infect Dis* 32: 289–301

27 Public Health Laboratory Service. Surveillance of hospital-acquired bacteraemia in English hospitals 1997–1999. 1–11. 2001. London, Public Health Laboratory Service

28 Cheong HJ, Yoo CW, Sohn JW, Kim WJ, Kim MJ, Park SC (2001) Bacteremia due to quinolone-resistant *Escherichia coli* in a teaching hospital in South Korea. *Clin Infect Dis* 33: 48–53

29 Cizman M, Orazem A, Krizan-Hergouth V, Kolman J (2001) Correlation between increased consumption of fluoroquinolones in outpatients and resistance of *Escherichia coli* from urinary tract infections. *J Antimicrob Chemother* 47: 502

30 Ena J, Lopez-Perezagua MM, Martinez-Peinado C, Cia-Barrio MA, Ruiz-Lopez I (1998) Emergence of ciprofloxacin resistance in *Escherichia coli* isolates after widespread use of fluoroquinolones. *Diagn Microbiol Infect Dis* 30: 103–107

31 Goettsch W, van Pelt W, Nagelkerke N, Hendrix MG, Buiting AG, Petit PL, Sabbe LJ, van Griethuysen AJ, de Neeling AJ (2000) Increasing resistance to fluoroquinolones in *Escherichia coli* from urinary tract infections in the netherlands. *J Antimicrob Chemother* 46: 223–228

32 Ena J, Amador C, Martinez C, Ortiz-de-la-Tabla V (1995) Risk factors for acquisition of urinary

tract infections caused by ciprofloxacin resistant *Escherichia coli*. *J Urol* 153: 117–120
33 Gupta K, Sahm DF, Mayfield D, Stamm WE (2001) Antimicrobial resistance among uropathogens that cause community-acquired urinary tract infections in women: a nationwide analysis. *Clin Infect Dis* 33: 89–94
34 Oethinger M, Conrad S, Kaifel K, Cometta A, Bille J, Klotz G, Glauser MP, Marre R, Kern WV (1996) Molecular epidemiology of fluoroquinolone-resistant *Escherichia coli* bloodstream isolates from patients admitted to European cancer centers. *Antimicrob Agents Chemother* 40: 387–392
35 Pena C, Albareda JM, Pallares R, Pujol M, Tubau F, Ariza J (1995) Relationship between quinolone use and emergence of ciprofloxacin-resistant *Escherichia coli* in bloodstream infections. *Antimicrob Agents Chemother* 39: 520–524
36 Paterson DL, Mulazimoglu L, Casellas JM, Ko WC, Goossens H, Von Gottberg A, Mohapatra S, Trenholme GM, Klugman KP, McCormack JG, Yu VL (2000) Epidemiology of ciprofloxacin resistance and its relationship to extended-spectrum beta-lactamase production in *Klebsiella pneumoniae* isolates causing bacteremia. *Clin Infect Dis* 30: 473–478 *(A good review of the clinical settings in which development of quinolone resistance is more common.)*
37 Wiener J, Quinn JP, Bradford PA, Goering RV, Nathan C, Bush K, Weinstein RA (1999) Multiple antibiotic-resistant *Klebsiella* and *Escherichia coli* in nursing homes. *JAMA* 281: 517–523
38 Allos BM (2001) *Campylobacter jejuni* Infections: update on emerging issues and trends. *Clin Infect Dis* 32: 1201–1206 *(A good review to summarize the epidemiology of quinolone resistant* Campylobacter *species in 1990s with the emphaize on the relationship between consumption of quinolone in food animal and the emergence of quinolone resistant* Campylobacter *species.)*
39 Aarestrup FM, Nielsen EM, Madsen M, Engberg J (1997) Antimicrobial susceptibility patterns of thermophilic *Campylobacter* spp from humans, pigs, cattle, and broilers in Denmark. *Antimicrob Agents Chemother* 41: 2244–2250
40 Thwaites RT, Frost JA (1999) Drug resistance in *Campylobacter jejuni*, *C. coli*, and *C. lari* isolated from humans in north west England and Wales, 1997. *J Clin Pathol* 52: 812–814
41 Saenz Y, Zarazaga M, Lantero M, Gastanares MJ, Baquero F, Torres C (2000) Antibiotic resistance in *Campylobacter* strains isolated from animals, foods, and humans in Spain in 1997–1998. *Antimicrob Agents Chemother* 44: 267–271
42 Gaudreau C, Gilbert H (1998) Antimicrobial resistance of clinical strains of *Campylobacter jejuni* subsp. *jejuni* isolated from 1985 to 1997 in Quebec, Canada. *Antimicrob Agents Chemother* 42: 2106–2108
43 Smith KE, Besser JM, Hedberg CW, Leano FT, Bender JB, Wicklund JH, Johnson BP, Moore KA, Osterholm MT (1999) Quinolone-resistant *Campylobacter jejuni* infections in Minnesota, 1992–1998. Investigation Team. *N Engl J Med* 340: 1525–1532 *(Molecular sub-typing of the strains showed that quinolone-resistant* C. jejuni *isolates from chicken products and from human were identical.)*
44 Rowe B, Ward LR, Threlfall EJ (1997) Multidrug-resistant *Salmonella typhi*: a worldwide epidemic. *Clin Infect Dis* 24 Suppl 1: S106–S109
45 Parry C, Wain J, Chinh NT, Vinh H, Farrar JJ (1998) Quinolone-resistant *Salmonella typhi* in Vietnam. *Lancet* 351: 1289
46 Murdoch DA, Banatvaia N, Bone A, Shoismatulloev BI, Ward LR, Threlfall EJ, Banatvala NA (1998) Epidemic ciprofloxacin-resistant *Salmonella typhi* in Tajikistan. *Lancet* 351: 339
47 Threlfall EJ, Ward LR (2001) Decreased susceptibility to ciprofloxacin in *Salmonella enterica* serotype Typhi, United Kingdom. *Emerg Infect Dis* 7: 448–450 *(This article showed that most quinolone resistant* S. typhi *in the United Kingdom were imported from India and Pakistan.)*
48 MacGowan AP, Wise R (2001) Establishing MIC breakpoints and the interpretation of *in vitro* susceptibility tests. *J Antimicrob Chemother* 48 Suppl 1: 17–28
49 National Committee for Clinical Laboratory Standards. Performance standards for antimicrobial susceptibility testing: eleventh informational supplement. [M100-S11]. 2001. Wayne, Pa, National Committee for Clinical Laboratory Standards
50 Umasankar S, Wall RA, Berger J (1992) A case of ciprofloxacin-resistant typhoid fever. *Commun Dis Rep CDR Rev* 2: R139–R140
51 Glynn MK, Bopp C, Dewitt W, Dabney P, Mokhtar M, Angulo FJ (1998) Emergence of multidrug-resistant *Salmonella enterica* serotype typhimurium DT104 infections in the United States. *N Engl J Med* 338: 1333–1338
52 Threlfall EJ, Ward LR, Rowe B (1998) Multiresistant *Salmonella typhimurium* DT 104 and sal-

monella bacteraemia. *Lancet* 352: 287–288
53 Molbak K, Baggesen DL, Aarestrup FM, Ebbesen JM, Engberg J, Frydendahl K, Gerner-Smidt P, Petersen AM, Wegener HC (1999) An outbreak of multidrug-resistant, quinolone-resistant *Salmonella enterica* serotype typhimurium DT104. *N Engl J Med* 341: 1420–1425 *(It described an outbreak of multidrug resistant typhimurium DT104 with reduced susceptibility to quinolone that resulted in significant morbidity and mortality.)*
54 Chiu CH, Wu TL, Su LH, Chu CS, Chia JH, Kuo AJ, Chien MS, Lin TY (2002) The emergence in Taiwan of fluoroquinolone resistance in *Salmonella enterica* serotype choleraesuis. *New England Journal of Medicine* 346: 413–419
55 Fridkin SK, Steward CD, Edwards JR, Pryor ER, McGowan JE, Archibald LK, Gaynes RP, Tenover FC (1999) Surveillance of antimicrobial use and antimicrobial resistance in United States hospitals: project ICARE phase 2. Project Intensive Care Antimicrobial Resistance Epidemiology (ICARE) hospitals. *Clin Infect Dis* 29: 245–252
56 Goldstein FW, Acar JF (1995) Epidemiology of quinolone resistance: Europe and North and South America. *Drugs* 49 Suppl 2: 36–42
57 Thomson CJ (1999) The global epidemiology of resistance to ciprofloxacin and the changing nature of antibiotic resistance: a 10 year perspective. *J Antimicrob Chemother* 43 Suppl A: 31–40. *(This review summarized trends in ciprofloxacin resistance among common bacteria in the ten years prior to 1995. Longitudinal and representative data from Europe, USA, Canada and UK were tabulated.)*
58 Jones RN, Croco MA, Kugler KC, Pfaller MA, Beach ML (2000) Respiratory tract pathogens isolated from patients hospitalized with suspected pneumonia: frequency of occurrence and antimicrobial susceptibility patterns from the SENTRY Antimicrobial Surveillance Program (United States and Canada, 1997) *Diagn Microbiol Infect Dis* 37: 115–125
59 Jones RN, Kugler KC, Pfaller MA, Winokur PL (1999) Characteristics of pathogens causing urinary tract infections in hospitals in North America: results from the SENTRY Antimicrobial Surveillance Program, 1997. *Diagn Microbiol Infect Dis* 35: 55–63
60 Felmingham D, Washington J (1999) Trends in the antimicrobial susceptibility of bacterial respiratory tract pathogens – findings of the Alexander Project 1992–1996. *J Chemother* 11 Suppl 15–21:-21
61 Kam KM, Lo KK, Chong LY, Au WF, Wong PY, Cheung MM (1999) Correlation between *in vitro* quinolone susceptibility of *Neisseria gonorrhoeae* and outcome of treatment of gonococcal urethritis with single-dose ofloxacin. *Clin Infect Dis* 28: 1165–1166
62 Rahman M, Alam A, Nessa K, Nahar S, Dutta DK, Yasmin L, Monira S, Sultan Z, Khan SA, Albert MJ (2001) Treatment failure with the use of ciprofloxacin for gonorrhea correlates with the prevalence of fluoroquinolone-resistant *Neisseria gonorrhoeae* strains in Bangladesh. *Clin Infect Dis* 32: 884–889
63 Ison CA, Dillon JA, Tapsall JW (1998) The epidemiology of global antibiotic resistance among *Neisseria gonorrhoeae* and *Haemophilus ducreyi*. *Lancet* 351 Suppl 3: 8–11
64 Tanaka M, Nakayama H, Haraoka M, Saika T (2000) Antimicrobial resistance of *Neisseria gonorrhoeae* and high prevalence of ciprofloxacin-resistant isolates in Japan, 1993 to 1998. *J Clin Microbiol* 38: 521–525
65 Ehret JM, Judson FN (1998) Quinolone-resistant *Neisseria gonorrhoeae*: the beginning of the end? Report of quinolone-resistant isolates and surveillance in the southwestern United States, 1989 to 1997. *Sex Transm Dis* 25: 522–526
66 Kilmarx PH, Knapp JS, Xia M, St Louis ME, Neal SW, Sayers D, Doyle LJ, Roberts MC, Whittington WL (1998) Intercity spread of gonococci with decreased susceptibility to fluoroquinolones: a unique focus in the United States. *J Infect Dis* 177: 677–682
67 Gordon SM, Carlyn CJ, Doyle LJ, Knapp CC, Longworth DL, Hall GS, Washington JA (1996) The emergence of *Neisseria gonorrhoeae* with decreased susceptibility to ciprofloxacin in Cleveland, Ohio: epidemiology and risk factors. *Ann Intern Med* 125: 465–470
68 Abellanosa I, Nichter M (1996) Antibiotic prophylaxis among commercial sex workers in Cebu City, Philippines. Patterns of use and perceptions of efficacy. *Sex Transm Dis* 23: 407–412
69 Division of Emerging and Other Communicable Disease Surveillance and Control. The medical impact of the use of antimicrobials in food animals: report and proceedings of a WHO meeting: Berlin, Germany, 13–17 October 1997. Geneve: World Health Organization, 1997. (Document no. WHO/EMC/ZOO/97.4.). *(This document is available at the WHO homepage, http: www.who.int/home-page. It summarizes the international consensus on medical problems arising*

from the use of antibiotics in livestock. Recommendations to contain the problem were made at the end and priorities for research identified. No reference for the text is a weak point.)

70 Division of Emerging and Other Communicable Disease Surveillance and Control. Use of quinolones in food animals and potential impact on human health: report of a WHO meeting: Geneva, Switzerland 2–5 June 1998. Geneve: World Health Organiztion, 1998. (Document no. WHO/EMC/ZDI/98.10)

71 Endtz HP, Ruijs GJ, van Klingeren B, Jansen WH, van der Reyden T, Mouton RP (1991) Quinolone resistance in campylobacter isolated from man and poultry following the introduction of fluoroquinolones in veterinary medicine. *J Antimicrob Chemother* 27: 199–208

72 Reina J, Borrell N, Serra A (1992) Emergence of resistance to erythromycin and fluoroquinolones in thermotolerant *Campylobacter* strains isolated from feces 1987–1991. *Eur J Clin Microbiol Infect Dis* 11: 1163–1166

73 Sam WI, Lyons MM, Waghorn DJ (1999) Increasing rates of ciprofloxacin resistant campylobacter. *J Clin Pathol* 52: 709

74 Bazile-Pham-Khac S, Truong QC, Lafont JP, Gutmann L, Zhou XY, Osman M, Moreau NJ (1996) Resistance to fluoroquinolones in *Escherichia coli* isolated from poultry. *Antimicrob Agents Chemother* 40: 1504–1507

75 Garau J, Xercavins M, Rodriguez-Carballeira M, Gomez-Vera JR, Coll I, Vidal D, Llovet T, Ruiz-Bremon A (1999) Emergence and dissemination of quinolone-resistant *Escherichia coli* in the community. *Antimicrob Agents Chemother* 43: 2736–2741

76 Winokur PL, Vonstein DL, Hoffman LJ, Uhlenhopp EK, Doern GV (2001) Evidence for Transfer of CMY-2 AmpC beta-Lactamase Plasmids between *Escherichia coli* and *Salmonella* Isolates from Food Animals and Humans. *Antimicrob Agents Chemother* 45: 2716–2722

77 Shoemaker NB, Vlamakis H, Hayes K, Salyers A (2001) Evidence for extensive resistance gene transfer among *Bacteroides* spp and among *Bacteroides* and other genera in the human colon. *Appl Environ Microbiol* 67: 561–568

78 Martinez-Martinez L, Pascual A, Jacoby GA (1998) Quinolone resistance from a transferable plasmid. *Lancet* 351: 797–799

79 Anderson VE, Osheroff N (2001) Type II topoisomerases as targets for quinolone antibacterials: turning Dr. Jekyll into Mr. Hyde. *Curr Pharm Des* 7: 337–353

80 Jones ME, Sahm DF, Martin N, Scheuring S, Heisig P, Thornsberry C, Kohrer K, Schmitz FJ (2000) Prevalence of gyrA, gyrB, parC, and parE mutations in clinical isolates of *Streptococcus pneumoniae* with decreased susceptibilities to different fluoroquinolones and originating from Worldwide Surveillance Studies during the 1997–1998 respiratory season. *Antimicrob Agents Chemother* 44: 462–466

81 Kaatz GW, Seo SM (1997) Mechanisms of fluoroquinolone resistance in genetically related strains of *Staphylococcus aureus*. *Antimicrob Agents Chemother* 41: 2733–2737

82 Richardson DC, Bast D, McGeer A, Low DE (2001) Evaluation of susceptibility testing to detect fluoroquinolone resistance mechanisms in *Streptococcus pneumoniae*. *Antimicrobial Agents and Chemotherapy* 45: 1911–1914

83 Pickerill KE, Paladino JA, Schentag JJ (2000) Comparison of the fluoroquinolones based on pharmacokinetic and pharmacodynamic parameters. *Pharmacotherapy* 20: 417–428

84 Hyatt JM, Schentag JJ (2000) Pharmacodynamic modeling of risk factors for ciprofloxacin resistance in *Pseudomonas aeruginosa*. *Infect Control Hosp Epidemiol* 21: S9–11

85 Thomas JK, Forrest A, Bhavnani SM, Hyatt JM, Cheng A, Ballow CH, Schentag JJ (1998) Pharmacodynamic evaluation of factors associated with the development of bacterial resistance in acutely ill patients during therapy. *Antimicrob Agents Chemother* 42: 521–527

86 Manges AR, Johnson JR, Foxman B, O'Bryan TT, Fullerton KE, Riley LW (2001) Widespread distribution of urinary tract infections caused by a multidrug-resistant *Escherichia coli* clonal group. *N Engl J Med* 345: 1007–1013

87 Doern GV, Pfaller MA, Erwin ME, Brueggemann AB, Jones RN (1998) The prevalence of fluoroquinolone resistance among clinically significant respiratory tract isolates of *Streptococcus pneumoniae* in the United States and Canada – 1997 results from the SENTRY Antimicrobial Surveillance Program. *Diagn Microbiol Infect Dis* 32: 313–316

88 Jones RN, Pfaller MA (2000) *In vitro* activity of newer fluoroquinolones for respiratory tract infections and emerging patterns of antimicrobial resistance: data from the SENTRY antimicrobial surveillance program. *Clin Infect Dis* 31 Suppl 2: S16–23

89 Jones RN, Pfaller MA, Doern GV (1998) Comparative antimicrobial activity of trovafloxacin test-

ed against 3049 *Streptococcus pneumoniae* isolates from the 1997–1998 respiratory infection season. *Diagn Microbiol Infect Dis* 32: 119–126
90 Odland BA, Jones RN, Verhoef J, Fluit A, Beach ML (1999) Antimicrobial activity of gatifloxacin (AM-1155, CG5501), and four other fluoroquinolones tested against 2,284 recent clinical strains of *Streptococcus pneumoniae* from Europe, Latin America, Canada, and the United States. The SENTRY Antimicrobial Surveillance Group (Americas and Europe). *Diagn Microbiol Infect Dis* 34: 315–320
91 Gorbach SL (2001) Antimicrobial use in animal feed – time to stop. *N Engl J Med* 345: 1202–1203
92 Schmitz FJ, Verhoef J, Fluit AC (1999) Comparative activity of 27 antimicrobial compounds against 698 *Streptococcus pneumoniae* isolates originating from 20 European university hospitals. SENTRY Participants Group. *Eur J Clin Microbiol Infect Dis* 18: 450–453
93 Pfaller MA, Jones RN, Doern GV, Sader HS, Kugler KC, Beach ML (1999) Survey of blood stream infections attributable to Gram-positive cocci: frequency of occurrence and antimicrobial susceptibility of isolates collected in 1997 in the United States, Canada, and Latin America from the SENTRY Antimicrobial Surveillance Program. SENTRY Participants Group. *Diagn Microbiol Infect Dis* 33: 283–297
94 Marshall SA, Wilke WW, Pfaller MA, Jones RN (1998) *Staphylococcus aureus* and coagulase-negative staphylococci from blood stream infections: frequency of occurrence, antimicrobial susceptibility, and molecular (mecA) characterization of oxacillin resistance in the SCOPE program. *Diagn Microbiol Infect Dis* 30: 205–214
95 Schmitz FJ, Verhoef J, Fluit A (1999) Geographical distribution of quinolone resistance among *Staphylococcus aureus*, *Escherichia coli* and *Klebsiella spp* isolates from 20 European university hospitals. SENTRY Participants Group. *J Antimicrob Chemother* 43: 431–434

Fluoroquinolone Antibiotics
ed. by A.R. Ronald and D.E. Low

Improved safety profile of newer fluoroquinolones

Lionel A. Mandell

Division of Infectious Disease, McMaster University, Henderson Hospital, 5th floor, 40 Wing, 711 Concession St., Hamilton, Ontario, L8V 1C3, Canada

Introduction

Since their introduction to clinical use over half a century ago, antibiotics have become among the most commonly used drugs in a physician's therapeutic armamentarium. There are, however, adverse effects that may be associated with these compounds and that range from mild, transient phenomena which may only be detectable by laboratory tests to severe life-threatening events such as anaphylaxis, seizures and on occasion ventricular arrhythmias. Fortunately these events are uncommon but it is incumbent upon physicians to be aware of them and to understand as much as possible about their pathogenesis. This paper reviews the general mechanisms of antibiotic toxicity, and focuses on the fluoroquinolone-related adverse events.

As we are dealing with safety and not efficacy data it has been difficult to obtain information exclusively from randomized controlled trials. When information was taken from such studies the safety data did not represent the primary end points and in some cases there may not have been sufficient power to discriminate between the experimental drug and the comparator.

A variety of sources have been used including animal studies, case reports, controlled trials and reviews. Consequently the results are not as robust as one would find when analyzing efficacy studies.

General mechanisms of antibiotic toxicity

Adverse events have been described with virtually every class of antibiotic. The varied untoward effects which one may see with drugs as diverse as the beta-lactams, the aminoglycosides, the macrolides and the fluoroquinolones can be explained by one of five mechanisms. These are: (1) direct effects; (2) hypersensitivity; (3) changes in microbial flora; (4) drug interactions; and (5) microbial lysis.

Direct effects

Direct effects of an antibiotic resulting in laboratory and/or clinical toxicity are well described. Direct toxicity can affect a variety of tissues or organ systems such as the blood, kidney, nervous system and gastrointestinal (GI) tract, to name a few. Selected examples include: hemolytic anemia in patients with G6PD deficiency who have been given sulphonamides, azotemia resulting from tubular damage as a result of polymyxin or colistin administration, and deafness secondary to injury to the inner hair cells of the Organ of Corti following neomycin or kanamycin injection [1].

Hypersensitivity

Hypersensitivity is a term that is usually used when an immune response occurs either in an exaggerated or inappropriate form resulting in tissue and/or organ damage. There are classically four types of hypersensitivity reactions. Type I or immediate hypersensitivity refers to mast cell degranulation resulting in the release of histamine following an encounter between a mast cell and bound IgE and an antigen. Type II refers to antibody-dependent cytotoxicity; Type III refers to the deposition of immune complexes in tissue; and Type IV refers to the release of lymphokines from antigen-sensitized T-cells following a secondary contact with the same antigen.

Unfortunately, the terms allergy and hypersensitivity are frequently used inappropriately and patients often refer to an allergy when in fact what they experienced was an adverse event resulting from the direct toxic effect of a drug. A common example is GI upset occurring with macrolides. Patients will state that they are allergic to a macrolide such as erythromycin when what they actually suffered was a direct mediated adverse event causing GI irritation and hypermotility.

The reaction of greatest concern to physicians is Type I hypersensitivity since there is a risk that this may go on to full-blown anaphylaxis. Other examples which are thought to be mediated by a hypersensitivity mechanism are a Coombs' positive hemolytic anemia, serum sickness and the Stevens-Johnson syndrome and erythema nodosum.

Changes in microbial flora

Humans and animals are colonized by bacteria that form the host's "normal flora." The relationship between host and microbe is often mutually beneficial and one of the best examples of this is the synthesis of vitamin K by human enteric bacteria.

If an individual is given a course of antibiotics, particularly one with a broad-spectrum of activity, the risk is that much of the normal flora will be eradicated. This can result in clinical infection such as *Candida* vaginitis. A more extreme example is fungal superinfection following a course of antimicrobials for a known bacterial infection. For example, *Aspergillus pneumonia* may develop in a patient who has recently completed a course of treatment for bacterial peritonitis.

Drug interaction

Ingestion of two or more antibiotics may result in unexpected adverse reactions, or unexpected unfortunate sequelae. One possibility is that one drug may render the other useless or ineffectual by interfering with its absorption while in other cases, drugs may display additive or synergistic toxicity resulting in adverse events which neither drug alone would produce. An example of the former interaction is seen with the ingestion of fluoroquinolones or tetracyclines and antacids. Chelation by cations will seriously impair the absorption of the antimicrobial. Additive or synergistic toxicity has been described with tolbutamide and chloramphenicol resulting in severe hypoglycemia, and cephaloradine and furosemide causing nephrotoxicity [2].

Microbial lysis

On occasion, patients have been known to deteriorate suddenly following the administration of an antibiotic and it was thought that this was occasionally secondary to the release of toxic products following microbial lysis. Two well-known reactions have been described for which adequate explanations are still unavailable. One is the Jarisch-Herxheimer reaction seen when patients with tertiary syphilis, particularly with brain involvement, are treated with intravenous penicillin [3]. The other is erythema nodosum leprosum which is noted in up to one-half of patients with lepromatous leprosy treated with dapsone [4]. In such cases, the appearance of disseminated, tender, inflamed nodules with fever and in some cases polyneuritis, glomerulonephritis and severe joint pain have been described.

The fluoroquinolones: structure/adverse event relationships

The fluoroquinolones are a heterogeneous group of synthetic compounds each having a bicyclic nucleus with various substituents contributing to the antimicrobial activity, pharmacokinetic properties and adverse effects. Their serendipitous discovery was the result of attempts to synthesize chloroquine which resulted ultimately in the discovery of nalidixic acid, the progenitor of the fluoroquinolone class.

The first generation quinolones provided coverage primarily of the *Enterobacteriaceae*. The second generation compounds witnessed the introduction of the fluorine atom at the C6 position and cyclopropyl at N1, while the third generation compounds saw the addition of more complex amines at R7 and the use of a difluorophenyl at the N1 position. As the various generations were developed, we noted the introduction of agents with broader activity, increased potency against selected pathogens, and markedly improved pharmacokinetic and pharmacodynamic properties [5, 6].

Just as structure-activity relationships define the antimicrobial properties of a compound, so do structure-side-effect relationships determine the adverse events that one may witness with a particular drug or class of drugs (Fig. 1). While any radical may potentially cause an adverse effect, selected substituents of the fluoroquinolone molecule such as R1, R7 and X8 deserve special consideration and mention. The R1 substituents usually seen in fluoroquinolones are ethyl, cyclopropyl or 2,4- difluorophenyl. The R1 cyclopropyl increases theophylline interactions and clastogenicity. The 2,4- difluorophenyl group has not been associated with any specific adverse events in terms of

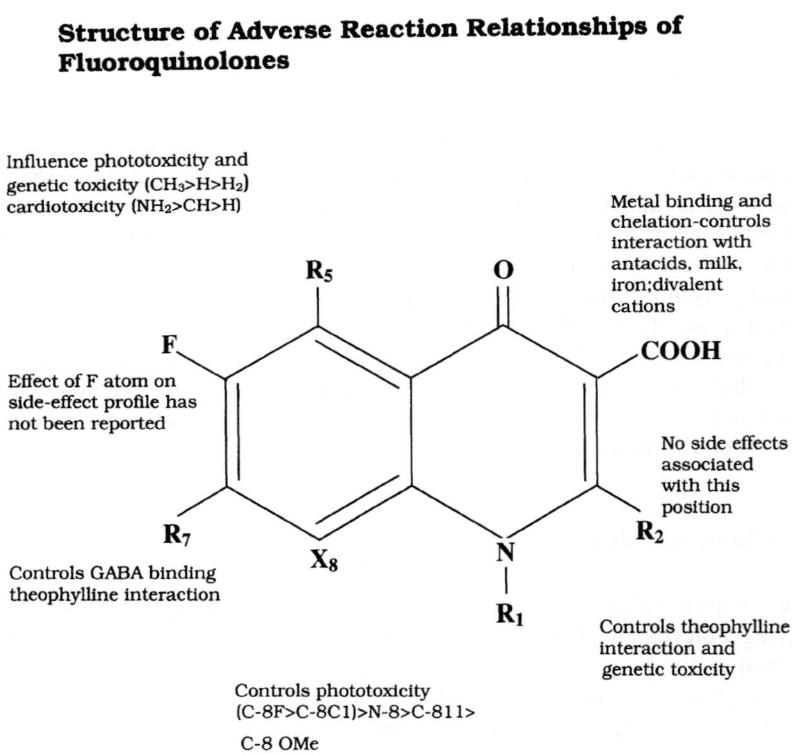

Figure 1. Structure of adverse reaction relationships of fluoroquinolones

cause and effect, however, temafloxacin trovafloxacin and tosufloxacin have this same substituent at the R1 position. Temofloxacin and trovafloxacin have been associated with severe hemolysis and hepatotoxicity respectively [7, 8]. Substituents at the R7 site have the greatest effect upon gamma-amino butyric acid (GABA) binding inhibition and therefore are most likely to be involved with central nervous system (CNS) toxicity, specifically convulsions [9]. It also is important for NSAID potentiated central nervous system (CNS) effects and fluoroquinolone-theophylline interactions [9]. A halogen at the 8 position is the single most important variable for phototoxicity and may play a role in genetic toxicity as well. Positions 3 and 4 are related to metal binding and chelation, and there are data to suggest that R5 substituents may influence photo and genetic toxicity. The phototoxicity seen with grepafloxacin for example may be attributable to the C5 methyl group since there is no halogen at the 8 position.

Organ system toxicity

While adverse events can affect virtually any organ system or body site, the most frequently involved are the GI tract, skin, CNS and hypersensitivity reactions [8, 10]. The overall incidence of adverse events associated with fluoroquinolones on the basis of data from the United States and Europe is given in Table 1.

Table 1. Overall incidence (%) of adverse events associated with fluoroquinolones on the basis of US and European data

Fluoroquinolone	Total adverse effects	Gastrointestinal effects	CNS effects	Skin effects
Ciprofloxacin po	5.8	3.4	1.1	0.7
Norfloxacin	9.1	3.9	4.4	0.5
Pefloxacin	8	5.6	0.9	2.2
Ofloxacin	4.2	2.6	0.89	0.53
Levofloxacin	2–9.9 (3.3)	5.1	0.2–1.1	0.2
Lomefloxacin	NS 5.1	5.5	2.4	
Fleroxacin (400 mg/200 mg)	21	11	9	3
Sparfloxacin (400 mg/200 mg	Overall:32 related:25.3	10	0.3	1.9[a]
Sparfloxacin RTI (400 mg/200 mg)	Total:40.9; related:13.7	11.4	4.2	5.1
Grepafloxacin (600 mg)	Related:47	15	5	2
Trovafloxacin RTI (100 mg/200 mg)	Related:12.7	6.1	4.4	0.2
Trovafloxacin (100 mg/200 mg)	27	4–7	-	1
Moxifloxacin (400 mg)	Related:27 comparators:24.5	8	5.4	2

Gastrointestinal tract

Virtually all antibiotics have been associated with varying degrees of GI upset. With some classes such as beta-lactams this can be minimal, whereas with drugs such as erythromycin, GI toxicity can be a use-limiting feature. With the fluoroquinolones there are no obvious structure adverse event relationships and the GI upset is thought to be due either to a direct irritative effect or to be mediated *via* a central mechanism [9].

The overall incidence ranges from 2–20% and most frequently includes nausea and vomiting but on occasion, anorexia and dyspepsia have been reported as well [11, 12]. Taste perversion has been seen most frequently with grepafloxacin, a fluoroquinolone which was recently discontinued because of concerns related to cardiac toxicity. Pseudomembranous colitis has been described with fluoroquinolone use but is unusual. The rank order of fluoroquinolone agents for GI adverse effects is: fleroxacin, grepafloxacin > trovafloxacin > sparfloxacin > pefloxacin > ciprofloxacin, levofloxacin > norfloxacin > enoxacin > ofloxacin [12].

Central nervous system

Toxicity involving the CNS is the second most common type of adverse effect and generally ranges in incidence between 1–2%. A wide range of events have been described varying from drowsiness and sleep disorders to dizziness, acute psychotic reactions and convulsions. These effects can result from one of two types of mechanisms. One is the direct action of a fluoroquinolone on receptors in the CNS, and the other is the result of the interaction between the fluoroquinolone and a second pharmacologic agent administered to the patient at the same time.

The direct actions on receptors can be further broken down into two subtypes. In one, the fluoroquinolone acts by binding to the GABA receptor and preventing the inhibitory neurotransmitter GABA from interacting with its own receptor and mediating its effect, thereby indirectly resulting in CNS stimulation. In another, the fluoroquinolone exerts a primarily excitatory effect by interaction with the N-methyl D-aspartate (NMDS) receptor, one of three excitatory inotropic receptors with glutamate as its natural ligand [13].

Binding of the fluoroquinolone to the GABA receptor can be enhanced by the presence of 4-biphenyl acetic acid (BPAA), an active metabolite of the NSAID fenbufen [14]. This drug interaction was clinically demonstrated when seven Japanese patients experienced seizures while taking the fluoroquinolone enoxacin and the non-steroidal agent fenbufen [15].

The GABA receptor interaction is not unique to the fluoroquinolones and has been described with certain beta-lactams as well such as penicillins, cephalosporins and carbacephams.

Interaction between a fluoroquinolone and a second pharmacological agent is probably best exemplified by the interaction between fluoroquinolones and theophylline. The latter agent is metabolized by cytochrome P450 enzymes which in turn may be inhibited by some but not all fluoroquinolones. A patient who is taking theophylline and a fluoroquinolone which inhibits the cytochrome P450 pathway would experience theophylline toxicity as the levels increased and could culminate in seizures [16]. The rank order of fluoroquinolones associated with CNS adverse reactions is: fleroxacin > trovafloxacin > grepafloxacin > norfloxacin > sparfloxacin > ciprofloxacin > enoxacin > ofloxacin > pefloxacin > levofloxacin [12].

Liver

Adverse effects involving the liver can range from mild clinically inapparent elevations of liver enzymes to end stage liver failure requiring transplantation. The juxtaposition of severe hepatic toxicity and the vagaries of drug adverse reactions were highlighted recently by trovafloxacin. This broad spectrum fluoroquinolone was for all intents and purposes withdrawn from the market because of severe liver toxicity and some deaths, and is discussed in a separate section dealing with unexpected adverse events.

A mild transient increase in liver function tests usually unassociated with any clinical manifestations is seen in 2–3% of patients who are treated with a fluoroquinolone. Since many drugs are concentrated in the liver, hepatotoxicity may occur as the result of a direct chemical effect or secondary to a hypersensitivity reaction.

Skin

Adverse reactions caused by photosensitivity and occasionally by hypersensitivity are expressed in the skin. The term photosensitivity includes photoallergy and phototoxicity. Photoallergy, which is quite rare, requires a prior encounter with the causative fluoroquinolone, the presence of photohaptens and the manifestations usually appear 1–2 days following such exposure [17]. This is in contrast to phototoxic reactions which may occur even with the initial drug exposure as long as there is sufficient UVA (320–420NM) contact and the drug is one which is known to cause such events. These are considerably more frequent than photoallergic phenomena.

When a fluoroquinolone is exposed to UVA radiation, one of three things may occur. It may decompose, it may return to its ground state, or it may pass the light energy on to oxygen resulting in the creation of toxic products such as singlet oxygen. Such toxic radicals and products can damage cell membranes and thus elicit an inflammatory response [18, 19]. The resultant clinical manifestations may vary in severity from the equivalent of a mild sunburn to severe bullous reactions. Fluoroquinolones which attain high concentrations in skin are more likely to result in phototoxicity, but the most important determinant is the presence of a halogen, particularly fluorine at the 8 position [9, 12]. As already mentioned, a methyl group at R5 (grepafloxacin) may contribute to phototoxicity as well.

The rank order for phototoxicity among the fluoroquinolones is: lomefloxacin, fleroxacin > sparfloxacin > enoxacin > pefloxacin > ciprofloxacin, grepafloxacin > norfloxacin, ofloxacin, levofloxacin, trovafloxacin [12].

Allergic or hypersensitivity reactions secondary to fluoroquinolone use occurs with an overall incidence of 0.5–3% and varies in severity from a mild rash to a severe exfoliative dermatitis. In extreme cases, anaphylaxis may occur. While this is certainly more likely to happen with a beta-lactam compound, both anaphylactoid and anaphylactic reactions have been described in up to 1.2/100,000 patients (0.0012%) treated with a fluoroquinolone [11].

Cardiac

The cardiac effect of greatest concern is prolongation of the rate corrected QT interval (QTc). This phenomenon is well-known with the macrolide class of antibiotics and has been associated with over 50 drugs of various classes currently listed in the compendium of pharmaceutical agents used by U.S. physicians (*Physician's Desk Reference*). The prolongation described with fluoroquinolones is felt to be a class effect, but the mechanism by which it occurs is unknown and it is thought to probably be multifactorial in nature. Even with a drug known to be as safe as ciprofloxacin, ventricular tachycardia can be induced when it is given rapidly intravenously at high doses (300 mg/kg) [20].

The main concern is that QTc prolongation may ultimately result in a malignant form of ventricular tachycardia known as Torsades de Pointes. In general, fluoroquinolones should probably be avoided in patients with known QT interval prolongation, patients with uncorrected hypokalemia, and patients receiving Class IA or III anti-arrhythmics.

Musculoskeletal

The adverse events of concern are either arthropathy or tendonitis. Cartilaginous lesions have been described in the weight-bearing diarthrodial joints of juvenile animals which had been exposed to prolonged high doses of fluoroquinolones. This is what led to the moratorium on the use of fluoroquinolones in children. In humans, it typically seems to involve weight-bearing joints of patients less than 30 years of age occurring with an overall incidence of 1% and resolving when the fluoroquinolone is discontinued [21].

The arthropathy described in animals is a class effect and virtually all fluoroquinolones tested have induced changes in immature cartilage of all animals studied. The cartilage lesions typically seen are fissures, blisters and erosions resulting from necrosis of the chondrocytes and disruptions of the extracellular matrix [22]. The exact mechanism is unknown and no definite structure adverse event relationship has been established. Some data however, suggest that the fluoroquinolones chelate magnesium ions resulting in disruption of the signal transduction from chondrocyte surface integrin receptors thought to play a role in maintaining the integrity of the cartilage matrix [23]. To date there is no evidence which categorically links fluoroquinolone use to arthropathy in humans and the long held restrictions appear to be lifting.

Tendonitis and tendon rupture are rare events associated with fluoroquinolone use but when they occur, the Achilles tendon is typically involved either unilaterally or bilaterally. Predisposing factors include steroid use, renal disease, hemodialysis and transplantation [8]. It is a class effect and inflammation may persist for several months in 10% of patients who develop this problem [24].

Renal

Adverse effects involving the kidney include hematuria, crystalluria, interstitial nephritis and acute renal failure resulting either from direct damage or hypersensitivity. Typically patients are older with the average age being over 65 years [12, 25].

Unexpected adverse events

We have learned that prelaunch clinical trial data may not be sufficient to highlight adverse events that occur with a very low incidence. For example, if a particular adverse event effects 1 in 30,000 people, trial data based on 15,000 individuals may not demonstrate the event of concern. It is now clear that post-marketing surveillance data involving much larger numbers of patients are needed to truly illustrate the range of toxicities that may occur with a particular drug.

Temafloxacin (Abbott) and trovafloxacin (Pfizer) are two fluoroquinolones of interest because of such unexpected events. Temafloxacin was launched in the United States in January 1992 and was withdrawn worldwide in June 1992 because of a constellation of adverse events known as the "temafloxacin syndrome." This was defined as hemolytic anemia or involvement of at least two of the following three systems in the absence of hemolysis: renal, hepatic and coagulation [7]. The typical patient presented with fever, discoloured urine, nausea, vomiting, jaundice, abdominal pain, myalgia and/or back pain and, in most cases, these findings resolved within days to weeks after the fluoroquinolone was discontinued.

Of the cases reviewed, 95 met the criteria for hemolysis and 19 met the criteria for multi-system disease [7]. The mean time to onset of hemolysis was

6.4 days but no correlation was noted with the dose of the drug. Fifty-eight percent of the hemolysis cases received doses of 600 mg bid, while 39% received 400 mg bid. Of the patients who developed hemolysis, renal dysfunction developed in 54 and 34 required dialysis. Biopsy studies revealed acute tubular necrosis together with "pigmented casts" and evidence of "hemoglobin plugging." Forty-eight of the 95 cases (51%) had evidence of hepatic dysfunction, and 33 (35%) had evidence of coagulopathy. Four patients experienced CNS complications including seizures secondary to cardiovascular accidents, and two patients with hemolysis died of ischemic colitis and disseminated intravascular coagulation and of renal failure.

The pathogenesis of the temafloxacin syndrome is not understood and a number of questions remained unanswered. They are: (1) Was the hemolysis the result of direct toxicity or was it immune mediated? (2) Did hemolysis lead to renal, hepatic and coagulation abnormalities or was there some underlying process which was responsible for all of the manifestations? (3) What is it about the temafloxacin molecule that caused any or all of these problems?

It has been suggested that temafloxacin induced an immune hemolytic anemia secondary to immune complex formation and that the hemolysis lead to the involvement of the other systems [7]. The structural aspect of interest is the difluorophenyl substituent at the N1 position, the same structure seen with tosufloxacin trovafloxacin and temafloxacin.

Interestingly, trovafloxacin has been associated with unexpected toxicity as well. Following its much-anticipated release as a broad-spectrum fluoroquinolone with 14 approved indications, post-marketing surveillance revealed a surprisingly high incidence of hepatotoxicity. Of 2.5 million patients treated with trovafloxacin, 140 cases of serious hepatic toxicity with 14 cases of acute liver failure were described [26, 27]. Most patients who experienced toxicity recovered but five required liver transplantation and five patients died.

Liver biopsies revealed that six patients has eosinophilic hepatitis and 30% of patients with toxicity had peripheral eosinophilia raising the question of a hypersensitivity reaction. In a small number of cases, the toxicity followed exposure to a second course of treatment with trovafloxacin or with another fluoroquinolone.

Grepafloxacin is another agent that has been withdrawn from the market. It was felt that because of QT prolongation associated with this drug, some patients might be at unduly high risk of Torsades de Pointes if treated with this agent. As discussed earlier, however, QTc prolongation is probably a class effect and is not necessarily an unexpected phenomenon, although some of the agents such as grepafloxacin and sparfloxacin, a fluorinated fluoroquinolone at the 8 position, seem to be associated with more of an effect than other members of this class.

Gemifloxacin is a fluoroquinolone that until very recently was under development by GSK. It has two features which arguably suggest that adverse events might be encountered. These are a nitrogen at the 8 position making the molecule a naphthyridone and 2-4 difluorophenyl at the 1 position. Because of its enhanced affinity for topoisomerase IV it has potent activity against most Gram positive cocci particularly *S. pneumoniae* and it is 30-fold more active than ciprofloxacin against this pathogen [28].

In a randomized controlled trial gemifloxacin was found to be significantly superior to trovafloxacin for treatment of community acquired pneumonia and preliminary results from clinical trials in acute exacerbations of chronic bronchitis, sinusitis and urinary tract infection suggested that the drug was effective and well tolerated [29–32].

The safety data suggest that there were no obvious problems with hepatotoxicity, photosensitivity, CNS events or QTc prolongation. Rash was reported in 3.3% of gemifloxacin patients as opposed to 0.7% of patients treated with a comparator (data on file with GSK). GSK has decided not to pursue their association with the drug and instead LG Chemical will try to market the compound.

Of the currently available fluoroquinolones the agents most frequently used are ciprofloxacin, moxifloxacin, gatifloxacin and levofloxacin. Ciprofloxacin is a second generation fluoroquinolone in use for over a dozen years while the others are referred to as the respiratory fluoroquinolones. Moxifloxacin and gatifloxacin are two new agents with increased Gram positive coccal activity while levofloxacin is the active L-isomer of ofloxacin and as such is not a new drug.

Each of these agents has been associated with adverse drug reactions. Typically these are mild but occasionally they are moderate and rarely severe. The same can be said however, of virtually any drug in any class that is used often in clinical practice. Toxicity has been described with the macrolides, the beta lactams and the aminoglycosides to name just a few but as with all of these, the toxicity is usually mild.

Generally the fluoroquinolones are safe and well tolerated and the incidence of adverse events must be kept in its proper perspective. For example an incidence of 140 cases of hepatotoxicity in 2.5 million patients treated with trovafloxacin is only 0.0056%, which is certainly uncommon and is similar to the rates of hepatotoxicity reported for beta-lactams such as flucloxacillin and amoxicillin-clavulanate [33, 34].

In order to better understand the adverse events associated with fluoroquinolones further additional efforts are needed in a number of areas. We must further define the drugs themselves and their various substituents that could predispose to toxicity. Examples include the radicals at the 1 and 7 positions, and whether being a naphthyridone makes a difference.

Host related factors such as age, drug clearance or genetic predisposition must be explored and risk factors in general should be delineated. This may be accomplished with the use of regression analysis of large data sets as well as subset analyses.

These can be summarized as:

1. Structure adverse event relationships
2. Host factors
3. Risk factors

References

1 Braude, AI (1976) Harmful reactions, incompatibilities and interactions of antimicrobial drugs. *In*: LH Smith (ed.) *Antimicrobial drug therapy* vol. VIII. Saunders Co. Philadelphia, pp 100–147
2 Christensen LK, Skovsted L (1969) Inhibition of drug metabolism by chloramphenicol. *Lancet* 1397–1399
3 Sheldon WH, Heyman A (1949) Morphologic changes in syphilitic lesions during Jarisch-Herxheimer reaction. *Am J Syph Gonor Ven Dis* 33: 213–224
4 Wemambu SN, Turk JL, Walters MF, Rees RJ (1969) Erythema nodosum leprosum: a clinical manifestation of the arthus phenomenon. *Lancet* 2: 933–935
5 Gootz TD, Brighty KE (1998) Chemistry and mechanism of action of the quinolone antibacterials. *In*: VT Andriole (ed.) *The Quinolones*, 2nd Edition. Academic Press, San Diego, pp 29–80
6 Hooper DC (2000) New uses for new and old quinolones and the challenge of resistance. *Clin Infect Dis* 30: 243–254
7 Blum MD, Graham DJ, McCloskey CA (1994) Temafloxacin syndrome: review of 95 cases. *Clin Infect Dis* 18: 946–950
8 Ball P, Mandell L, Niki Y, Tillotson G (1999) Comparative tolerability of the newer fluoroquinolone antibacterials. *Drug Safety* 21(S): 407–421
9 Domagala JM (1994) Structure-activity and structure-side-effect relationships for the quinolone antibacterials. *J Antimicrob Chemother* 33: 685–706
10 Zhanel GG, Walkty A, Vercaigne L, Karlowsky JA, Embil J, Gin AS, Hoban DJ (1999) The new fluoroquinolones: A critical review. *Can J Infect Dis* 10: 207–238
11 Ball P, Tillotson G (1995) Tolerability of fluoroquinolone antibiotics: past, present and future. *Drug Saf* 13: 343–358
12 Lipsky BA, Baker CA (1999) Fluoroquinolone toxicity profiles: A review focusing on newer agents. *Clin Inf Dis* 28: 352–364
13 Schmuck G, Schurmann A, Schluter G (1998) Determination of the excitatory potencies of fluoroquinolones in the central nervous system by an *in vitro* model. *Antimicrob Agents Chemother* 42: 1831–1836
14 Akahane K, Kimura Y, Tsutomi Y, Hayakawa I (1994) Possible intermolecular interaction between quinolones and biphenylacetic acid inhibits gamma-aminobutyric acid receptor sites. *Antimicrob Agents Chemother* 38: 2323–2329
15 Hori S, Shimada J, Saito A, Matsuda M, Miyailara T (1989) Comparison of the inhibitory effects of new quinolones on gamma-aminobutyric acid receptor binding in the presence of anti-inflammatory drugs. *Rev Infect Dis* 11 Suppl. 5: S1397–S1398
16 Janknegt R (1989) Drug interactions with quinolones. *J Antimicrob Chemother* 11: 33–43
17 Tokura Y (1998) Quinolone photoallergy: photosensitivity dermatitis induced by systemic administration of photohaptenic drugs. *J Dermatol Sci* 18: 1–10
18 Robertson DG, Epling GA, Kiely JS, Bailey DL, Song B (1991) Mechanistic studies on the phototoxic potential of PD 117596, a quinolone antibacterial compound. *Toxicology and Applied Pharmacology* 1111: 221–232
19 Matsumoto M, Kajima K, Nagano H, Matsubara S, Yokota T (1992) Photostability and biological activity of fluoroquinolones substituted at the 8-position after UV irradiation. *Antimicrob Agents and Chemother* 36: 1715–1719
20 Anon (1996) Grepafloxacin clinical investigators brochure. Greenford, UK: GlaxoWellcome research and development
21 Hayem G, Carbon C (1995) A reappraisal of quinolone tolerability: the experience of their musculoskeletal adverse effects. *Drug Saf* 13: 338–342
22 Stahlmann R, Merker HJ, Hinz N, Chahoud I, Webb J, Heger W, Neubert D (1990) Ofloxacin in juvenile non-human primates and rats. Arthropathia and drug plasma concentrations. *Arch Toxicol* 64: 193–204
23 Hynes RQ (1992) Integrins: Versatility, modulation and signaling in cell adhesion. *Cell* 69: 11–25
24 Royer RJ, Pierfitte C, Netter P (1994) Features of tendon disorders with fluoroquinolones. *Therapie* 49: 75–76
25 Paton JH, Reeves DS (1992) Adverse reactions to the fluoroquinolones. *Adverse Drug Reaction Bulletin* 153: 575–578
26 FDA Talk paper (1999) FDA issues public health advisory on liver toxicity associated with the antibiotic Trovan. Rockville (MD): US Department of Health and Human Service, Food and Drug

Administration 6 June
27 Press release, 15770/99, London: European Agency for the Evaluation of Medicinal Products. 20 May 1999
28 Lowe MN, Lamb, HM (2000) Gemifloxacin. *Drugs* 59(5): 1137–1148
29 File TM, Schlemmer B, Garau J, Cupo M, Young C and the 049 Clinical Study Group (2001) Efficacy and safety of gemifloxacin in the treatment of community-acquired pneumonia: A randomized, double-blind comparison with trovafloxacin. *JAC* 48: 67–74
30 Ball P, Wilson R, Mandell LA, Tremoliers F, Langan C, Henkel TJ and the Gemifloxacin 069 Study Group (2000) Effective short course therapy of acute exacerbation of chronic bronchitis (AECB) with once daily gemifloxacin. 3rd European Congress of Chemotherapy, Madrid, May 2000
31 Gehanno P, Poole MD, Wald ER, Weich-Jung C, Baran C, Henkel TJ and the Gemifloxacin 010 Study Group (2000) Efficacy of 7 days of gemifloxacin in patients with acute bacterial sinusitis (ABS). 3rd European Congress of Chemotherapy, Madrid, May 2000
32 Gruneberg RN, Schaeffer A, Goldstein F, Young C, and the gemifloxacin 014 study group (2000) Effective once daily gemifloxacin for the therapy of cmplicated UTI and pyelonephritis. 3rd European Congress of Chemotherapy, Madrid, May 2000
33 Olsson R, Wiholm BE, Sand C, Zettergren L, Hultcrantz R, Myrhed M (1992) Liver damage from flucloxacillin, cloxacillin and dysloxacillin. *J Hepatol* 15: 154–161
34 Garcia-Rodriguez L, Stricker BIH, Zimmerman HJ (1996) Risk of acute liver injury associated with the combination of amoxicillin and clavulanic acid. *Arch Inter Med* 156: 1327–1332

Fluoroquinolone Antibiotics
ed. by A.R. Ronald and D.E. Low

Pharmacokinetics and pharmacodynamics (PK/PD) of fluoroquinolones: tools for combating bacteria and preventing resistance

George G. Zhanel and Ayman M. Noreddin

Department of Medical Microbiology, Faculty of Medicine, University of Manitoba; Departments of Clinical Microbiology and Medicine, Health Sciences Centre, Winnipeg, Manitoba, Canada

Introduction

High rates of penicillin-resistant and multi-drug resistant organisms are influencing the empiric treatment of respiratory infections and allowing the new fluoroquinolones (FQs) (e.g., gatifloxacin, gemifloxacin, levofloxacin and moxifloxacin) to serve as important treatment alternatives. Selection of the optimal fluoroquinolone dosing regimen, however, requires careful consideration of not only organism and patient-specific factors but also pharmacokinetics (PK) and pharmacodynamic (PD) characteristics. The newer FQs display excellent bioavailability and have longer serum half lives than ciprofloxacin. In addition, they have the ability to concentrate in respiratory tract tissues and fluids at levels that exceed serum-drug concentrations. The broad spectrum of activity including against antibiotic resistant organisms as well as favorable pharmacokinetics makes the new FQs attractive therapeutic alternatives to traditional agents for common respiratory infections. Understanding the PK/PD of fluoroquinolone (FQ) antibiotics can facilitate selection of optimal regimens to hasten response, prevent treatment failures, and minimize the development of resistance. Although this paper will discuss all recently developed fluoroquinolones, the focus will be on recent data with agents currently used or soon to be available for clinical use (e.g., ciprofloxacin, gatifloxacin, gemifloxacin, levofloxacin and moxifloxacin). This review describes the PK and PD characteristics of the new FQs and discusses its implication on adequate therapy of patients with respiratory infections.

Pharmacokinetics

The newer FQs exhibit improved PK properties as compared to the older agents such as ciprofloxacin. First, their serum half-lives are significantly longer, allowing for once daily dosing. Second, these agents achieve higher peak serum concentrations (Cmax), resulting in higher Cmax/MIC ratios, which result in excellent bacterial killing. Third, an increased volume of distribution of the newer FQs results in extensive tissue penetration [1, 2, 2a]. The pharmacokinetic parameters of the new FQs following a single dose are summarized in Table 1 [2–59].

Absorption

All of the new fluoroquinolones are well absorbed after oral administration, with bioavailability ranging from approximately 70% for grepafloxacin to 99% for levofloxacin (Tab. 1). The majority of the new fluoroquinolones are absorbed quickly, attaining their maximum concentration in plasma (Cmax) within approximately 1 to 2 h after oral administration (Tab. 1). A number of investigations into the effect of food on the pharmacokinetics of the new fluoroquinolones have demonstrated that although food intake can slow absorption, it does not cause clinically significant alterations in the extent of absorption (area under the plasma concentration time curve [AUC]) or overall bioavailability of gatifloxacin, gemifloxacin, levofloxacin and moxifloxacin [60, 13, 20, 33, 41]. Therefore, all of these new fluoroquinolones can be given orally without regard to food intake.

Distribution

The new fluoroquinolones have volumes of distribution, ranging from 1.1 to 7.7L/kg and protein binding ranging from 5–73% (Tab. 1). Their distribution into selected fluids and tissues is summarized in Table 2 [5, 6, 8, 12, 13, 15, 22, 27, 31, 33, 58, 61–78]. The limited data on the penetration of the new fluoroquinolones into cerebrospinal fluid suggest that it is not as extensive as that of ciprofloxacin (Tab. 2), with the exception of trovafloxacin. Overall, the new fluoroquinolones display good penetration into alveolar macrophages, bronchial mucosa, epithelial lining fluid, and saliva. Specifically, grepafloxacin and moxifloxacin display superior penetration into alveolar macrophages and epithelial lining fluid in comparison to ciprofloxacin (Tab. 2). Concerning inflammatory fluid penetration, the new fluoroquinolones all demonstrate fluid to serum ratios in the range of 0.9 to 1.3 (Tab. 2). Limited data on gemifloxacin suggests that it is well distributed into inflammatory fluid, prostatic fluid and saliva similar to other fluoroquinolones (Tab. 2). This is not surprising as gemifloxacin demonstrates a large volume of distribution (3.5 L/Kg) (Tab. 1).

Elimination

All of the new fluoroquinolones exhibit longer half-lives than that of ciprofloxacin (Tab. 1). Gatifloxacin and levofloxacin are excreted in the urine

Table 1. Pharmacokinetic parameters of the new fluoroquinolones following a single oral dose

Drug	Dosage[a] (mg)	% F	Cmax (µg/mL)	Tmax (h)	AUC (mg*h/L)	T1/2 (h)	Vd/F (L/kg)	% Protein binding	% Excreted unchanged	Dose renal	Adjustment[b] hepatic	References
Ciprofloxacin	500	70	2.30	1.2	10.1	3.5	3.5	30	34	Yes	No	[3, 4–7]
	750	70	3.00	1.2	14.0	3.5	3.5	30	34	Yes	No	
Clinafloxacin	200	90	2.10	1.2	10.0	5.9	2.3	5	50	Yes	n.d.	[8–12]
Gatifloxacin	400	96	3.86	1.5	33.8	8.0	1.8	20	76	Yes	No	[13–19]
Gemifloxacin	320	n.d.	1.19	1.2	7.3	8.0	3.5	60	27	Yes*	No	[20–24]
	640	n.d.	2.29	1.2	15.9	8.0	3.5	60	27	Yes	No	
Grepafloxacin	200	72	0.64	2.3	6.6	11.1	7.7	50	8	No	Yes	[25–30]
	400	72	1.24	2.3	12.7	11.1	7.7	50	8	No	Yes	
	600	72	1.58	2.3	22.6	11.1	7.7	50	8	No	Yes	
Levofloxacin	500	99	5.08	1.7	48.0	6.9	1.1	31	83	Yes	n.d.	[6, 31–34]
	750	99	7.13	1.7	82.0	6.9	1.1	31	83	Yes	n.d.	
Moxifloxacin	200	86	1.16	1.7	15.4	12.1	3.3	47	19	No	No	[18, 35–40]
	400	86	3.34	1.7	33.8	12.1	3.3	47	19	No	No	
Sitafloxacin	25	>70	0.29	1.2	1.5	4.7	1.7	50	72	n.d.	n.d.	[41]
	50	>70	0.51	1.2	2.6	4.7	1.7	50	72	n.d.	n.d.	
	100	>70	1.00	1.2	5.6	4.7	1.7	50	72	n.d.	n.d.	
	200	>70	1.86	1.2	12.0	4.7	1.7	50	72	n.d.	n.d.	
Sparfloxacin	200	90	0.77	4.4	20.8	18.7	4.7	56	9	Yes	No	[5, 42–51]
	400	90	1.17	4.4	33.5	18.7	4.7	56	9	Yes	No	
Trovafloxacin	100	88	1.17	1.7	10.1	11.0	1.3	73	6	No	No	[52–58]
	200	88	2.48	1.7	26.2	11.0	1.3	73	6	No	No	

n.d. = no data; F = bioavailability; Cmax = peak concentration reached in the plasma/serum; Tmax = time to reach Cmax; AUC = area under the concentration time curve; T1/2 = half life; Vd = volume of distribution. a: Dosage only applies to Cmax and AUC. The other parameters represent an average of the values available in the literature irrespective of dosage. The dosages reported are based on the dosages commonly used in clinical trials for these drugs. b: dose adjustment refers to whether or not the fluoroquinolone requires any dosage adjustments in patients with impaired renal or hepatic function. Only adjust in severe renal impairment (creatinine clearance ≤ 29 ml/min).

Table 2. Penetration of the new fluoroquinolones into selected fluids and tissues

Site	Tissue/serum or fluid/serum ratio [reference]							
	Sampling time post dose							
	Ciprofloxacin 1 to 6 h	Clinafloxacin 1 to 5 h	Gatifloxacin 2 to 3 h	Grepafloxacin 2 to 5 h	Levofloxacin 1 to 6 h	Moxifloxacin 1 to 24 h	Sparfloxacin 2 to 6 h	Trovafloxacin 2 to 6 h
Aqueous humour	0.13 [61]	n.d.	n.d.	n.d.	0.23 [33][a]	n.d.	0.22 [44]	n.d.
Cerebrospinal fluid	0.37 [7]*	n.d.	n.d.	n.d.	0.16 [33]	n.d.	0.30 [44]	0.20 [33][b]
Gall bladder								
Tissue	n.d.	n.d.	n.d.	6.22 [64]*	1.53 [33, 68]	n.d.	7.1 [44]*[c]	n.d.
Bile	5.08 [61]	n.d.	n.d.	56.4 [64]*	1.28 [33, 68]	12–27% [71a]	9.6 [44]*[c]	n.d.
Inflammatory (blister) fluid	1.17 [31]	0.93 [8]	1.17 [13]	1.33 [15]	0.96 [69]*	0.84 [38, 70]	1.17 [42]	0.62 [58]
Male genital tissues								
Epididymis	n.d.	n.d.	n.d.	4.88 [65]	1.22 [33]	n.d.	n.d.	n.d.
Testis	n.d.	n.d.	n.d.	4.95 [65]	1.63 [33]	n.d.	n.d.	n.d.
Prostate								
Prostatic fluid	[7]	n.d.	n.d.	1.23 [66]	n.d.	n.d.	1.5 [44]	n.d.
Tissue	1.86 [61]	n.d.	n.d.	3.60 [65]	1.28 [33]	n.d.	1.4 [44][d]	0.96 [34]*
Respiratory tract								
Alveolar macrophages	10.6 [5]	10.13 [63]	26.5 [13a]	194.52 [67]*	18.5 [33a]	24.5 [71, 72]	65.5 [5][b] [62]	13.32 [75]
Bronchial mucosa	1.1 [62]*[e]	1.72 [63]	1.65 [13a]	3.13 [67]*	1.55 [71a]	2.07 [71]	3.3 [62][e]	1.07 [75]
Epithelial lining fluid	1.1 [62]	1.76 [63]	1.67 [13a]	12.21 [67]*	2.0 [33b]	6.95 [71, 42]	63 [5][b] [62]	2.27 [75]
Saliva	n.d.	n.d.	0.80 [12]	n.d.	0.73 [33]	0.83 [70]	0.68 [44][d]	n.d.
Sputum	0.58[e] [7]	n.d.	1.27 [13a]	n.d.	1.37 [33]	n.d.	1.4 [44][d]	0.79 [76]*
Skin	1.9 [61]	n.d.	n.d.	n.d.	1.44 [33]	n.d.	1.2 [44]	n.d.

Specific dosages and sampling times for all of the above data were not provided due to lack of space – see appropriate reference for further details (found in brackets beside values). No data were available for gemifloxacin and sitafloxacin, hence they were excluded from this table. Inflammatory fluid to serum ratio was determined by taking the ratio of the AUC values (sampling time not applicable). All others were determined by taking the ratio of tissue concentration to serum concentration (or the ratio of the mean tissue concentration to the mean serum concentration).

*Multiple doses of the fluoroquinolone were administered to subjects before sample was taken. All other data was collected after a single administration of the study drug.

n.d. = no data, a = sampling time of 2 to 9 h post dose, b = sampling time of 1 to 24 h post dose, c = sampling time of 18 h post dose, d = sample taken at Cmax (time not specified in reference), e = sampling time not specified

Gemifloxacin: Inflammatory (blister fluid) 0.61 [81c]; Prostatic fluid 0.70 [81a]; Saliva 0.41 [81b].

as the parent compound (>50%), indicating that these agents primarily undergo renal elimination (Tab. 1). Conversely, gemifloxacin and moxifloxacin are eliminated predominantly by non-renal pathways (Tab. 1). In patients with renal impairment, the dosages of gatifloxacin and levofloxacin require dosage adjustments [33, 77]. Dosage adjustment is also required for gemifloxacin in patients with severe renal impairment, even though this agent displays predominantly non-renal elimination (Tab. 1). Allen et al. demonstrated that in severely renal impaired patients (CrCl 10–29 ml/min), the total plasma clearance of gemifloxacin was reduced by approximately 50% and the half-life was prolonged to approximately double that compared to subjects with normal renal function [24]. Based on these findings, it is recommended to reduce the dose of gemifloxacin by half when administering it to patients with severe renal impairment [24].

A number of investigators have studied the pharmacokinetics of the new fluoroquinolones in special populations. In the elderly, it has been demonstrated that the pharmacokinetics (e.g., bioavailability) of levofloxacin, gatifloxacin and moxifloxacin are not appreciably affected [15, 21, 33, 79]. The pharmacokinetics of levofloxacin remains unchanged in patients with Acquired Immunodeficiency Syndrome (AIDS) in relation to healthy adults [80]. Levofloxacin also displays similar pharmacokinetics in asymptomatic Human Immunodeficiency Virus (HIV)-infected individuals compared to healthy subjects [81].

Pharmacodynamics

The pharmacodynamic parameters of antibiotics describe the relationship between the drug's serum concentration and its corresponding pharmacological and toxicological effects [82]. Optimal therapy requires the consideration of all of the available data from *in vitro* and animal models on pharmacodynamics as well as clinical trials and translation of these data into an antibiotic regimen that maximizes clinical efficacy and minimizes toxicity [83]. Evaluation of the *in vitro* activity of fluoroquinolones and other antibiotics is usually performed through measurement of MIC values, and less frequently minimum bactericidal concentration (MBC) [82, 84]. MICs measure the net drug effect when a standard bacterial inoculum is exposed to a fixed and constant drug concentration for 18 to 24 h [85]. Although MIC and MBC measurements reveal useful information on the inhibition or killing of a pathogen at the measured endpoint, they are static measurements that do not provide data on the time-course of antimicrobial action, including the duration of drug exposure necessary for bacterial eradication, the rate of bactericidal activity or persistent effects of antimicrobial agents [82, 84]. Similarly, pharmacokinetic parameters considered alone provide some clues to the clinical outcome, but do not sufficiently predict the true clinical response [79]. Assessment of pharmacodynamic activity of antimicrobial agents based on the integration of microbiologic activity, pharmacokinetics, and achievable serum and tissue concentrations is necessary for the best prediction of *in vivo* potency and efficacy [86, 87].

Inherent in a drug's antimicrobial activity is binding or interacting with specific targets in the respective pathogen and occupying the necessary number of critical binding sites for a minimum period of time. As such, the mathematical description of bacterial killing can be described as a function of the relationship between the peak serum drug concentration (Cmax) and time of exposure, expressed as the area under the plasma concentration-time curve (AUC) [83]. Pharmacodynamic properties can be used to predict the therapeutic response of microorganisms to antimicrobials by correlating measures of drug exposure (peak serum concentration [Cmax] or area under the plasma concentration-time curve over 24 h of dosing [AUC_{24}]) to measures of drug potency (MIC), or by evaluating the time the drug concentration remains above the MIC [79]. Thus the pharmacokinetic/pharmacodynamic parameters of interest in predicting clinical outcomes are the Cmax/MIC, the AUC_{24}/MIC (also sometimes referred to as the area under the inhibitory plasma concentration-time curve [AUIC]), and the time above the MIC (T/MIC) [82].

It has been clearly documented that antibiotics display two types of antibacterial activity, either concentration-dependent killing or time-dependent killing [85]. In time-dependent (or concentration-independent) killing, once the antibiotic concentration exceeds two to five times the MIC for a particular organism, the rate of killing becomes saturated and further increases in concentration do not increase the speed or extent of microbial death [82, 83]. The extent of bacterial killing for antibiotics in this group (β-lactams, vancomycin, clindamycin, and the macrolides) correlates poorly with the peak serum concentration and instead the best predictor of clinical success is the duration that serum antibiotic concentrations exceed the MIC of the microorganism [82, 83]. Since the primary parameter influencing *in vivo* success of these agents is T/MIC [82], small frequent doses will optimize clinical success [79]. Conversely, for antimicrobial agents that kill bacteria in a concentration-dependent manner, the rate and extent of bactericidal activity increases proportionately as the drug concentrations are increased, even at levels substantially above the MIC of the targeted organism [82, 83]. Aminoglycosides and fluoroquinolones display concentration-dependent killing [82, 83, 86–89]. However, although this theory was proven for Gram-negative pathogens, Dalhoff has demonstrated that sparfloxacin and ciprofloxacin exhibit concentration-independent effects *versus* Gram-positive isolates, while retaining concentration-dependent killing for Gram-negative bacteria [84]. In contrast, moxifloxacin displayed concentration-dependent activity for both Gram-positive and -negative organisms, a possible indication of higher intrinsic activity for Gram-positive species or modified target specificity over some of the older agents [84].

Despite the above findings, overall fluoroquinolones are still considered to possess concentration-dependent activity and the AUC_{24}/MIC and Cmax/MIC ratios have correspondingly shown to be the major parameters predictive of bacteriological eradication and clinical efficacy [90]. In order to optimize clinical outcomes in bacterial infections treated with fluoroquinolones, a number of investigators have studied which of these pharmacodynamic ratios display higher correlation with therapeutic success and the optimal target ratios to maximize bacterial eradication. *In vitro* models have provided conflicting reports, some indicating that the AUC_{24}/MIC provides the best correlation with bacteriological eradication [91, 92], while others suggest that Cmax/MIC is more predictive of eradication [93]. The characterization of whether one parameter provides greater predictive correlation with bacteriological and/or clinical cure than the other is difficult as interrelation of the variables is inevitable and neither stands alone as the sole determinant of antibacterial effects [91, 94]. Further increasing the complexity of the results, *in vitro* studies evaluating the activity of ciprofloxacin, gatifloxacin and levofloxacin against strains of *S. pneumoniae* have shown that the AUC_{24}/MIC and the T/MIC may better predict bacteriological eradication than Cmax/MIC [95], potentially due to time-dependent bactericidal activity of some fluoroquinolones for Gram-positive species, as discussed above.

Hoang et al. have reported concentration-independent killing of levofloxacin *versus S. pneumoniae* [95a]. Data from human studies exhibit similar controversies. In the treatment of infections with levofloxacin, the Cmax/MIC predicted clinical outcomes and microbiologic eradication better than the AUC_{24}/MIC, although the two parameters were highly correlated [96]. Clinical trials of intravenous ciprofloxacin and oral grepafloxacin in the treatment of respiratory tract infections have demonstrated that the AUC_{24}/MIC appears to be the most important parameter predicting the probability of both clinical and bacteriologic cures and the time to bacterial eradication [97–99]. However, these trials also showed that a high Cmax/MIC helps prevent selection of resistant bacterial strains, and thus may be the more important parameter if there is a significant risk of emergence of resistant subpopulation [99]. Recent explanations suggest that if the Cmax/MIC ratio is greater than 10:1 it will be the most important parameter in determining outcomes, whereas at Cmax/MIC ratios of less than 10:1, the AUC_{24}/MIC ratio will better predict therapeutic results [91, 96].

In terms of optimal target ratios, it has been shown that attainment of peak serum concentration (Cmax) to MIC ratios of >10:1 for fluoroquinolones increases the probability of successful clinical and microbiological outcomes and prevents the emergence of resistant mutants during therapy [82, 96, 97]. A landmark clinical study by Forrest et al. reported that the optimal AUC_{24}/MIC ($AUIC_{24}$) with ciprofloxacin of greater than or equal to 125 was associated with bacterial eradication in critically ill patients with nosocomial lower respiratory tract infections caused by Gram-negative bacilli (e.g., *Pseudomonas aeruginosa*) [97]. This critical breakpoint represented the minimum necessary ratio for rapid bacterial eradication and prevention of regrowth of resistant subpopulations; lower values resulted in clinical and bacteriological cure rates less than 50% [97]. A further evaluation of optimal AUC_{24}/MIC ($AUIC_{24}$) in the same patient population with nosocomial lower respiratory tract infections demonstrated a breakpoint for preventing resistance on therapy at approximately 100 [100]. However, in clinical trials in outpatients with community acquired respiratory infections such as acute exacerbations of chronic bronchitis performed with oral grepafloxacin, bacteriologic and clinical cures resulted at optimal AUC_{24}/MIC ratios of 75 or above [98], a much lower breakpoint than the minimum recommended in nosocomial infection. This is most likely a result of differences in the immunocompetence of subjects in the respective in-patient and out-patient settings [86]. The authors did report, however, that AUC_{24}/MIC ratios greater than 175 were associated with more rapid bacterial killing [98]. *In vitro* analyses have demonstrated that the minimum AUC_{24}/MIC ratio can be significantly lower for Gram-positive pathogens, as gatifloxacin and levofloxacin display bacterial eradication against *S. pneumoniae* and decreased regrowth of the resistant pneumococcus with $AUC_{24}/MIC \geq 25$ (Tab. 3) [95, 101–104, 105a]. However, an investigation into the activity of moxifloxacin against *S. aureus* and β-haemolytic streptococci reported optimal antibacterial effects with AUC_{24}/MIC ratios of 150–200 [105]. Complicating the determination of optimal target AUC_{24}/MIC ratios, longer-acting fluoroquinolones have been shown to display comparable antimicrobial effects at much lower ratios, most likely a result of their longer half-lives [106]. *In vitro* models have predicted that the breakpoints of trovafloxacin and gatifloxacin equivalent to ciprofloxacin's AUC_{24}/MIC ratio of 125 are 71 and 102, respectively [107, 108].

In summary, clinical data indicate that a peak serum concentration to MIC ratio of 10:1 or greater and AUC_{24}/MIC ratios in the range of 100 to 125 maximize bacterial eradication and prevent resistance in critically ill patients with nosocomial lower respiratory infections caused by Gram-negative bacilli (e.g.,

Table 3. Fluoroquinolone pharmacokinetic/pharmacodynamic parameters *versus S. pneumoniae*

Fluoroquinolone	Cpmax (μg/ml)	AUC_{24} total (μg.h/ml)	AUC_{24} free (μg.h/ml)	MIC_{90} (μg/ml)	AUC_{24}/MIC total	AUC_{24}/MIC free
Ciprofloxacin[a]	2.3	20	14	2	10	7
Ciprofloxacin[b]	3.0	28	20	2	14	10
Gatifloxacin	3.9	34	27	0.5	68	54
Gemifloxacin	1.2	10	4	0.03	333	133
Grepafloxacin	1.6	23	12	0.25	92	48
Levofloxacin	5.1	48	34	1	48	34
Moxifloxacin	3.3	34	18	0.25	136	72
Trovafloxacin	2.5	26	7	0.12	217	58

Single doses simulated: ciprofloxacin 500 mg BID[a], ciprofloxacin 750 mg BID[b], gatifloxacin 400 mg OD, gemifloxacin 320 mg OD, grepafloxacin 600 mg OD, levofloxacin 500 mg OD, moxifloxacin 400 mgOD and trovafloxacin 200 mg OD.

P. aeruginosa) [97, 100]. However, in outpatients with community acquired respiratory infections such as acute exacerbations of chronic bronchitis and community acquired pneumonia caused by *S. pneumoniae*, animal, *in vitro* and clinical data support AUC_{24}/MIC of ≥ 25 as being predictive of bacterial eradication [95, 96, 101, 102, 105a]. Perhaps these different pharmacodynamic targets reflect the fact that the new fluoroquinolones display concentration-dependent killing against Gram-negative bacilli and concentration-independent killing against Gram-positive cocci. In Table 3 the pharmacodynamic parameters of fluoroquinolones *versus S. pneumoniae* are depicted following single oral dosing. As can be seen all of the new fluoroquinolones achieve free AUC_{24}/MIC > 25. With *H. influenzae*, all of the new fluoroquinolones (gatifloxacin, gemifloxacin, levofloxacin and moxifloxacin) as well as ciprofloxacin achieve AUC_{24}/MIC > 1000 [86].

A further pharmacodynamic property that fluoroquinolones exhibit is continued suppression of an organism's growth that persists after antimicrobial exposure, known as the post-antibiotic effect (PAE) [82, 85]. Although all antibiotics produce PAEs *in vitro versus* susceptible Gram-positive pathogens, fluoroquinolones also display prolonged PAEs for Gram-negative bacilli [82, 109–111]. The PAEs for fluoroquinolones for both Gram-positive and -negative isolates are generally in the range of 1.5–2.5 h [109–113]. This phenomenon of persistent antibacterial activity becomes important when the concentration of the drug falls below the MIC.

Closely related to the PAE properties of fluoroquinolones is another pharmacodynamic phenomenon known as the post-antibiotic sub-MIC effect (PA SME), which is similar to the PAE except that subinhibitory concentrations of the antibiotic are present in the environment, in contrast to when the antibiotic is virtually eliminated [114]. This property has been reported for both ciprofloxacin and levofloxacin against *S. pneumoniae*, inhibiting inoculum regrowth during the early, sub-MIC dosing intervals [102, 114a]. As well sub-MIC effects of fluoroquinolones have been well described [114].

Post-antibiotic leukocyte enhancement (PALE) is also important in the persistence of antimicrobial action as it describes the observed characteristic increase in the susceptibility of bacteria to leukocyte phagocytosis that occurs in the post-antibiotic phase. This added bacterial susceptibility to intracellular killing doubles the duration of the PAE of fluoroquinolones for Gram-negative bacilli [82]. Overall, these supplemental pharmacodynamic properties allow infrequent dosing of large doses of fluoroquinolones because prolonged PAEs protect against bacterial regrowth during troughs when serum levels decline below the MIC value [82].

Since fluoroquinolones exhibit concentration-dependent killing, these large-dose regimens administered once daily (resulting in the achievement of high AUC and Cmax levels) contribute to high initial speed of killing, maximal bactericidal effects, optimal eradication times and decreased selection of resistant bacteria [87, 91]. In clinical practice, optimization of these variables by the achievement of high concentrations must then be balanced with the risk of toxicity and potentially serious adverse drug effects [87].

Recently, a new methodology for evaluating fluoroquinolone's potency has received considerable attention, namely the Mutant Prevention Concentration (MPC). Utilizing this new concept may provide a novel method for preventing resistance [115]. MPC is the drug concentration at which the selection of resistant mutants may be inhibited during antibiotic treatment [115]. Selection of resistant mutants occurs within a narrow concentration range. Below the low end of the concentration range, growth of the majority of drug-susceptible cells is suppressed. The upper boundary of the concentration range is the antibiotic concentration at which the growth of resistant, single-step mutants is inhibited [115]. This is designated the MPC as two simultaneous mutations must occur for cells to grow at this antibiotic concentration. The simultaneous acquisition of multiple mutations is a rare genetic event [115]. The mutational frequency of *S. pneumoniae* for fluoroquinolones is 10^{-7} to 10^{-10} [115a]. Based on a mutational frequency of 10^{-7}, an infection of more than 10^{14} *S. pneumoniae* would be required in order for two simultaneous fluoroquinolone-resistant mutations to occur [115, 115a, 115b]. Administering antibiotics at the MPC may thus prevent mutant selection [115]. Fortunately, it has been shown that many of the newer fluoroquinolones can be safely administered such that the serum and tissue drug concentrations remain above the MPC throughout the course of treatment [115].

Recent results suggest that the MPCs for *S. pneumoniae* vary amongst the fluoroquinolones and between different strains [115a, 115b]. Mutant prevention concentration was evaluated in relation to the actual drug concentration (MPC) and as a function of the fold MIC increase (MP_{MIC}). The MPC demonstrates whether administering the necessary dose is clinically achievable. The MP_{MIC} permits a comparison of the antibiotics' intrinsic abilities to prevent the formation of resistant mutants [115b]. Table 4 compares fluoroquinolone pharmacodynamics against *S. pneumoniae* using MPC instead of MIC values. As can be seen fluoroquinolone free AUC_{24}/MIC (Tab. 3) compare favorably with free AUC_{24}/MPC (Tab. 4). Whether dosing at or above MPC levels will truly prevent the selection of antibiotic-resistant mutants remains to be determined [115]. Thus, further MPC studies need to be conducted. The possibility of curtailing the selection of antibiotic-resistant mutants by altering dosing strategies is a new, important area of study.

Conclusion

Fluoroquinolones are a valuable addition to our antibiotic armamentarium. The broader spectrum and favorable pharmacokinetics of the newer FQs therefore makes these drugs an attractive therapeutic alternative to traditional agents for common respiratory pathogens. However, it is essential that *in vitro* susceptibility be considered alongside the specific PK/PD properties of the antibi-

Table 4. Fluoroquinolone pharmacokinetic/pharmacodynamic parameters *versus S. pneumoniae* (single-step mutants)

Fluoroquinolone	Cpmax (µg/ml)	AUC_{24} Total (µg.h/ml)	AUC_{24} Free (µg.h/ml)	MPC (µg/ml)	Cpmax/MPC	AUC_{24}/MPC (Total)	AUC_{24}/MPC (Free)
Ciprofloxacin	2.3	20	14	16	0.1	1.3	0.9
Gatifloxacin	3.9	34	27	1	3.9	34	27
Gemifloxacin	1.2	10	4	0.13	9.2	76.9	30.8
Levofloxacin	5.1	48	34	2	2.6	24	17
Moxifloxacin	3.3	34	18	1	3.3	34	18

Single doses simulated: ciprofloxacin 500 mg BID, gatifloxacin 400 mg OD, gemifloxacin 320 mg OD, levofloxacin 500 mg OD and moxifloxacin 400 mgOD. MPC's obtained from reference 115b.

otic chosen for therapy. Utilization of PK/PD concepts can be used to design regimens that maximize bacteriological eradication while minimizing the emergence of resistant organisms and preventing treatment failure.

Key research issues that need to be resolved with the new FQ over the next 5 years include: 1) Is a higher AUC_{24}/MIC for *S. pneumoniae* with a particular FQ associated with faster bacteriological eradication and faster clinical resolution of respiratory infection? 2) Is a higher AUC_{24}/MIC for *S. pneumoniae* with a particular FQ associated with less emergence of resistance? 3) Will optimizing the PD of FQ that preferentially bind to GyrA in *S. pneumoniae* (gatifloxacin and moxifloxacin) *versus* ParC (levofloxacin and gemifloxacin) lead to lower likelihood of resistance development? 4) What FQ AUC_{24}/MIC with *S. pneumoniae* is required to kill one step ParC or GyrA mutants or efflux mutants? 5) What will be the pharmacodynamic effect on the bowel flora of using new FQ with anaerobic activity for outpatient and inpatient respiratory infections?

Acknowledgement

The secretarial assistance of M. Wegrzyn is highly appreciated

References

1 Blondeau JM (1999) Expanded activity and utility of the new fluoroquinolones. A review. *Clin Ther* 21: 3 *(A thorough review of the activity of new fluoroquinolones.)*

2 Zhanel GG, Ennis K, Vercaigne L, Walkty A, Gin AS, Embil J, Smith H, Hoban DJ (2002) A critical review of the fluoroquinolones: Focus on respiratory infections. *Drugs* 62(1): 13–59 *(This is a comprehensive review of the chemistry, microbiology, pharmacokinetics, pharmacodynamics, clinical trials and adverse effects of new fluoroquinolones.)*

2a Schentag JJ, Scully BE (1999) Quinolones. *In*: VL Yu, TC Merigan Jr, Barriere S (eds): *Antimicrobial therapy and vaccines*. Baltimore, Williams and Wilkins, 875

3 Davis R, Markham A, Balfour JA (1996) Ciprofloxacin. An updated review of its pharmacology, therapeutic efficacy and tolerability. *Drugs* 51(6): 1019–1074

4 Naber CK, Hammer M, Kinzig-Schippers M, Sauber C, Sorgel F, Bygate EA, Fairless AJ, Machka K, Naber KG (1999) Urinary excretion and bactericidal activity of intravenous ciprofloxacin compared with oral ciprofloxacin. *Eur J Clin Microbiol Infect Dis* 18(11): 783–789

5 Schuler P, Zemper K, Borner K, Koeppe P, Schaberg T, Lode H (1997) Penetration of sparfloxacin and ciprofloxacin into alveolar macrophages, epithelial lining fluid, and polymorphonuclear leucocytes. *Eur Respir J* 10(5): 1130–1136

6 Compendium of Pharmaceuticals and Specialties. 35th ed. (2000) Ottawa: Canadian Pharmacists Association 322–5: 838–841

7 Vance-Bryan K, Guay DR, Rotschafer JC (1990) Clinical pharmacokinetics of ciprofloxacin. *Clin Pharmacokinet* 19(6): 434–461

8 Bron NJ, Dorr MB, Mant TG, Webb CL, Vassos AB (1996) The tolerance and pharmacokinetics of clinafloxacin (CI-960) in healthy subjects. *J Antimicrob Chemother* 38(6): 1023–1029

9 Wise R, Jones S, Das I, Andrews JM (1998) Pharmacokinetics and inflammatory fluid penetration of clinafloxacin. *Antimicrob Agents Chemother* 42(2): 428–430

10 Randinitis EJ, Brodfuehrer J, Vassos AB (1998) Pharmacokinetics of clinafloxacin following oral and intravenous single and multiple dosing in volunteers [abstr]. *In*: 38th Interscience Conference on Antimicrobial Agents and Chemotherapy San Diego, CA

11 Randinitis EJ, Koup JR, Rausch G, Abel R, Bron NJ, Hounslow NJ, Vassos AB, Sedman AJ (1998) Single-dose clinafloxacin pharmacokinetics in subjects with various degrees of renal

function [abstr]. *In*: 38th Interscience Conference on Antimicrobial Agents and Chemotherapy. San Diego, CA
12 Wise R, Ashby JP, Andrews JM (1988) *In vitro* activity of PD 127,391, an enhanced-spectrum quinolone. *Antimicrob Agents Chemother* 32(8): 1251–1256
13 Nakashima M, Uematsu T, Kosuge K, Kusajima H, Ooie T, Masuda Y, Ishida R, Uchida H (1995) Single and multiple-dose pharmacokinetics of AM-1155, a new 6-fluoro-8- methoxy quinolone, in humans. *Antimicrob Agents Chemother* 39(12): 2635–2640
13a Package Insert Gatifloxacin (2001) Bristol Myers Squibb. Connecticut, USA
14 Wise R, Andrews JM, Ashby JP, Marshall J (1999) A study to determine the pharmacokinetics and inflammatory fluid penetration of gatifloxacin following a single oral dose. *J Antimicrob Chemother* 44(5): 701–704
15 LaCreta FP, Kaul S, Kollia GD, Duncan G, Randall DM, Grasela DM (2000) Interchangeability of 400-mg intravenous and oral gatifloxacin in healthy adults [in process citation]. *Pharmacotherapy* 20(6 Pt 2): 59S-66S
16 LaCreta FP, Kollia GD, Duncan G, Behr D, Grasela DM (2000) Age and gender effects on the pharmacokinetics of gatifloxacin [in process citation]. *Pharmacotherapy* 20(6 Pt 2): 67S-75S
17 Grasela DM, Christofalo B, Kollia GD, Duncan G, Noveck R, Manning JAJr LaCreta FP (2000) Safety and pharmacokinetics of a single oral dose of gatifloxacin in patients with moderate to severe hepatic impairment [in process citation]. *Pharmacotherapy* 20(6 Pt 2): 87S-94S
18 Abramowicz ME (2000) Gatifloxacin and moxifloxacin: two new fluoroquinolones. *The Medical Letter* 42(1072): 15–17
19 Lober S, Ziege S, Rau M, Schreiber G, Mignot A, Koeppe P, Lode H (1999) Pharmacokinetics of gatifloxacin and interaction with an antacid containing aluminum and magnesium. *Antimicrob Agents Chemother* 43(5): 1067–1071
20 Allen A, Bygate E, Clark D, Lewis A, Pay V (2000) The effect of food on the bioavailability of oral gemifloxacin in healthy volunteers [poster]. *In*: 3rd European Congress of Chemotherapy. Madrid, Spain
21 Allen A, Bygate E, Faessel H, Isaac L, Lewis A (2000) The effect of ferrous sulphate and sucralfate on the bioavailability of oral gemifloxacin in healthy volunteers [poster]. *In*: 3rd European Congress of Chemotherapy. Madrid, Spain
22 Saliba F, Isaac L, Barker PJ, Bird N, Allen A, Montague T, Romain D (2000) The pharmacokinetics and tolerability of a single oral dose of gemifloxacin in patients with mild or moderate hepatic impairment [poster]. *In*: 3rd European Congress of Chemotherapy. Madrid, Spain
23 Sörgel F, Allen A, Pay V, Bygate E, Kinzig-Shippers M, Bulitta C, Bird N, Naber K (2000) Distribution of gemifloxacin into saliva, sweat, tears and nasal secretion in healthy volunteers [poster]. *In*: 3rd European Congress of Chemotherapy. Madrid, Spain
24 Allen A, Walls CM, McDonnel D, Bird N, Lewis A, Romain D, Pay V, Bygate E, Rouvaix B, Moulin B (2000) Pharmacokinetics of gemifloxacin administered to patients with severe renal impairment and patients on dialysis [poster]. *In*: 3rd European Congress of Chemotherapy. Madrid, Spain
25 Efthymiopoulos C, Bramer SL, Maroli A, Gambertoglio JG (1997) Effect of renal impairment on the pharmacokinetics of grepafloxacin. *Clin Pharmacokinet* 33(Suppl 1): 32–38
26 Child J, Andrews JM, Wise R (1995) Pharmacokinetics and tissue penetration of the new fluoroquinolone grepafloxacin. *Antimicrob Agents Chemother* 39(2): 513–515
27 Efthymiopoulos C, Bramer SL, Maroli A (1997) Pharmacokinetics of grepafloxacin after oral administration of single and repeat doses in healthy young males. *Clin Pharmacokinet* 33(Suppl 1): 1–8
28 Kozawa O, Uematsu T, Matsuno H, Niwa M, Nagashima S, Kawamara M (1996) Comparative study of pharmacokinetics of two new fluoroquinolones, balofloxacin and grepafloxacin, in elderly subjects. *Antimicrob Agents Chemother* 40(12): 2824–2828
29 Efthymiopoulos C, Bramer SL, Maroli A, Flaherty JFJr Wolfe E, Bass N, Somberg K (1997) Grepafloxacin pharmacokinetics in individuals with hepatic dysfunction. *Clin Pharmacokinet* 33(Suppl 1): 25–31
30 Efthymiopoulos C, Bramer SL, Maroli A (1997) Effect of food and gastric pH on the bioavailability of grepafloxacin. *Clin Pharmacokinet* 33(Suppl 1): 18–24
31 Chien SC, Rogge MC, Gisclon LG, Curtin C, Wong F, Natarajan J, Williams RR, Fowler CL, Cheung WK, Chow AT (1997) Pharmacokinetic profile of levofloxacin following once-daily 500-milligram oral or intravenous doses. *Antimicrob Agents Chemother* 41(10): 2256–2260

32 Chien SC, Chow AT, Natarajan J, Williams RR, Wong FA, Rogge MC, Nayak RK (1997) Absence of age and gender effects on the pharmacokinetics of a single 500-milligram oral dose of levofloxacin in healthy subjects. *Antimicrob Agents Chemother* 41(7): 1562–1565
33 Fish DN, Chow AT (1997) The clinical pharmacokinetics of levofloxacin. *Clin Pharmacokinet* 32(2): 101–119 *(An extensive review of the pharmacokinetics of levofloxacin.)*
33a Gotfried MH, Danzinger LH, Rodvold K (2001) Steady state plasma and intrapulmonary concentrations of levofloxacin and ciprofloxacin in healthy adult subjects. Chest 119: 1114–1122 *(Detailed study reporting the high concentrations achieved in epithelial lining fluid and alveolar macrophages with new fluoroquinolones.)*
33b Andrews JM, Honeybourne D, Jevons G, Brenwald NP, Cunningham B, Wise R (1997) Concentration of levofloxacin (HR 355) in the respiratory tract following a single dose in patients undergoing fibre-optic bronchoscopy. *J Antimicrob Chemother* 40: 573–577
34 Chien SC, Wong FA, Fowler CL, Callery-D'Amico SV, Williams RR, Nayak R, Chow AT (1998) Double-blind evaluation of the safety and pharmacokinetics of multiple oral once-daily 750-milligram and 1-gram doses of levofloxacin in healthy volunteers. *Antimicrob Agents Chemother* 42(4): 885–888
35 Stass H, Kubitza D (1999) Pharmacokinetics and elimination of moxifloxacin after oral and intravenous administration in man. *J Antimicrob Chemother* 43 Suppl B: 83–90
36 Stass H, Kubitza D, Schuhly U (1998) Pharmacokinetics, safety, and tolerability of ascending single doses of moxifloxacin, a new 8-methoxy quinolone, administered to healthy subjects. *Antimicrob Agents Chemother* 42(8): 2060–2065
37 Sullivan JT, Woodruff M, Lettieri J, Agarwal V, Krol GJ, Leese PT, Watson S, Heller AH (1999) Pharmacokinetics of a once-daily oral dose of moxifloxacin (Bay 12-8039), a new enantiomerically pure 8-methoxy quinolone. *Antimicrob Agents Chemother* 43(11): 2793–2797
38 Wise R, Andrews JM, Marshall G, Hartman G (1999) Pharmacokinetics and inflammatory-fluid penetration of moxifloxacin following oral or intravenous administration. *Antimicrob Agents Chemother* 43(6): 1508–1510
39 Stass H, Halabi A, Delesen H (1998) No dose adjustment needed for patient's with renal impairment receiving oral BAY 12-8039 [abstr]. *In*: 38th Interscience Conference on Antimicrobial Agents and Chemotherapy. San Diego, CA
40 Stass H, Kubitza D, von Bergmann Halabi A, Kuhlmann J, Sudhop T (1999) No dose adjustment is needed for moxifloxacin in subjects suffering from hepatic impairment [abstr]. *In*: 9th European Congress of Clinical Microbiology and Infectious Disease. Berlin
41 Nakashima M, Uematsu T, Kosuge K, Umemura K, Hakusui H, Tanaka M (1995) Pharmacokinetics and tolerance of DU-6859a, a new fluoroquinolone, after single and multiple oral doses in healthy volunteers [published erratum appears in *Antimicrob Agents Chemother* 1995 Apr; 39(4): 1015]. *Antimicrob Agents Chemother* 39(1): 170–174
42 Johnson JH, Cooper MA, Andrews JM, Wise R (1992) Pharmacokinetics and inflammatory fluid penetration of sparfloxacin. *Antimicrob Agents Chemother* 36(11): 2444–2446
43 Montay G, Bruno R, Vergniol JC, Ebmeier M, Le Roux Y, Guimart C, Frydman A, Chassard D, Thebault JJ (1994) Pharmacokinetics of sparfloxacin in humans after single oral administration at doses of 200, 400, 600, and 800 mg. *J Clin Pharmacol* 34(11): 1071–1076
44 Shimada J, Nogita T, Ishibashi Y (1993) Clinical pharmacokinetics of sparfloxacin. *Clin Pharmacokinet* 25(5): 358–369
45 Montay G (1996) Pharmacokinetics of sparfloxacin in healthy volunteers and patients: a review. *J Antimicrob Chemother* 37 Suppl A: 27–39
46 Kamberi M et al (1998) Sparfloxacin pharmacokinetics in healthy volunteers: the influence of acidification and alkalinization. *Eur J Clin Pharmacol* 54(8): 633–637
47 Johnson R, Geary W, Jenssen B (1996) The absolute oral bioavailability of sparfloxacin in healthy male subjects [abstr]. *In*: 36th Interscience Conference on Antimicrobial Agents and Chemotherapy. New Orleans
48 Zix JA et al (1997) Pharmacokinetics of sparfloxacin and interaction with cisapride and sucralfate. *Antimicrob Agents Chemother* 41(8): 1668–1672
49 Fillastre JP, Montay G, Bruno R, Etienne I, Dhib M, Vivier N, Le Roux Y, Guimart C, Gay G, Schott D (1994) Pharmacokinetics of sparfloxacin in patients with renal impairment. *Antimicrob Agents Chemother* 38(4): 733–737
50 Ritz M, Lode H, Fassbender M, Borner K, Koeppe P, Nord CE (1994) Multiple-dose pharmacokinetics of sparfloxacin and its influence on fecal flora. *Antimicrob Agents Chemother* 38(3):

455–459
51 Mugnier P, Taubert AM, Wyld PJ, Nimmo WS, Hayes P, Grange X, Amiot E, Singlas E (1994) Pharmacokinetics of sparfloxacin in patient's with hepatic failure [abstr]. *In*: 34th Interscience Conference on Antimicrobial Agents and Chemotherapy. Washington, DC
52 Melnik G, Schwesinger WH, Teng R, Dogolo LC, Vincent JRelated Articles Links (1998) Hepatobiliary elimination of trovafloxacin and metabolites following single oral doses in healthy volunteers. *Eur J Clin Microbiol Infect Dis* 17(6): 424–426
53 Vincent J, Dogolo L, Baris BA, Willavize SA, Teng R (1998) Single- and multiple-dose administration, dosing regimens, and pharmacokinetics of trovafloxacin and alatrofloxacin in humans. *Eur J Clin Microbiol Infect Dis* 17(6): 427–430
54 Teng R, Dogolo LC, Willavize SA, Friedman HL, Vincent J (1997) Oral bioavailability of trovafloxacin with and without food in healthy volunteers. *J Antimicrob Chemother* 39 Suppl B: 87–92
55 Teng R, Liston TE, Harris SC (1996) Multiple-dose pharmacokinetics and safety of trovafloxacin in healthy volunteers. *J Antimicrob Chemother* 37(5): 955–963
56 Teng R, Harris SC, Nix DE, Schentag JJ, Foulds G, Liston TE (1995) Pharmacokinetics and safety of trovafloxacin (CP-99, 219), a new quinolone antibiotic, following administration of single oral doses to healthy male volunteers. *J Antimicrob Chemother* 36(2): 385–394
57 Vincent J, Teng R, Dalvie DK, Friedman HL (1998) Pharmacokinetics and metabolism of single oral doses of trovafloxacin. *Am J Surg* 176(6A Suppl): 8S-13S
58 Wise R, Mortiboy D, Child J, Andrews JM (1996) Pharmacokinetics and penetration into inflammatory fluid of trovafloxacin (CP-99, 219). *Antimicrob Agents Chemother* 40(1): 47–49
59 Vincent J, Venitz J, Teng R, Baris BA, Willavize SA, Polzer RJ, Friedman HL (1997) Pharmacokinetics and safety of trovafloxacin in healthy male volunteers following administration of single intravenous doses of the prodrug, alatrofloxacin. *J Antimicrob Chemother* 39 Suppl B: 75–80
60 Gajjar DA, LaCreta FP, Uderman HD, Kollia GD, Duncan G, Birkhofer MJ, Grasela DM (1998) Effect of a high-fat meal on the bioavailability of gatifloxacin in healthy volunteers [abstr]. *In*: 38th Interscience Conference on Antimicrobial Agents and Chemotherapy. San Diego, CA
61 Wilson APR, RNGruneberg (1997) Ciprofloxacin: 10 years of clinical experience, Maxim Medical: Somerset. 67
62 Wise R, Honeybourne D (1996) A review of the penetration of sparfloxacin into the lower respiratory tract and sinuses. *J Antimicrob Chemother* 37 Suppl A: 57–63
63 Honeybourne D, Andrews JM, Cunningham B, Jevons G, Wise R (1999) The concentrations of clinafloxacin in alveolar macrophages, epithelial lining fluid, bronchial mucosa and serum after administration of single 200 mg oral doses to patients undergoing fibre-optic bronchoscopy. *J Antimicrob Chemother* 43(1): 153–155
64 Tanimura H, Uchiyama K, Kashiwagi H (1995) Gallbladder tissue concentrations, biliary excretion and pharmacokinetics of OPC-17116. *Drugs* 49(Suppl 2): 341–343
65 Takahashi Y, Itoh Y, Dot T, Kuryaama M, Kawada Y (1991) Penetration of OPC-17116, a new quinolone compound, into male genital tracts and its *in vitro* antibacterial activity [abstr]. *In*: 31st Interscience Conference on Antimicrobial Agents and Chemotherapy. Chicago, IL
66 Suzuki K, Horiba M (1991) Penetration of OPC-17116, a new quinolone derivative, into human prostatic fluid [abstr]. *In*: 31st Interscience Conference on Antimicrobial Agents and Chemotherapy. Chicago, IL
67 Cook PJ, Andrews JM, Wise R, Honeybourne D, Moudgil H (1995) Concentrations of OPC-17116, a new fluoroquinolone antibacterial, in serum and lung compartments. *J Antimicrob Chemother* 35(2): 317–326
68 Ohnishi H et al (1993) Excretion of levofloxacin into bile and gallbladder tissue [abstr]. *Drugs* 45(Suppl 3): 260–261
69 Child J, Mortiboy D, Andrews JM, Chow AT, Wise R (1995) Open-label crossover study to determine pharmacokinetics and penetration of two dose regimens of levofloxacin into inflammatory fluid. *Antimicrob Agents Chemother* 39(12): 2749–2751
70 Muller M, Stass H, Brunner M, Moller JG, Lackner E, Eichler HG (1999) Penetration of moxifloxacin into peripheral compartments in humans. *Antimicrob Agents Chemother* 43(10): 2345–2349
71 Soman A, Honeybourne D, Andrews J, Jevons G, Wise R (1999) Concentrations of moxifloxacin in serum and pulmonary compartments following a single 400 mg oral dose in patients undergo-

ing fibre-optic bronchoscopy. *J Antimicrob Chemother* 44(6): 835–838
71a Wise R (1999) A review of the clinical pharmacology of moxifloxacin, a new 8-methoxy quinolone and its potential relationship to therapeutic efficacy. *Clin Drug Invest* 17(5): 365–387
72 Andrews J, Wise R, Jennifer M, Marshall G abd Hartmann G (1998) Penetration of Bay 12-8039 into bronchial mucosa, epithelial lining [abstr]. *In*: Interscience Conference on Antimicrobial Agents and Chemotherapy. San Diego, CA
73 Cutler NR, Vincent J, Jhee SS, Teng R, Wardle T, Lucas G, Dogolo LC, Sramek JJ (1997) Penetration of trovafloxacin into cerebrospinal fluid in humans following intravenous infusion of alatrofloxacin. *Antimicrob Agents Chemother* 41(6): 1298–1300
74 Childs S et al (1997) Penetration of trovafloxacin into prostatic tissue following multiple dosing in man [abstr]. *In*: 37th Interscience Conference on Antimicrobial Agents and Chemotherapy. Toronto, ON
75 Andrews JM, Honeybourne D, Brenwald NP, Bannerjee D, Iredale M, Cunningham B, Wise R (1997) Concentrations of trovafloxacin in bronchial mucosa, epithelial lining fluid, alveolar macrophages and serum after administration of single or multiple oral doses to patients undergoing fibre-optic bronchoscopy. *J Antimicrob Chemother* 39(6): 797–802
76 Peleman RA, Van De Velde V, Germonpre PR, Fleurinck C, Rosseel MT, Pauwels RA (2000) Trovafloxacin concentrations in airway fluids of patients with severe community-acquired pneumonia. *Antimicrob Agents Chemother* 44(1): 178–180
77 Abramowicz M (2000) Gatifloxacin, moxifloxacin: two new fluoroquinolones. *Med Lett Drugs Ther* 42(1072): 15–17
78 Bradley JS, Kearns GL, Reed MD, Capparelli EV, Vincent J (2000) Pharmacokinetics of a fluoronaphthyridone, trovafloxacin (CP 99,219), in infants and children following administration of a single intravenous dose of alatrofloxacin. *Antimicrob Agents Chemother* 44(5): 1195–1199
79 Nightingale CH (2000) Moxifloxacin, a new antibiotic designed to treat community-acquired respiratory tract infections: a review of microbiologic and pharmacokinetic-pharmacodynamic characteristics [in process citation]. *Pharmacotherapy* 20(3): 245–256 (*Extensive review of moxifloxacin pharmacokinetics and pharmacodynamics*)
80 Lacy MK, Nicolau DP, Nightingale CH, Geffken A, Teng R, Vincent J, Quintiliani R (1999) Oral bioavailability and pharmacokinetics of trovafloxacin in patients with AIDS. *Antimicrob Agents Chemother* 43(12): 3005–3007
81 Goodwin SD, Gallis HA, Chow AT, Wong FA, Flor SC, Bartlett JA (1994) Pharmacokinetics and safety of levofloxacin in patients with human immunodeficiency virus infection. *Antimicrob Agents Chemother* 38(4): 799–804
81a Naber CK, Steghafner M, Kinzig-Schippers M, Sauber C, Sorgel F, Stahlberg HJ, Naber KG (2001) Pharmacokinetics and penetration of gemifloxacin *versus* ofloxacin into prostate secretions and ejaculate after single oral dosing in volunteers [abstr]. *In*: 11th European Congress Clinical Microbiology and Infectious Diseases. Istambul, Turkey
81b Wise R, Gee T, Andrews JM, Ashby JP, Marshall G (2001) The pharmacokinetics and inflammatory fluid penetration of gemifloxacin [abstr]. *In*: 11th European Congress Clinical Microbiology and Infectious Diseases. Istambul, Turkey
82 Craig WA (1998) Pharmacokinetic/pharmacodynamic parameters: rationale for antibacterial dosing of mice and men. *Clin Infect Dis* 26(1): 1–10 (*State of the art review of pharmacodynamics by the father of pharmacodynamics.*)
83 Ambrose PG, Owens RC (2000) New antibiotics in pulmonary and critical care medicine: focus on advanced generation quinolones and cephalosporins. *Sem Resp Crit Care Med* 21(1): 19–32
84 Dalhoff A (1999) Pharmacodynamics of fluoroquinolones. *J Antimicrob Chemother* 43 Suppl B: 51–59 (*Excellent review of pharmacodynamics of fluoroquinolones.*)
85 Vogelman B, Craig WA (1996) Kinetics of antimicrobial activity. *J Pediatr* 108: 835–840 (*This is a classic study describing the pharmacokinetics/pharmacodynamics of antibiotics.*)
86 Pickerill KE, Paladino JA, Schentag JJ (2000) Comparison of the fluoroquinolones based on pharmacokinetic and pharmacodynamic parameters. *Pharmacotherapy* 20(4): 417–428 (*This paper reviews the key pharmacodynamic and pharmacokinetic parameters of fluoroquinolones.*)
87 Stein GE (1996) Pharmacokinetics and pharmacodynamics of newer fluoroquinolones. *Clin Infect Dis* 23 Suppl 1: S19–24
88 Schentag JJ, Nix DX, Forrest A (1993) Pharmacodynamics of the fluoroquinolones. *In*: DC Hooper, JS Wolfson (eds): *Quinolone antimicrobial agents*, 2nd ed. American Society for Microbiology: Washington, DC 259–271

89 Rotschafer JC, Zabinski RA, Walker KJ (1992) Pharmacodynamic factors of antibiotic efficacy. *Pharmacother* 12: 64S-70S

90 Hyatt JM, McKinnon PS, Zimmer GS, Schentag JJ (1995) The importance of pharmacokinetic/pharmacodynamic surrogate markers to outcome: focus on antibacterial agents. *Clin Pharmacokinet* 28: 143–160

91 Bowker KE, Wootton M, Rogers CA, Lewis R, Holt HA, MacGowan AP (1999) Comparison of *in vitro* pharmacodynamics of once and twice daily ciprofloxacin. *J Antimicrob Chemother* 44(5): 661–667

92 Madaras-Kelly KJ, Ostergaard BE, Hovde LB, Rotschafer JC (1996) Twenty-four hour area under the concentration-time curve/MIC ratio as a generic predictor of fluoroquinolone antimicrobial effect by using three strains of *Pseudomonas aeruginosa* and an *in vitro* pharmacodynamic model. *Antimicrob Agents Chemother* 40: 627–632

93 Blaser J, Stone BB, Groner MC, Zinner SH (1987) Comparative study with enoxacin and netilimicin in a pharmacodynamic model to determine importance of ratio of antibiotic peak concentration to MIC for bacterial activity and emergence of resistance. *Antimicrob Agents Chemother* 31: 1054–1060

94 MacGowan AP, Bowker KE, Wootton M, Holt HA (1999) Activity of moxifloxacin, administered once a day, against *Streptococcus pneumoniae* in an *in vitro* pharmacodynamic model of infection. *Antimicrob Agents Chemother* 43(7): 1560–1564

95 Hershberger E, Rybak MJ (2000) Activities of trovafloxacin, gatifloxacin, clinafloxacin, sparfloxacin, levofloxacin, and ciprofloxacin against penicillin-resistant *Streptococcus pneumoniae* in an *in vitro* infection model. *Antimicrob Agents Chemother* 44(3): 598–601 *(Pharmacodynamic comparison of the new fluoroquinolones against various resistant phenotypes of* S. pneumoniae.*)*

95a Hoang AD, Raddatz JK, Hovde LB, Rotschafer JC (1997) An *in vitro* pharmacodynamic evaluation of levofloxacin against four strains of penicillin resistant *S. pneumoniae* [abstr]. *In*: 78th American Society for Microbiology. Miami, FL

96 Preston SL, Drusano GL, Berman AL, Fowler CL, Chow AT, Dornseif B, Reichl V, Natarajan J, Corrado M (1998) Pharmacodynamics of levofloxacin: a new paradigm for early clinical trials [see comments]. *JAMA* 279(2): 125–129 *(A critical study that correlated pharmacodynamics of new fluoroquinolones with clinical outcome.)*

97 Forrest A, Nix DE, Ballow CH, Goss TF, Birmingham MC, Schentag JJ (1993) Pharmacodynamics of intravenous ciprofloxacin in seriously ill patients. *Antimicrob Agents Chemother* 37(5): 1073–1081

98 Forrest A, Chodosh S, Amantea MA, Collins DA, Schentag JJ (1997) Pharmacokinetics and pharmacodynamics of oral grepafloxacin in patients with acute bacterial exacerbations of chronic bronchitis. *J Antimicrob Chemother* 40 Suppl A: 45–57 (*Study reporting that* $AUC_{24}/MIC < 125$ *is required for eradication of* S. pneumoniae *in outpatient respiratory infections.*)

99 Tran JQ, Ballow CH, Forrest A, Hyatt JM, Sands MF, Peloquin CA, Schentag JJ (2000) Comparison of the abilities of grepafloxacin and clarithromycin to eradicate potential bacterial pathogens from the sputa of patients with chronic bronchitis: influence of pharmacokinetic and pharmacodynamic variables. *J Antimicrob Chemother* 45: 9–17

100 Thomas JK, Forrest A, Bhavnani SM, Hyatt JM, Cheng A, Ballow CH, Schentag JJ (1998) Pharmacodynamic evaluation of factors associated with the development of bacterial resistance in acutely ill patients during therapy. *Antimicrob Agents Chemother* 42(3): 521–527 *(A study showing that achieving* $AUC_{24}/MIC > 100$ *against Gram-negative bacilli is required to prevent resistance from developing to fluoroquinolones.)*

101 Lacy MK, Lu W, Xu X, Tessier PR, Nicolau DP, Quintiliani R, Nightingale CH (1999) Pharmacodynamic comparisons of levofloxacin, ciprofloxacin, and ampicillin against *Streptococcus pneumoniae* in an *in vitro* model of infection. *Antimicrob Agents Chemother* 43(3): 672–677

102. Lister PD and Sanders CC (2000) Pharmacodynamics of levofloxacin and ciprofloxacin against *Streptococcus pneumoniae. J Antimicrob Chemother* 43(1): 79–86 *(This study showed that levofloxacin was more effective than ciprofloxacin at eradicating* S. pneumoniae.*)*

103 Lister PD, Sanders CC (1999) Pharmacodynamics of trovafloxacin, ofloxacin, and ciprofloxacin against *Streptococcus pneumoniae* in an *in vitro* pharmacokinetic model. *Antimicrob Agents Chemother* 43(5): 1118–1123

104 Coyle EA, Rybak MJ (1999) Evaluation of the activity of the newer fluoroquinolones against ciprofloxacin-resistant *Streptococcus pneumoniae* (SP) [abstr]. *In*: 39th Interscience Conference

on Antimicrobial Agents and Chemotherapy. San Francisco, CA
105 MacGowan AP, Bowker KE, Wootton M, Holt HA (1999) Exploration of the *in vitro* pharmacodynamic activity of moxifloxacin for *Staphylococcus aureus* and Streptococci of Lancefield groups A and G. *J Antimicrob Chemother* 44(6): 761–766
105a Zhanel GG, Walters M, Laing N, Hoban DJ (2001) *In vitro* pharmacodynamic modeling simulating free serum concentrations of fluoroquinolones against multi-drug resistant *Streptococcus pneumoniae. J Antimicrob Chemother* 47: 435-440 *(Study reporting that* $AUC_{24}/MIC > 35$ *is associated with bacterial killing by new fluoroquinolones* versus S. pneumoniae.*)*
106 Vostrov SN, Kononenko OV, Lubenko IY, Zinner SH, Firsov AA (2000) Comparative pharmacodynamics of gatifloxacin and ciprofloxacin in an *in vitro* dynamic model: prediction of equiefficient doses and the breakpoints of the area under the curve/MIC ratio. *Antimicrob Agents Chemother* 44(4): 879–884
107 Firsov AA, Vasilov RG, Vostrov SN, Kononenko OV, Lubenko IY, Zinner SH (1999) Prediction of the antimicrobial effects of trovafloxacin and ciprofloxacin on staphylococci using an *in vitro* dynamic model. *J Antimicrob Chemother* 43: 483–490
108 Pankuch GA, Jacobs MR, Appelbaum PC (1999) Post-antibiotic and post-antibiotic subMIC effect of gatifloxacin against Gram-positive and -negative bacteria. *In*: Interscience Conference on Antimicrobial Agents and Chemotherapy. San Francisco, CA
109 Boswell FJ, Andrews JM, Wise R (1997) Pharmacodynamic properties of BAY 12-8039 on Gram-positive and Gram-negative organisms as demonstrated by studies of time-kill kinetics and postantibiotic effect. *Antimicrob Agents Chemother* 41(6): 1377–1379
110 Moore T, Coleman K, Donald B, Rittenhouse S (1999) Postantibiotic effect (PAE) of gemifloxacin (SB-265805) and ciprofloxacin against Gram-positive and Gram-negative organisms. *In*: 39th Interscience Conference on Antimicrobial Agents and Chemotherapy. San Francisco, CA
111 Mackenzie FM, Gould IM (1993) The post-antibiotic effect. *J Antimicrob Chemother* 32: 519–537
112 Davies TA, Kelly LM, Pankuch GA, Credito KL, Jacobs MR, Appelbaum PC (1999) Post-antibiotic effect (PAE) of gemifloxacin (SB 265805) compared with five other quinolones against pneumococci. *In*: 39th Interscience Conference on Antimicrobial Agents and Chemotherapy. San Francisco, CA
113 Cars O, Odenholt-Tornqvist I (1993) The post-antibiotic sub-MIC effect *in vitro* and *in vivo. J Antimicrob Chemother* 31(Suppl. D): 159–166
114 Zhanel GG, Hoban DJ, Harding GKM (1992) Subinhibitory antimicrobial concentrations: A review of *in vitro* and *in vivo* data. Can *J Infect Dis* 3(4): 193–201
114a Licata L, Smith CE, Goldschmidt RM, Barrett JF, Frosco M (1997) Comparisons of the post-antibiotic and post-antibiotic sub-MIC effects of levofloxacin and ciprofloxacin on *Staphylococcus aureus* and *Streptococcus pneumoniae. Antimicrob Agents Chemother* 41: 950–955
115 Drlica K (2001) A strategy for fighting antibiotic resistance. *ASM News* 67: 27–33 *(A review of the principles that govern mutant prevention concentration.)*
115a Blondeau JM, Xilin A, Hansen G, Drlica K (2001) A mutant prevention concentrations of fluoroquinolones for clinical isolates of *Streptococcus pneumoniae. Antimicrob Agents Chemother* 45(2): 433–438 *(An assessment of mutant prevention concentration of fluoroquinolones* versus *various phenotypes of* S. pneumoniae.*)*
115b Smith HJ, Nichol KA, Walkty A, Zhanel GG, Hoban DJ (2001) Molecular characterization and mutant prevention concentration (MPC) determination of single-step fluoroquinolone resistant mutants of *S. pneumoniae* [poster]. *In*: 2001 Meeting of Canadian Association for Clinical Microbiology and Infectious Disease, Victoria, BC

Fluoroquinolone Antibiotics
ed. by A.R. Ronald and D.E. Low

Fluoroquinolones in urinary tract infection

James R. Johnson

VA Medical Center and Department of Medicine, University of Minnesota, Minneapolis, MN, USA

Introduction

Urinary tract infection (UTI) is one of the most common infectious diseases for which antibiotic therapy is prescribed. Many characteristics of the fluoroquinolones make them ideal agents for the management of UTI [1–12]. As a class, the fluoroquinolones traditionally have been highly active *in vitro* against nearly all significant urinary pathogens. Most are renally excreted, hence achieve high concentrations in the urine. They penetrate the prostrate well. Their high oral bioavailability allows oral therapy for infections that traditionally would be treated with intravenous antibiotics, and their long half-lives allow convenient once- or twice-daily dosing. The currently marketed fluoroquinolones have favorable adverse effect profiles and few significant drug-drug interactions. Consequently, fluoroquinolones have been and probably will continue to be used extensively in the treatment and prevention of UTI in a wide variety of clinical contexts, as reviewed below. To what extent emerging drug resistance will compromise the utility of fluoroquinolones for UTI therapy in coming years remains to be seen, but is a significant concern.

UTI syndromes and host status

The appropriate role for fluoroquinolones in UTI management depends on the patient's gender, age, and clinical syndrome, and on the presence or absence of underlying host conditions such as urinary tract abnormalities, instrumentation, or systemic illnesses that predispose to UTI or interfere with cure [1, 8–10]. Infections that occur in patients with such complicating factors are designated "complicated", whereas those that occur in patients without such conditions are designated "uncomplicated" [13, 14]. Treatment of uncomplicated UTI will be considered first (separately for women, men, and children), followed by treatment of complicated UTI, then prophylaxis.

Treatment of uncomplicated UTI

Women

Uncomplicated cystitis

Acute bacterial cystitis, i.e., symptomatic infection of the urinary bladder, is the most frequently encountered symptomatic UTI syndrome [9, 15, 16]. It occurs most commonly, and has been studied most extensively, in reproductive-age women.

Guidelines for the management of acute uncomplicated cystitis in women were recently proposed by the Infectious Diseases Society of America, based on a systematic review and meta-analysis of the available randomized clinical trials that met strict *a priori* inclusion criteria [17]. The main conclusions of this review with respect to the fluoroquinolones were fourfold. First, when different drug classes are compared at the same duration of therapy, with respect to efficacy the fluoroquinolones are comparable to trimethoprim-sulfamethoxazole and trimethoprim alone but are significantly better than beta-lactam agents, whereas with respect to adverse effects there are no significant differences among drug classes. Second, for most fluoroquinolones multi-day therapy yields significantly better efficacy than single-dose therapy. Exceptions include the long half-life agents pefloxacin and rufloxacin (which currently are not available in the U.S.) [18–20]. These two drugs achieve eradication rates of approximately 95% even with single-dose therapy, but also may cause increased adverse effects (40%, pefloxacin), particularly those involving the central nervous system (CNS) (rufloxacin). Third, with the fluoroquinolones treatment durations longer than 3 days provide no advantage over 3-day therapy. An exception may be lomefloxacin, which in the only evaluable study yielded significantly higher eradication rates with 7-d (98%) than with 3-day therapy (92%) [21]. Fourth, when directly compared the various fluoroquinolone agents do not differ significantly with respect to eradication or recurrence rates. They also are largely similar with respect to the frequency of adverse effects. Exceptions to the latter statement would be the higher incidence of adverse effects noted above with pefloxacin and rufloxacin single-dose therapy, and as noted with lomefloxacin (35%) *versus* norfloxacin (24%) when given for 3 or 7 days [21, 22].

These conclusions have been largely borne out by several more recent studies [23–28]. In two of these studies, patient-initiated therapy using an oral fluoroquinolone was found to be a highly effective management approach for women with frequent recurrences of uncomplicated cystitis [23, 26]. The significantly increased incidence of phototoxicity associated with sparfloxacin (which is no longer marketed) that was demonstrated in two of these studies illustrates the importance of agent-specific adverse effects that may become apparent only in post-marketing evaluations [27, 28].

These data indicate that according to clinical parameters 3-day therapy with renally cleared fluoroquinolone agents such as ciprofloxacin, ofloxacin, levofloxacin, and probably gatifloxacin is optimal for acute uncomplicated cystitis in women [11, 17]. However, the concern that routine use of fluoroquinolones might hasten the emergence of bacterial resistance prompted the IDSA guidelines committee to recommend that TMP-SMZ or TMP alone should be preferred for empiric therapy of uncomplicated cystitis unless resistance to these drugs is anticipated, e.g., in communities where the prevalence of TMP-SMZ resistance among uropathogens is >10–20% [17]. Of note, although data regarding the impact of TMP-SMZ resistance on clinical outcomes in cystitis are scarce, resistance appears to be associated with a failure rate of approximately 50% [25, 29–31]. A recent cost-benefit analysis generally supported the prevalence threshold suggested by the IDSA guidelines, yielding a calculated break-even point of 22% for the community prevalence of TMP-SMZ resistance at which empiric therapy with a fluoroquinolone would become more cost-effective than empiric TMP-SMZ therapy [32]. Other data suggest that older age, male sex, recent hospitalization, diabetes mellitus, history of recurrent UTI, and recent exposure to antibiotics (particularly TMP or TMP-SMZ) predict an increased likelihood of TMP-SMZ resistance [29, 33–35]. These historical features thus conceivably could be used as patient-specific indicators for use of a non-TMP-SMZ empiric regimen, including a fluoroquinolone.

Unfortunately, levels of resistance to TMP-SMZ at or above the proposed 10–20% threshold are increasingly prevalent in many locales [29, 36–44], prompting many physicians to adopt fluoroquinolone-based regimens for routine empiric therapy of cystitis [29]. However, as discussed further below, emerging resistance to fluoroquinolones among *Escherichia coli* and other uropathogens is already threatening the reliability of fluoroquinolones as an alternative to TMP-SMZ. This development introduces troubling new questions with respect to optimal drug selection for cystitis.

Uncomplicated pyelonephritis

Few comparative trials are available on which to base recommendations for therapy of acute pyelonephritis. A recent trial demonstrated that acute uncomplicated pyelonephritis of mild-to-moderate severity in women can be treated quite effectively (i.e., 99% microbiological cure, 96% clinical cure) in the ambulatory setting with 7 days of oral ciprofloxacin, with or without an initial intravenous dose [45]. Of note, in this study population the prevalence of ciprofloxacin resistance was low (<0.5%). In contrast, TMP-SMZ resistance was encountered in 18% of urine isolates, and was associated with 50% bacteriological failure and 65% clinical failure if the patient was treated with TMP-SMZ [45]. Since in the outpatient context it is inconvenient to modify the antibiotic regimen after the initial encounter when resistance is later discovered, routine use of empiric fluoroquinolone therapy (if the isolate is not already known to be susceptible to TMP-SMZ) is recommended by the IDSA guidelines [17].

For patients with pyelonephritis who are sufficiently ill as to require hospital admission, fluoroquinolones are one of several reasonable alternative initial therapeutic regimens [17]. For inpatients who can tolerate oral medications, treatment outcomes for pyelonephritis appear to be as good when therapy is given orally as when given intravenously, with considerable cost savings [46]. For patients who initially require an intravenous regimen, rapid conversion to oral therapy can be done using a fluoroquinolone, possibly even prior to the availability of susceptibility results (depending on local susceptibility data). This attractive "oral step-down" feature of the fluoroquinolones, and the option of switching to a less-costly agent once susceptibility results are known, are not always taken advantage of by physicians, which suggests that additional in-hospital cost savings may be possible [47].

Men

Cystitis

Few data are available regarding the optimal management of cystitis in men [48, 49]. Authorities recommend longer courses of therapy than in women, e.g., 7 to 14 days, because single-dose and short-course therapy have not been shown to be effective [49]. Drug selection can be individualized if susceptibilities for the patient's organism are known, but for empiric therapy population-based susceptibility data and patient-specific risk factors can be used to select an appropriate agent, as discussed above for cystitis in women. Fluoroquinolones are highly effective when given for 7 to 10 days [48, 50]. If enterococci, which cause an appreciable minority of UTIs in men [48], are suspected or documented, amoxicillin may be preferable to a fluoroquinolone. Recurrent bacteriuria in a man after a course of appropriate antibiotic therapy for presumed cystitis usually reflects prostate involvement [49], for which cure rates exceeding 90% can be achieved with a 6-week course of fluoroquinolone therapy (see below) [2, 49].

Pyelonephritis and febrile UTI

Even fewer data or authoritative recommendations are available regarding the management of uncomplicated pyelonephritis or febrile UTI in men [48, 49]. Fluoroquinolones would be expected to be ideal empirical agents. A recent trial of twice-daily oral ciprofloxacin for men with febrile UTI showed comparable success rates with 2 *versus* 4 weeks of therapy (short-term microbiological cure, 89% *versus* 97%; cumulative clinical cure after 1 year, 72% *versus* 82%) (P. Ulleryd, personal communication). Interestingly, >80% of men with febrile UTI have an elevated prostate-specific antigen level that declines with effective treatment of the UTI and have ultrasonographically demonstrable enlargement of the prostate gland and/or seminal vesicles [51]. These manifestations typically occur in the absence of prostatic tenderness or symptoms referable to the prostate gland and, in contrast to the experience with overt acute bacterial prostatitis (see below), are not associated with a high rate of clinical failure or of complications if fluoroquinolone therapy is limited to 14 days (P. Ulleryd, personal communication).

Prostatitis

Bacterial prostatitis occurs in an acute and a chronic form, both of which require antimicrobial therapy [49]. Bacterial prostatitis of either variety must be distinguished from nonbacterial prostatitis (also known as chronic pelvic pain syndrome), which is associated with negative cultures of urine and expressed prostatic secretions and responds unpredictably to antibiotic therapy [49, 52]. Acute bacterial prostatitis causes intense symptoms as well as constitutional findings [49]. Chronic bacterial prostatitis has a more insidious onset, less pronounced prostatic inflammation, and no constitutional manifestations; patients instead typically have irritative or obstructive genitourinary symptoms and relapsing or persistent UTI [49].

Fluoroquinolones are the drugs of choice for both acute and chronic bacterial prostatitis. The data favoring the fluoroquinolones over alternatives such as TMP-SMZ in acute prostatitis are compelling [1, 2, 53]. Treatment should be given for 3 to 4 weeks to avoid complications such as abscess formation or chronic bacterial prostatitis [49, 53]. Chronic bacterial prostatitis requires at least 4 to 6 weeks of appropriate antibiotic therapy. Here again the superiority of fluoroquinolones over alternative agents is clear, with success rates of 60% to 90% obtained with fluoroquinolones as compared with 30% to 40% with TMP-SMZ [49, 54, 55]. To prevent relapse, antibiotic therapy for chronic prostatitis should be continued for at least 3 months. If this fails, low dose suppressive therapy can be used (e.g., daily or thrice weekly ofloxacin or ciprofloxacin, 100 mg; TMP-SMZ, one regular strength tablet; or nitrofurantoin, 100 mg) [49]. Removal of prostatic stones or prostatectomy may be needed for cure in selected patients.

Children

Fluoroquinolones traditionally have been avoided in children because of concerns regarding induction of arthropathy, which are based on data from immature animals [56–58]. Hence, fluoroquinolones usually are not recommended for treatment of pediatric UTI [59]. However, increasing human clinical experience suggests that fluoroquinolones actually are safe to use in children, including for extended treatment courses [10, 60–66]. (Of note, published data regarding repeated courses of fluoroquinolones therapy in children and use of fluoroquinolones below age 5 years are scant to nil.) Thus, although not yet approved for pediatric use in the U.S., fluoroquinolone therapy could reasonably be considered for children over age 5 with UTIs due to multi-resistant organisms that otherwise would require intravenous therapy, or if alternative agents are otherwise contraindicated [10, 66]. As a precaution, if a fluoroquinolone is to be used in a child the physician should inform parents of the animal arthropathy data, obtain informed consent for off-label use of the drug, and be alert for signs or symptoms suggesting possible arthropathy so that therapy can be promptly discontinued if problems are detected.

Treatment of complicated UTI

Therapy for complicated UTI (i.e., UTI occurring in the presence of a significant underlying medical condition, an anatomical or functional urinary tract abnormality, or urinary tract instrumentation) has been comparatively little studied [13, 67]. In addition, the available trials have used highly heterogeneous inclusion criteria, and most have not stratified outcomes according to underlying complicating condition, gender, or severity of illness [13, 67, 68]. Notwithstanding these limitations, the available data, which derive mostly from adults, suggest that for many patients with complicated UTI oral fluoroquinolones are as or more effective than alternative agents, including traditional intravenous regimens [9, 11, 12, 69–72]. Likewise, few clinically significant differences are evident among the various renally excreted fluoroquinolones, with the possible exception of increased adverse effects with lomefloxacin [71]. Thus, fluoroquinolones can be considered drugs of choice for complicated UTI for empiric therapy and also for pathogen-specific therapy, if the urine organism is susceptible and other considerations (e.g., bacterial resistance, drug allergy, or drug-drug interactions) exclude less expensive alternatives such as TMP-SMZ [12]. For severe infections due to less susceptible pathogens such as *Pseudomonas aeruginosa*, intensified dosing has been proposed with ciprofloxacin (750 mg PO bid) or levofloxacin (500 mg PO bid) [12].

Although newer fluoroquinolones with enhanced Gram-positive activity (e.g., gatifloxacin and gemifloxacin) may offer an advantage in complicated UTI, more episodes of which are due to Gram-positive bacteria than is true with uncomplicated UTI [73], any such superiority remains to be demonstrated clinically [12, 73]. Dosing of ciprofloxacin for complicated UTI is best done twice daily rather than once-daily [74], despite kinetic considerations suggesting that for highly susceptible organisms once-daily dosing might suffice [75].

Prophylaxis

Recurrent uncomplicated cystitis in women

Fluoroquinolones have been used successfully for prevention of recurrent cystitis in women both as low-dose continuous prophylaxis [76, 77] and as postcoital prophylaxis [78]. The long half-life agents pefloxacin and fleroxacin allow continuous prophylaxis with once-weekly dosing [79]. Emergence of resistant organisms during continuous prophylaxis not been reported to date, although this remains a future concern as the prevalence of fluoroquinolone-resistant *E. coli* rises generally (see later). An alternative management approach for recurrent cystitis is patient-initiated therapy, which may be preferred by women who have relatively infrequent recurrences that are not associated with coitus [23, 26, 80].

Complicated UTI

Fluoroquinolones, the agents of choice for treatment of complicated UTI, also have been used to prevent complicated UTI in diverse clinical contexts, with consistently positive results. Prophylaxis trials have included patients with spinal cord injury [81], acute urinary catheterization [82], and other underlying conditions [83]. However, the absence of demonstrated clinical benefit and the documented emergence of resistant bacteria have tempered enthusiasm for routine systemic antibiotic prophylaxis in spinal cord injured and catheterized patients [84–88]. Nonetheless, in carefully selected patients with frequent or severe recurrent episodes of complicated UTI, a trial of fluoroquinolone prophylaxis could be considered, with the recognition that this may result in the loss of this drug class for therapy of break-through symptomatic infections.

Urological procedures

For prophylaxis against post-operative bacteriuria in patients undergoing prostate biopsy or transurethral surgery, oral fluoroquinolones are as effective as are oral TMP-SMZ or intravenous first or third generation cephalosporins [89–95]. Multiple doses offer no significant advantage over a single pre-operative oral dose [89, 93]. Although the incidence of a positive urine culture is significantly lower with antibiotic prophylaxis than with placebo, this is mostly due to a reduction in asymptomatic bacteriuria; no significant reduction in symptomatic UTI or febrile complications has been demonstrated, nor has even a consistent trend [93–95]. However, since the available studies have been under-powered for excluding small differences, definitive conclusions are not possible. Of note, in one prophylaxis study cefotaxime was associated with a significantly increased incidence of adverse events as compared with placebo, whereas ciprofloxacin was not [94]. This suggests that even if fluoroquinolones provide no definite benefit when used as prophylaxis for minor urological or uroradiological procedures they may be less toxic than alternative antibiotics.

Bacterial resistance to fluoroquinolones

When fluoroquinolones were first introduced in the 1980s nearly all urine organisms from patients with UTI, whether uncomplicated or complicated, were susceptible *in vitro*. Even today, fluoroquinolones remain among the most active oral agents among urine isolates overall [29, 36, 41, 42, 44, 96, 97]. However over the past decade a growing number of locales have reported a substantial prevalence of fluoroquinolone resistance among urine isolates in general and specifically among *E. coli*, and the prevalence of fluoroquinolone resistance at individual locales has progressively risen [97–103].

Fluoroquinolone resistance levels among *E. coli* urine isolates as high as 25% have been reported from Latin America [97], where even susceptible isolates commonly have single point mutations in *gyrA* that presage progression to full resistance with additional mutations [104]. Of concern, in San Juan, Costa Rica, 70% of *E. coli* urine isolates from intensive care unit patients are resistant to ciprofloxacin [105].

The observed widespread emergence of fluoroquinolone resistance poses two quandaries for practitioners, one pertaining to provision of optimal therapy for today's patient, the other to prevention of future resistance. With respect to current management, the clinical implications of *in vitro* fluoroquinolone resistance among patients with UTI are unknown. However, based on the observation that *in vitro* resistance to TMP-SMZ predicts an approximately 50% failure rate with TMP-SMZ therapy despite this agent's high urine concentrations and long half-life [25, 29–31, 34, 45], clinical failures can be expected also with fluoroquinolone resistance. Consequently, as the prevalence of fluoroquinolone resistance increases, so also does the calculated threshold for the prevalence of TMP-SMZ resistance at which empiric fluoroquinolone therapy becomes the preferred strategy for uncomplicated UTI [32]. That is, the appeal of fluoroquinolones as alternatives to TMP-SMZ diminishes as fluoroquinolone resistance increases. In addition, if the prevalence of resistance to both fluoroquinolones and TMP-SMZ is substantial, it may be preferable to consider a different drug altogether rather than to rely on "the lesser of two evils." Nitrofurantoin and fosfomycin have been less well studied in the treatment of UTI than the fluoroquinolones and TMP-SMZ, and are somewhat less efficacious (unless nitrofurantoin is given for a longer course, e.g., 7 days for cystitis) [17]. Still, resistance to these alternative agents has not been observed to nearly the extent noted with fluoroquinolones and TMP-SMZ, making them attractive considerations for empiric therapy if resistance is prevalent to both fluoroquinolones and TMP-SMZ.

In addition, even if in a locale with substantial TMP-SMZ resistance the prevalence of fluoroquinolone resistance is not yet so high as to oblige non-fluoroquinolone therapy, consideration of non-fluoroquinolone alternatives to TMP-SMZ still may be prudent, as a way to limit selection pressure for emergence of fluoroquinolone resistance. This strategy would in effect keep fluoroquinolones "in reserve," available to be used when alternative drugs predictably would not suffice, as in pyelonephritis, bacteremia, or prostatitis, or with organisms known to be resistant to the alternative. However, the utility of such a "fluoroquinolone-sparing" strategy is uncertain. It is unknown what proportion of total fluoroquinolone use is for UTI therapy, hence how great an impact even complete avoidance of fluoroquinolones for UTI therapy might have. It is likely that as clinical indications for fluoroquinolones expand, e.g., to include respiratory tract infections [106, 107], infections in children [63], and prophylaxis following exposure to *Bacillus anthracis* [108], the proportion of fluoroquinolones use accounted for by UTI therapy will shrink, thereby diminishing the resistance-retarding effect of fluoroquinolone avoidance for UTI therapy.

Unfortunately, levels of resistance to nitrofurantoin have already been documented among urine isolates in certain settings (e.g., in San Juan, Costa Rica: 19% among all outpatient urine isolates, 43% among ICU *E. coli* urine isolates [105]. This suggests that the currently available alternative agents may provide only temporary relief from the emerging drug resistance problem, an example of the so-called "squeezing the balloon" phenomenon [109]. Thus, the future role of fluoroquinolones in UTI therapy will be strongly influenced by how the antibiotic resistance story evolves, which remains to be seen.

References

1 Naber KG (1989) Use of quinolones in urinary tract infections and prostatitis. *Rev Infect Dis* 11 (suppl 5): S1321–S1327

2 Naber KG (1993) Role of quinolones in treatment of chronic bacterial prostatitis *In*: DC Hooper, JS Wolfson (eds): *Quinolone antimicrobial agents* (2nd ed.). Washington, DC, American Society for Microbiology, 285–297

3 Sable CA, Scheld WM (1993) Fluoroquinolones: how to use (but not overuse) these antibiotics. *Geriatrics* 48: 41–51

4 Blondeau JM (2001) Clinical utility of the new fluoroquinolones for treating respiratory and urinary tract infections. *Expert Opin Invest Drugs* 10: 213–237

5 Martin SJ, Jung R, Garvin CG (2001) A risk-benefit assessment of levofloxacin in respiratory, skin and skin structure, and urinary tract infections. *Drug Safety* 24: 199–222

6 Blondeau JM (2000) A review of clinical trials with fluoroquinolones with an emphasis on new agents. *Expert Opin Invest Drugs* 9: 383–413

7 Cunha BA (1994) The fluoroquinolones for urinary tract infections: a review. *Adv Ther* 11: 277–296

8 Hooton TM, Stamm WE (1997) Diagnosis and treatment of uncomplicated urinary tract infection. *Infect Dis Clin North Am* 11: 551–582

9 Stamm WE, Hooton TM (1993) Management of urinary tract infections in adults. *N Engl J Med* 329: 1328–1334

10 Van Wijk JAE, de Jon TPVM, Vanbool JD (1992) Using quinolones in urinary tract infections in children. *Adv Antimicrob Antineopl Chemother* 11 (suppl. 2): 157–161

11 Langtry HD (1998) Levofloxacin. Its use in infections of the respiratory tract, skin, soft tissues and urinary tract. *Drugs* 56: 487–515

12 Naber KG (2001) Which fluoroquinolones are suitable for the treatment of urinary tract infections? *Int J Antimicrob Agents* 17: 331–341

13 Ronald AR, Harding GKM (1997) Complicated urinary tract infections. *Infect Dis Clin North Am* 11: 583–592

14 Preheim LC (1985) Complicated urinary tract infections. *Am J Med* 79: 62–66

15 Foxman B, Barlow R, D'Arcy H, Gillespie B, Sobel JD (2000) Urinary tract infection: self-reported incidence and associated costs. *Ann Epidemiol* 10: 509–515

16 Stull TL, Li Puma JL (1991) Epidemiology and natural history of urinary tract infections in children. *Med Clin North Am* 75: 287–298

17 Warren JW, Abrutyn E, Hebel JR, Johnson JR, Schaffer AJ, Stamm WE (1999) Guidelines for antimicrobial therapy of uncomplicated acute bacterial cystitis and acute pyelonephritis in women. *Clin Infect Dis* 29: 745–758

18 Del Rio G, Dalet F, Aguilar L, Caffaratti J, Dalre R (1996) Single-dose rufloxacin *versus* three day norfloxacin treatment of uncomplicated cystitis. *Antimicrob Agents Chemother* 40: 408–412

19 Jardin A, Cesana M (1995) French Multicenter Urinary Tract Infection – Rufloxacin Group. Randomized, double-blind comparison of single-dose regimens of rufloxacin and pefloxacin for acute uncomplicated cystitis in women. *Antimicrob Agents Chemother* 39: 215–220

20 van Balen FA, Touw-Otten FW, de Melker RA (1990) Single-dose pefloxacin *versus* five-days treatment with norfloxacin in uncomplicated cystitis in women. *J Antimicrob Agents Chemother*

6: 153–1660
21 Neringer R, Forsgren A, Hansson C, Ode B (1992) South Swedish Lolex Study Group. Lomefloxacin *versus* norfloxacin in the treatment of uncomplicated urinary tract infections: three-day *versus* seven-day treatment. *Scand J Infect Dis* 24: 773–780
22 Nicolle LE, Dubois J, Martel AY, Harding GKM, Shafran SD, Conly JM (1995) Treatment of acute uncomplicated urinary tract infections with 3 days of lomefloxacin compared with treatment with 3 days of norfloxacin. *Antimicrob Agents Chemother* 37: 574–579
23 Gupta K, Hooton TM, Roberts PL, Stamm WE (2001) Patient-initiated treatment of uncomplicated recurrent urinary tract infections in young women. *Ann Intern Med* 135: 9–16
24 Iravani A, Klimberg I, Briefer C, Munera C, Kowalsky SF, Echols RM (1999) A trial comparing low-dose, short-course ciprofloxacin and standard 7 day therapy with co-trimoxazole or nitrofurantoin in the treatment of uncomplicated urinary tract infection. *J Antimicrob Chemother* 43 (suppl A): 67–75
25 McCarty JM, Richard G, Huck W et al (1999) A randomized trial of short-course ciprofloxacin, ofloxacin, or trimethoprim/sulfamethoxazole for the treatment of acute urinary tract infection in women. Ciprofloxacin Urinary Tract Infection Group. *Am J Med* 106: 292–299
26 Schaeffer AJ, Stuppy BA (1999) Efficacy and safety of self-start therapy in women with recurrent urinary tract infections. *J Urol* 161: 207–211
27 Henry DC, Nenad RC, Iravani A et al (1999) Comparison of sparfloxacin and ciprofloxacin in the treatment of community-acquired acute uncomplicated urinary tract infection in women. Sparfloxacin Multicenter Uncomplicated Urinary Tract Infection Study Group. *Clin Ther* 21: 966–981
28 Henry DC, Ellison W, Sullivan J et al (1998) Treatment of community-acquired uncomplicated urinary tract infection with sparfloxacin *versus* ofloxacin. The Sparfloxacin Multi Center UUTI Study Group. *Antimicrob Agents Chemother* 42: 2262–2266
29 Gupta K, Hooton TM, Stamm WE (2001) Increasing antimicrobial resistance and the management of uncomplicated community-acquired urinary tract infections. *Ann Intern Med* 135: 41–50
30 Masterton RG, Bochsler JA (1995) High-dosage co-amoxiclav in a single dose *versus* 7 days of co-trimoxazole as treatment of uncomplicated lower urinary tract infection in women. *J Antimicrob Chemother* 35: 129–137
31 Raz R, Chazan B, Kennes Y et al (2002) Empiric use of trimethoprim-sulfamethoxazole (TMP-SMZ) in the treatment of women with uncomplicated urinary tract infections, in a geographical area with a high prevalence of TMP-SMZ-resistant uropathogens. *Clin Infect Dis* 34(9): 1165–1169
32 Le TP, Miller LG (2001) Empirical therapy for uncomplicated urinary tract infections in an era of increasing antimicrobial resistance: a decision and cost analysis. *Clin Infect Dis* 33: 615–621
33 Steinke DT, Seaton RA, Phillips G, MacDonald TM, Davey PG (1999) Factors associated with trimethoprim-resistant bacteria isolated from urine samples. *J Antimicrob Chemother* 43: 841–843
34 Wright SW, Wrenn KD, Haynes JL (1999) Trimethoprim-sulfamethoxazole resistance among urinary coliform isolates. *J Gen Intern Med* 14: 606–609
35 Sotto A, de Boever CM, Fabbro-Peray P, Gouby A, Sirot D, Jourdan J (2001) Risk factors for antibiotic-resistant *Escherichia coli* isolated from hospitalized patients with urinary tract infections: a prospective study. *J Clin Microbiol* 39: 438–444
36 Gupta K, Scholes D, Stamm WE (1999) Increasing prevalence of antimicrobial resistance among uropathogens causing acute uncomplicated cystitis in women. *JAMA* 281: 736–738
37 Gupta K, Sahm DF, Mayfield D, Stamm WE (2001) Antimicrobial resistance among uropathogens that cause community-acquired urinary tract infections in women: a nationwide analysis. *Clin Infect Dis* 33: 89–94
38 Enne VI, Livermore DM, Stephens P, Hall LCM (2001) Persistence of sulphonamide resistance in *Escherichia coli* in the UK despite national prescribing restriction. *Lancet* 357: 1325–1328
39 Young H-K, Jesudason MV, Koshi G, Amyes SGB (1986) Trimethoprim resistance amongst urinary pathogens in South India. *J Antimicrob Chemother* 17: 615–621
40 Andrasevic AT, Tambic T, Kalenic S, Jankovid V (2002) The Working Group of the Croatian Committee for Antibiotic Resistance Surveillance. Surveillance for antimicrobial resistance in Croatia. *Emerg Infect Dis* 8: 14–18
41 Felmingham D, Arakawa S (2001) Resistance among urinary tract pathogens. Experience outside the USA. *Clin Drug Invest* 21 (suppl 1): 7–11
42 Kahlmeter G (2000) The ECO-SENS project: a prospective, multinational, multicenter epidemio-

logical survey of the prevalence and antimicrobial susceptibility of urinary tract pathogens – interim report. *J Antimicrob Chemother* 46 (suppl S1): 15–22
43 Murray BE, Alvarado T, Kim KH et al (1985) Increasing resistance to trimethoprim-sulfamethoxazole among isolates of *Escherichia coli* in developing countries. *J Infect Dis* 152: 1107–1113
44 Karlowsky JA, Jones JE, Thornsberry C, Critchley I, Kelly LJ, Sahm DF (2001) Prevalence of antimicrobial resistance among urinary tract pathogens isolated from female outpatients across the US in 1999. *Int J Antimicrob Agents* 18: 121–127
45 Talan DA, Stamm WE, Hooton TM et al (2000) Comparison of ciprofloxacin (7 days) and trimethoprim-sulfamethoxazole (14 days) for acute uncomplicated pyelonephritis in women. *JAMA* 283: 1583–1590
46 Moribelli G, Pezzoli R, Pinoja-Lutz G, Monotti R, Marone C, Franciolli M (1999) Oral *versus* intravenous ciprofloxacin in the initial empirical management of severe pyelonephritis or complicated urinary tract infections: a prospective randomized clinical trial. *Arch Intern Med* 159: 53–58
47 Dydek CJ, Souney PF, Matthews SJ (1992) DUE of ciprofloxacin in the treatment of urinay tract infections in hospitalized patients. *Hosp Formulary* 27: 185–191
48 Lipsky BA (1989) Urinary tract infections in men: epidemiology, pathophysiology, diagnosis, and treatment. *Ann Intern Med* 110: 138–150
49 Lipsky BA (1999) Prostatitis and urinary tract infection in men: what's new; what's true? *Am J Med* 106: 327–334
50 Schaeffer AJ (1987) Multiclinic study of norfloxacin for treatment of urinary tract infections. *Am J Med* 82 (suppl 6B): 53–58
51 Ulleryd P, Zackrisson B, Aus G, Bergdahl S, Hugosson J, Sandberg T (1999) Prostatic involvement in men with febrile urinary tract infection as measured by serum prostate-specific antigen and transrectal ultrasonography. *B J U International* 84: 470–474
52 Nickel JC, Downey J, Johnston B, Clark J, Group TC (2001) The Canadian Prostatitis Research Group. Predictors of patient response to antibiotic therapy for the chronic prostatis/pelvic pain syndrome: a prospective multicenter clinical trial. *J Urol* 165: 1539–1544
53 Falagas ME (1995) Practice guidelines: prostatitis, epididymitis, and urethritis. *Infect Dis Clin Pract* 4: 325–333
54 Pewitt EB, Schaeffer AJ (1997) Urinary tract infection in urology, including acute and chronic prostatitis. *Infect Dis Clin North Am* 11: 623–646
55 Falagas ME, Gorbach SL (1995) Practice guidelines: urinary tract infections. *Infect Dis Clin Pract* 4: 241–257
56 Ingham B (1977) Arthropathy induced by antibacterial fused n-alkyl-4-pyridone-3carboxylic acids. *Toxicol Lett* 1: 21–26
57 Schluter G (1986) Toxicology of ciprofloxacin [Abstract First International Ciprofloxacin Workshop, Proceedings (Amsterdam). *Exerpta Medica* 61–70
58 Amacher DE, Schomaker SJ, Gootz TD, McGuirk PR (1989) Proteoglycan and procollagen synthesis in rat embryo limb bud cultures treated with quinolone antibacterials. *Altern Methods Toxicol* 7: 307–312
59 Johnson CE (1999) New advances in childhood urinary tract infections. *Pediatr Rev* 20: 335–342
60 Fanos VC, L (2000) Fluoroquinolones in pediatrics and their nephrotoxicity in adults: minireview. *J Chemother* 12: 228–231
61 Ogle JW (1999) Antimicrobial therapy for ambulatory pediatrics. *Pediatr Ann* 28: 434–444
62 Redmond AO (1997) Risk-benefit experience of ciprofloxacin use in pediatric patients in the United Kingdom. *Pediatr Infect Dis J* 16: 147–149
63 Hampel B, Hullmann R, Schmidt H (1997) Ciprofloxacin in pediatrics: worldwide clinical experience based on compassionate use – safety report. *Pediatr Infect Dis J* 16: 160–162
64 Schaad UB (1992) Role of the new quinolones in pediatric practice. *Pediatr Infect Dis J* 11: 1043–1046
65 Green SD (1996) Indications and restrictions of fluoroquinolone use in children. *Br J Hosp Med* 56: 420–423
66 Fujii R, Meguro H, Arimasu O et al (1990) Evaluation of norfloxacin in the pediatric field. Pediatric Study Group for Norfloxacin. *Jpn J Antibiot* 43: 181–215
67 Ronald AR, Nicolle LE, Stamm WE et al (2001) Urinary tract infection in adults: research priorities and strategies. *Int J Antimicrob Agents* 17: 343–348
68 Ronald AR, Nicolle LE, Harding GK (1992) Standards of therapy for urinary tract infections in adults. *Infection* 20 (suppl 3): S164–S170

69 Johnson JR, Stamm WE (1989) Urinary tract infections in women: diagnosis and treatment. *Ann Intern Med* 111: 906–917
70 Peng MY (1999) Randomized, double-blind, comparative study of levofloxacin and ofloxacin in the treatment of complicated urinary tract infections. *J Microbiol Immunol Infect* 32: 33–39
71 Klimberg IW, Cox CEn Fowler CL, King W, Kim SS, Callery-D'Amico S (1998) A controlled trial of levofloxacin and lomefloxacin in the treatment of complicated urinary tract infection. *Urol* 51: 610–615
72 Raz R, g NK, Raizenberg C et al (2000) Ciprofloxacin 250 mg twice daily *versus* ofloxacin 200 mg twice daily in the treatment of complicated urinary tract infections in women. *Eur J Clin Microbiol Infect Dis* 19: 327–331
73 Naber KG, Hollauer K, Kirchbauer D, Witte W (2000) *In vitro* activity of gatifloxacin compared with gemifloxacin, moxifloxacin, trovafloxacin, ciprofloxacin and ofloxacin against uropathogens cultured from patients with complicated urinary tract infections. *Int J Antimicrob Agents* 16: 239–243
74 Krcmery S, Naber KG (1999) Ciprofloxacin once *versus* twice daily in the treatment of complicated urinary tract infections. German Ciprofloxacin UTI Study Group. *Int J Antimicrob Agents* 11: 133–138
75 Naber KG, Theuretzbacher U, Moneva-Koucheva G, Stass H (1999) Urinary excretion and bactericidal activity of intravenous ciprofloxacin compared with oral ciprofloxacin. *Eur J Clin Microbiol Infect Dis* 18: 783–789
76 Nicolle LE, Harding GKM, Thompson M, Kennedy J, Urias B, Ronald AR (1989) Prospective, randomized, placebo-controlled trial of norfloxacin for the prophylaxis of recurrent urinary tract infection in women. *Antimicrob Agents Chemother* 33: 1032–1035
77 Raz R, Boger S (1991) Long-term prophylaxis with norfloxacin *versus* nitrofurantoin in women with recurrent urinary tract infection. *Antimicrob Agents Chemother* 35: 1241–1242
78 Pfau A, Sacks TG (1994) Effective postcoital quinolone prophylaxis of recurrent urinary tract infections in women. *J Urol* 152: 136–138
79 Krcmery S, Hromec J, Tvrdikova M, Hassan M, Gulla D (1999) Newer quinolones in the long-term prophylaxis of recurrent urinary tract infections (UTI). *Drugs* 58 (Suppl 2): 99–102
80 Wong ES, McKevitt M, Running K, Counts GW, Turck M, Stamm WE (1985) Management of recurrent urinary tract infections with patient-administered single-dose therapy. *Ann Intern Med* 102: 302–307
81 Biering-Sorensen F, Hoiby N, Nordenbo A, Ravnborg M, Bruun B, Rahm V (1994) Ciprofloxacin as prophylaxis for urinary tract infection: prospective, randomized, cross-over, placebo controlled study in patients with spinal cord lesion. *J Urology* 151: 105–108
82 van der Wall E (1992) Prophylactic ciprofloxacin for catheter-associated urinary-tract infection. *Lancet* 339: 946–951
83 Sheehan GJ, Harding GKM, Haase DA et al (1988) Double-blind randomized comparison of 24 weeks of norfloxacin and 12 weeks of norfloxacin followed by 12 weeks of placebo in the therapy of complicated urinary tract infection. *Antimicrob Agents Chemother* 32: 1292–1293
84 Cardenas DD, Hooton TM (1995) Urinary tract infection in persons with spinal cord injury. *Arch Phys Med Rehabil* 76: 272–280
85 Warren JW (1997) Catheter-associated urinary tract infections. *Infect Dis Clin North Am* 11: 609–622
86 Warren J, Bakke A, Desgranchamps F et al (2001) Catheter-associated bacteriuria and the role of biomaterial in prevention. *In*: KG Naber, JC Pechere, J Kumazawa, S Khoury, JL Gerberding, AJ Schaeffer (eds): *Nosocomial and health care associated infections in urology*. Health Publication Ltd., Plymouth, UK, 151–176
87 Bloch R (2000) Review: antimicrobial prophylaxis reduces asymptomatic bacteriuria in patients with neurogenic bladder. *ACP J Club* 4: 21
88 Lightner DJ (1998) Contemporary urologic management of patients with spinal cord injury. *Mayo Clin Proc* 73: 434–438
89 Janoff DM, Skarecky DW, McLaren CE, Ahlering TE (2000) Prostate needle biopsy infection after four or six dose ciprofloxacin. *Can J Urol* 7: 1066–1069
90 Christiano AP, Hollowell CM, Kim H et al (2000) Double-blind randomized comparison of single-dose ciprofloxacin *versus* intravenous cefazolin in patients undergoing outpatient endourologic surgery. *Urol* 55: 182–185
91 Shandera KC, Thibault GP, Deshon GEJ (1998) Efficacy of one dose fluoroquinolone before

prostate biopsy. *Urol* 52: 641–643
92 Isen K, Kupeli B, Sinik Z, Sozen S, Bozkirli I (1999) Antibiotic prophylaxis for transrectal biopsy of the prostate: a prospective randomized study of the prophylactic use of single dose oral fluoroquinolone *versus* trimethoprim-sulfamethoxazole. *Int Urol Nephrol* 31: 491–495
93 Aron M, Rajeev TP, Gupta NP (2000) Antibiotic prophylaxis for transrectal needle biopsy of the prostate: a randomized controlled study. *BJU International* 85: 682–685
94 Klimberg IW, Malek GH, Cox CE et al (1999) Single-dose oral ciprofloxacin compared with cefotaxime and placebo for prophylaxis during transurethral surgery. *J Antimicrob Chemother* 43 (suppl A): 77–84
95 Tsugawa M, Monden K, Nasu Y, Kumon H, Ohmori H (1998) Prospective randomized comparative study of antibiotic prophylaxis in urethrocystoscopy and urethrocystography. *Int J Urol* 5: 441–443
96 Sahm DF, Critchley IA, Kelly LJ et al (2001) Evaluation of current activities of fluoroquinolones against Gram-negative bacilli using centralized *in vitro* testing and electronic surveillance. *Antimicrob Agents Chemother* 45: 267–274
97 Gales AC, Jones RN, Gordon KA et al (2000) Activity, spectrum of 22 antimicrobial agents tested against urinary tract infection pathogens in hospitalized patients in Latin America: report from the second year of the SENTRYAntimicrobial Surveillance Program (1998) *J Antimicrob Chemother* 45: 295–303
98 Garau J, Xercavins M, Rodriguez-Carballeira M et al (1999) Emergence and dissemination of quinolone-resistant *Escherichia coli* in the community. *Antimicrob Agents Chemother* 43: 2736–2741
99 Perez-Trallero E, Urbeita M, Jimenez D, Garcia-Arenzana JM, Cilla G (1993) Ten-year survey of quinolone resistance in *Escherichia coli* causing urinary tract infections. *Eur J Clin Microbiol Infect Dis* 12: 349–351
100 Mirelis B, Miro E, Navarro F, Ogalla CA, Bonal J, Prats G (1993) Increased resistance to quinolones in Catalonia, Spain. *Diagn Microbiol Infect Dis* 16: 137–139
101 Cheong H-J, Yoo C-W, Sohn J-W, Kim W-J, Kim M-J, Park S-C (2001) Bacteremia due to quinolone-resistant *Escherichia coli* in a teaching hospital in South Korea. *Clin Infect Dis* 33: 48–53
102 van Belkum A, Glessens W, van der Schee C et al (2001) Rapid emergence of ciprofloxacin-resistant enterobacteriaceae containing multiple gentamicin resistance-associated integrons in a Dutch hospital. *Emerg Infect Dis* 7: 862–871
103 Hsueh P-R, Liu C-Y, Luh K-T (2002) Current status of antimicrobial resistance in Taiwan. *Emerg Infect Dis* 8: 132–137
104 Gales A, KAG, Wilke W, Pfaller M, Jones R (2000) Occurrence of single-point *gyrA* mutations among ciprofloxacin-susceptible *Escherichia coli* isolates causing urinary tract infections in Latin America. *Diagn Microbiol Infect Dis* 36
105 Sannes MR, San Roman M, Moya T et al (2003) Antimicrobial resistance among *Escherichia coli* causing urinary tract infections in Costa Rica: a clinical dilemma. *Int J Antimicrob Agents* 21: 79–82
106 Bartlett JG, Breiman RF, Mandell LA, File TM (1998) Community-acquired pneumonia in adults: guidelines for management. *Clin Infect Dis* 26: 811–838
107 Mandell LA, Marrie TJ, Grossman RF, Chow AW, Hyland RH (2000) The Canadian Community-Acquired Pneumonia Working Group. Canadian guidelines for the initial management of community-acquired pneumonia: an evidence-based update by the Canadian Infectious Diseases Society and the Canadian Thoracic Society. *Clin Infect Dis* 31: 383–421
108 (2001) Drugs and vaccines against biological weapons. *Med Lett Drugs Ther* 43: 87–89
109 Burke JP (1998) Antibiotic resistance – squeezing the balloon? *JAMA* 280: 1270–1271

Fluoroquinolone Antibiotics
ed. by A.R. Ronald and D.E. Low

The quinolones and sexually transmitted infections

Sarah A. Wyllie and Geoffrey L. Ridgway

Department of Clinical Microbiology, University College London Hospitals, London WC1E 6DB, England

Introduction

Chlamydia trachomatis serovars D-K and *Neisseria gonorrhoeae* are the major sexually transmitted bacteria worldwide. Genital mycoplasmas, in particular *Mycoplasma genitalium*, are thought to be important causes of sexually transmitted non-gonococcal, non-chlamydial urethritis and cervicitis, more commonly termed, non-specific genital infection (NSGI). In tropical countries sexually transmitted infections also include lymphogranuloma venereum caused by *Chlamydia trachomatis* serovars L1, L2 and L3, chancroid caused by *Haemophilus ducreyi* and granuloma inguinale caused by *Calymmatobacterium granulomatis*. Epididymo-orchitis in men and pelvic inflammatory disease in women are caused either by sexually transmitted bacteria or by ascending infection with normal rectal and genital flora as a result of sexual activity. The quinolones play an important role in the management of all the above sexually transmitted infections. Syphilis is the only bacterial sexually transmitted disease against which the fluoroquinolones to date have no useful activity.

Sexually transmitted infections are often polymicrobial. Between 20–60% of patients infected with gonorrhoea are concomitantly infected with *C. trachomatis* [1]. Antimicrobial chemotherapy must therefore be directed against *N. gonorrhoeae*, *C. trachomatis* and other genital pathogens as indicated from the presenting features. Quinolones have revolutionized the management of many sexually transmitted infections, particularly uncomplicated gonorrhoea. However their global clinical usefulness is being limited by increasing antimicrobial resistance.

Gonorrhoea

The incidence of gonorrhoea varies dramatically around the world with the highest incidence (between 5 and 10%) in the developing countries [2]. The incidence of gonorrhoea in the United States and Europe peaked in the mid 1970s and then declined dramatically reaching a nadir in the mid 1990s [3].

Over the past 5 years there has been a small resurgence with a rising trend in the diagnosis of many acute sexually transmitted diseases [4]. Accurate and timely diagnosis with appropriate successful treatment and effective surveillance programmes are necessary to control both the rising incidence of sexually transmitted infections and the increasing incidence of antimicrobial resistance. Empirical antimicrobial therapy is directed by local patterns of antimicrobial sensitivity. The aims of treatment are to eliminate infection in uncomplicated disease with a single antibiotic dose in at least 95% of those presenting in the local community [5]. In response to the increasing frequency of penicillin-, tetracycline-, and spectinomycin-resistant strains of *N. gonorrhoeae,* broad spectrum cephalosporins or fluoroquinolones were recommended for the primary treatment of uncomplicated gonorrhoea in 1989 [6]. Studies in the 1980s demonstrated that a single oral dose of fluoroquinolone is as effective as a single oral dose of amoxicillin-probenecid [7, 8] or as a single intra-muscular dose of ceftriaxone [9] for the treatment of uncomplicated gonococcal infection. In the study by Black et al. [7], a single 400 mg dose of ofloxacin orally was compared with a single 3 g dose of amoxicillin plus 1 g of probenecid. The cure rate for men treated with ofloxacin was 98% (47 of 48) and the cure rate for women was 100% (52 of 52). All 13 patients with positive rectal cultures and seven of eight with positive pharyngeal cultures were cured. In the study by Hook et al. [9] a single 250 mg dose of ciprofloxacin orally had a 100% cure rate including successful treatment of five cases of pharyngeal infection and 20 cases of rectal gonococcal infection. There is no significant difference in efficacy between single doses of 250 mg or 500 mg of ciprofloxacin [10]. In a worldwide review of 1180 patients with uncomplicated gonococcal urethritis who were given a single dose (between 100 mg and 2000 mg) of ciprofloxacin no dose response was detected [11]. The most common dose of ciprofloxacin used worldwide was 250 mg [11]. The current guidelines for treatment of sexually transmitted diseases produced in the United States [12], the United Kingdom [13], and in Europe [14] all recommend quinolones, either ciprofloxacin 500 mg orally or ofloxacin 400 mg orally as single-dose treatment of gonococcal infection of the urethra, cervix, rectum or pharynx as an alternative to ceftriaxone, spectinomycin, or amoxicillin-probenecid. A dose of 500 mg rather than 250 mg is recommended in an attempt to lessen the emergence of resistance and to treat effectively infection with *N. gonorrhoeae* with reduced susceptibility to ciprofloxacin. When infection has been acquired in South-East Asia, quinolone-resistance is anticipated and alternative therapy with ceftriaxone or spectinomycin is recommended [14].

Ciprofloxacin 500 mg intravenously every 12 h or ofloxacin 400 mg intravenously every 12 h are alternative recommendations to intravenous cephalosporin or intramuscular spectinomycin for the initial management of disseminated gonococcal infection [12–14]. Once symptoms have improved, therapy for disseminated gonococcal infection may be switched to ciprofloxacin 500 mg orally twice daily, ofloxacin 400 mg orally twice daily or cefixime 400 mg orally twice daily for a total treatment course of 7 days.

Clinical studies of the newer fluoroquinolones have shown sparfloxacin 200 mg orally to be as effective as ciprofloxacin 250 mg orally (99% *versus* 98% efficacy) in the treatment of acute gonococcal urethritis in men [15]. In this study, three of the four patients, from a total study population of 238, who were culture-positive for gonococci at follow-up admitted to having had unprotected sexual intercourse after treatment. Grepafloxacin 400 mg orally has been shown to be as effective as cefixime 400 mg orally (99% *versus* 100% efficacy) in the treatment of uncomplicated gonorrhoea in men [16]. Trovafloxacin 100 mg orally was equivalent in efficacy to ofloxacin 400 mg orally (99% *versus* 100% efficacy) for uncomplicated gonococcal urethritis (270 patients) and uncomplicated gonococcal cervicitis (355 patients) [17]. Recent *in vitro* testing of a new fluoroquinolone, gemifloxacin, against ciprofloxacin-resistant strains of *N. gonorrhoeae* found the MIC_{90} to be 0.12 mg/L [18]. This compared favourably with moxifloxacin and grepafloxacin (MIC_{90} 0.5 mg/L) and trovafloxacin (MIC_{90} 0.25 mg/L). However the vast majority (43 of 50) of the ciprofloxacin-resistant strains tested only had low level resistance to ciprofloxacin (MIC 0.12–0.25 mg/L) and as such would probably respond *in vivo* to a single oral 500 mg dose of ciprofloxacin. There does not appear to be any treatment advantage of these newer agents. The older fluoroquinolones, ciprofloxacin and ofloxacin, are still favoured because they have a better safety profile. Many new fluoroquinolones including clinafloxacin, gemifloxacin, grepafloxacin, sparfloxacin and trovafloxacin have been withdrawn from clinical use as a result of adverse toxicity. The *in vitro* activity of various quinolones against *N. gonorrhoeae* is shown in Table 1.

The National Committee for Clinical Laboratory Standards (NCCLS) in the United States defines *N. gonorrhoeae* as fluoroquinolone resistant if the MIC is $\geq$ 1.0 mg/L for ciprofloxacin or $\geq$ 2.0 mg/L for ofloxacin [20]. In addition, reduced susceptibility may be defined as MIC > 0.06 mg/L for ciprofloxacin

Table 1. Activity of various fluoroquinolones against *Neisseria gonorrhoeae* [18, 19]

Antibiotic	MIC_{90} (mg/L)
Clinafoxacin	0.002
Grepafloxacin	0.004
Ciprofloxacin	0.008
Gemifloxacin	0.008
Levofloxacin	0.008
Sitafloxacin	0.008
Gatifloxacin	0.015
Trovafloxacin	0.015
Ofloxacin	0.015
Moxifloxacin	0.03
Sparfloxacin	0.03

or >0.0125 mg/L for ofloxacin. These criteria are based on theoretical predictions of the MICs at which infection with *N. gonorrhoeae* may fail to respond to CDC-recommended doses of fluoroquinolones. The criteria have been further defined by comparison of antibiotic disc diffusion testing with agar dilution MIC testing [21]. Since different methods of antibiotic susceptibility testing are used in different countries and even in different areas within the same country, local susceptibility criteria need to be defined in comparison with control reference strains of known susceptibility [22].

Gonococci acquire resistance through mutations in the quinolone resistance-determining region (QRDR) of *gyrA* and *parC* [23]. Single *gyrA* mutations are associated with reduced susceptibility to ciprofloxacin (MIC 0.12 to 1 mg/L), whereas multiple mutations within *gyrA* and co-existing mutations of *parC* are associated with resistance (MIC > 1 mg/L) [24]. Ciprofloxacin and ofloxacin resistant strains also show reduced sensitivity to other newer quinolones including grepafloxacin, moxifloxacin, sitafloxacin, trovafloxacin and clinafloxacin [18, 25].

Treatment failures using single dose fluoroquinolone have been reported over the last decade from around the world including the United Kingdom [26], Australia [27], Canada [28], Singapore [29], the United States [30] and Southeast Asia [31]. Sensitivity testing of these isolates support the NCCLS definitions of resistance. However *in vitro* ciprofloxacin resistance does not always equate to treatment failure. In the study by Ng et al. [29], of 694 patients treated for *N gonorrhoeae*, 17 cases had ciprofloxacin resistant infection. Twelve of these 17 patients were treated with ciprofloxacin and four patients were cured despite evidence of *in vitro* resistance. In the study by Ivens et al. [32], 10% (28 of 292) of the gonococcal isolates from a London sexually transmitted infection clinic exhibited reduced susceptibility to ciprofloxacin. Of 20 patients who reattended for test of cure, none had failed treatment. All patients were however treated for co-existent chlamydial infection with doxycycline, which would have had an antimicrobial effect against all but one of the isolates. The highest levels of quinolone resistance are seen in the Far East where 72.6% of isolates of *N. gonorrhoeae* were found to be fluoroquinolone resistant in 1997 [33]. In the Philippines, high level ciprofloxacin resistance (MIC ≥ 4.0 mg/L) increased from 9% in 1994 to 49% by 1997 [31]. In this study, treatment failure was seen in a third (32.3%) of patients given ciprofloxacin *versus* only 3.8% of patients given cefixime. In Hong Kong treatment failure occurred in nearly a third (27.9%) of patients who were treated for gonorrhoea with a single 600 mg oral dose of ofloxacin [34]. In Hawaii there has been a dramatic increase in the number of ciprofloxacin resistant isolates of *N. gonorrhoeae* from 1.4% (4 of 290) in 1997 to 9.5% (22 of 231) in 1999 [35]. These isolates were characterized phenotypically by auxotype and serovar (A/S) class, genetically by identifying mutations within the quinolone resistance-determining regions (QRDRs) of *gyrA* and *parC* and also by plasmid profile analysis. In 1999, three-quarters (78.6%) of all the ciprofloxacin resistant isolates from Hawaii belonged to two strain phenotypes suggesting either endemic spread of a few strains, or that there is less strain variation of the imported isolates [35]. In Sydney, Australia, since 1984 when the first strain with reduced sensitivity to ciprofloxacin was isolated (MIC 0.25 mg/L), the percentage of resistant strains has risen to 3.1% of all isolates in 1997 [36]. Phenotypic characterization of these resistant isolates identified an outbreak associated with international commercial sex workers [36]. In Ohio, USA, the prevalence of gonococci with decreased susceptibility to ciprofloxacin rose from 2% in 1991 to 16% in 1994 [31]. These isolates had an MIC to ciprofloxacin of between 0.12 mg/L and 0.25 mg/L. No isolate was found to exhibit true resistance as defined by the NCCLS [21]. The evolution of antimicrobial resistance in *N. gonorrhoeae* in Durban, South Africa, over a 5-year period from 1995 to 2000 has been recently reported [37]. In South Africa, syndromic management of sexually transmitted infections was introduced in 1995, with recommendation to treat the "discharge syndrome" with ciprofloxacin 250 mg orally as a single dose plus doxycycline 200 mg orally once daily for 7 days and supplemented with metronidazole 2 g orally as a single dose in the non-pregnant female. In 1995, all gonococcal isolates were fully susceptible to both ciprofloxacin and ofloxacin. By 1999/2000, only 71% of isolates were fully susceptible to ciprofloxacin, with the remaining 29% exhibiting reduced susceptibility (MIC 0.015–0.06 mg/L). By 1999/2000, no strains were fully susceptible to ofloxacin and some had been found to be resistant (MIC ≥ 2.0 mg/L). Over the 5-year period a dramatic increase was seen in the number of isolates of *N. gonorrhoeae* exhibiting high-level resistance to tetracycline, from 3% in 1997 to 51% in 1998/9 [37]. This may be related to syndromic management recommendations meaning that gonococci are being exposed to tetracyclines and quinolones simultaneously. Since decreasing susceptibility was also identified with penicillin, azithromycin, erythromycin, ceftriaxone and spectinomycin, the emerging resistance may also be caused by selective pressure from widespread use in the community of all these antimicrobials.

Routine surveillance of gonococcal resistance to antimicrobials is critical to ensure effectiveness of treatment and prevention of spread of disease. Active surveillance is currently being carried out by the World Health Organisation in the Western Pacific region [38], by the Centers for Disease Control (CDC) in the United States, by the Communicable Disease Surveillance Center (CDSC) in England and Wales [39] and in many other countries around the world.

Chlamydia trachomatis and non-specific genital infection (NSGI)

Chlamydia trachomatis is the commonest cause of non-gonococcal urethritis (NGU) accounting for 30–50% of cases [13]. *Mycoplasma genitalium* is also strongly, and independently of *C. trachomatis,* associated with acute NGU [40]. The precise role of the other genital mycoplasmas (*Ureaplasma urealyticum* and *Mycoplasma hominis*) and anaerobes in the pathogenesis of NGU and NSGI remains uncertain [41, 42]. A causative organism is not identified in 20 to 30% of men with NGU. *In vitro* susceptibility testing techniques for chlamydia and mycoplasmas are not standardised, however the newer fluoroquinolones are considerably more active than ciprofloxacin. The activity of various quinolones against *C. trachomatis, M. hominis* and *U. urealyticum* is listed in Table 2. There is limited data on the activity of fluoroquinolones against *M. genitalium.* In one study the activity of sparfloxacin and moxifloxacin against *M. genitalium* was similar to that against *M. hominis* [44]. Clinical studies with ofloxacin administered orally have demonstrated high eradication rates with a dose of 200 mg twice daily or 400 mg once daily for 7 days [1]. An American study reported that ofloxacin 300 mg orally twice daily for 7 days had a greater than 95% bacteriological cure rate against chlamydial cervicitis [45]. In the United States, ofloxacin 300 mg orally twice daily for 7 days is recommended as an alternative to azithromycin or doxycycline for the treatment of uncomplicated chlamydial infection of the cervix, urethra, or rectum [12]. In the United Kingdom and Europe, ofloxacin 200 mg orally twice daily or 400 mg orally once daily for 7 days is a recommended treatment of *C. trachomatis* genital tract infection [13, 46]. Ofloxacin treatment is appropriate for concurrent gonococcal and chlamydial infections when given as a treatment course over 7 days. A single dose of ofloxacin is effective in treating quinolone-sensitive gonococcal infection but it is not adequate for treatment of chlamydial infection [47]. Ciprofloxacin is unreliable in the treatment of NSGI and should not be used for this purpose [48]. Of the newer fluoroquinolones, sparfloxacin 200 mg orally on day 1 followed by 100 mg daily for 6 additional days has been reported to be successful in the treatment of NGU in men [49], as has grepafloxacin 400 mg/day orally for 7 days [50]. Trovafloxacin 200 mg orally once daily for 5 days was equivalent in efficacy to doxycycline 100 mg orally twice daily for 7 days in women with uncom-

Table 2. Activity of various fluoroquinolones against *Chlamydia trachomatis*, *Mycoplasma hominis* and *Ureaplasma urealyticum* [20, 43]

Antibiotic	MIC_{90} (mg/L) *C. trachomatis*	MIC range (mg/L) *M. hominis*	*U. urealyticum*
Sitafloxacin	0.06	0.06 (MIC_{90})	0.12 (MIC_{90})
Grepafloxacin	0.06	0.015–0.06	0.12–1.0
Moxifloxacin	0.06	0.06 (MIC_{90})	0.12 (MIC_{90})
Trovafloxacin	0.06	0.015–0.03	0.12–0.5
Sparfloxacin	0.06	0.008–0.015	0.06–0.5
Clinafloxacin	0.06	0.015–0.06	0.06–2.0
Gatifloxacin	0.12	N/A	N/A
Levofloxacin	0.5	N/A	N/A
Ofloxacin	1.0	0.25–1.0	1.0–4.0
Ciprofloxacin	2.0	0.25–0.5	0.25–1.0

Key: N/A = not available

plicated cervicitis [51]. In this study, trovafloxacin was not as effective as doxycycline for the treatment of uncomplicated chlamydial urethritis in men. Sparfloxacin, grepafloxacin and trovafloxacin have all since been withdrawn from clinical use.

Quinolone resistance has been demonstrated in a laboratory-manipulated L2 strain of *C. trachomatis* [52]. Two mutant strains were isolated on subculture in subinhibitory concentrations of ofloxacin and sparfloxacin. These isolates showed cross-resistance against ciprofloxacin and pefloxacin and reduced susceptibility to norfloxacin. The resistance is characterised by a point mutation in *gyrA* resulting in the substitution of isoleucine for serine at codon 83. Serial passage of *C. trachomatis* isolates in sub-inhibitory concentrations of ciprofloxacin and ofloxacin have resulted in quinolone resistance with a final MIC greater than 256 times that of the original wild-type strain [53]. These mutant isolates again show the same point mutation in *gyrA*. The clinical significance of these *in vitro* findings is becoming apparent as reports of clinical treatment failure of drug-resistant *C. trachomatis* appear in the literature [54]. These clinical isolates had an MIC_{90} to ofloxacin of 2 and >4 mg/L as compared with an MIC_{90} of 0.5 mg/L for the control strain. In a study of 45 clinical isolates of *C. trachomatis*, Rice et al. [55] found that isolates with higher MICs belonged predominantly to serovar Ia which was more commonly associated with severe symptomatic chlamydial infection (pelvic inflammatory disease or mucopurulent cervicitis) compared with asymptomatic infection. Whether antibiotic resistance correlates to pathogenicity in chlamydial infection remains to be seen. Resistance to macrolides and tetracyclines has not been found to be associated with resistance to ciprofloxacin, ofloxacin or trovafloxacin [56].

Syphilis

There are, as yet, no reports of clinically useful activity of quinolones against *Treponema pallidum*.

Lymphogranuloma venereum

Lymphogranuloma venereum is caused by *Chlamydia trachomatis* serovars L1, L2 and L3. Quinolones are not used routinely to treat this uncommon disease [57].

Chancroid

Chancroid caused by *Haemophilus ducreyi* is a common cause of genital ulceration in many tropical areas including Africa, the Carribean and South West Asia. *Haemophilus ducreyi,* including beta-lactamase-producing and tetracy-

Table 3. Activity of the fluoroquinolones against *Haemophilus ducreyi* [59]

Antibiotic	MIC_{90} (mg/L)
Clinafoxacin	0.001
Sparfloxacin	<0.03
Ciprofloxacin	0.02
Ofloxacin	0.03
Fleroxacin	0.06

cline-resistant organisms, are highly susceptible to most fluoroquinolones [58]. Table 3 lists the activity of various quinolones against *Haemophilus ducreyi.* Ciprofloxacin 500 mg orally twice daily for 3 days is highly effective and is recommended as an alternative to a macrolide in the current American and European guidelines for the management of tropical genito-ulcerative disease [12, 60]. A single 500 mg oral dose of ciprofloxacin was compared with 500 mg of erythromycin given orally every 8 h for 7 days for the treatment of tropical genital ulceration in Kenya [61]. Of the patients enrolled who had culture- and/or PCR-confirmed infection with *H. ducreyi,* four out of 60 failed to respond to ciprofloxacin, and four out of 51 failed to respond to erythromycin. Treatment failures were associated with ulcers caused by *Herpes simplex* virus and *Treponema pallidum.* In India, 500 mg of ciprofloxacin given orally for 3 days cured genital ulceration caused by *H. ducreyi* in 15 patients, with clinical improvement observed in a further patient [62]. There were no treatment failures. Of the other fluoroquinolones, a single 400 mg dose orally of fleroxacin has been shown to be effective for the treatment of chancroid in Kenya [63]. In this study, culture proven failure occurred in only 1 of 36 patients treated with fleroxacin *versus* 11 of 37 patients treated for 3 days with oral trimethoprim-sulphamethoxazole (60/800 mg).

Donovanosis (granuloma inguinale)

Donovanosis is a chronic genital ulcerative diseases caused by *Calymmatobacterium granulomatis* seen predominantly in tropical countries. Few treatment studies have been conducted. Treatment recommendations include norfloxacin 400 mg orally twice daily or ciprofloxacin 500 mg orally twice daily until ulceration is healed [13, 64]. The CDC recommends ciprofloxacin 750 mg orally twice daily for a minimum of 3 weeks [12].

Epididymo-orchitis

In men younger than 35 years old, epididymo-orchitis is commonly caused by sexually transmitted bacteria, predominantly *Neisseria gonorrhoeae* and

Chlamydia trachomatis [6]. Current CDC guidelines recommend ofloxacin 300 mg orally twice daily for 10 days for the treatment of epididymitis [12]. In Europe and the UK, ofloxacin 200 mg orally twice daily for 14 days is recommended as an alternative to doxycycline [13, 65].

Pelvic inflammatory disease

Pelvic inflammatory disease (PID) refers to the clinical syndrome that results when infection ascends from the endocervix. Endometritis, salpingitis, pelvic peritonitis, or tubo-ovarian abcess may result. *Chlamydia trachomatis* and *Neisseria gonorrhoeae* have been identified as major causative agents [66]. Antimicrobial therapy must eradicate these organisms as well as enterobacteriaceae and possibly anaerobes. As noted above, the role of *M. hominis* remains uncertain. Ofloxacin 400 mg orally twice daily for 10 days was as effective as cefoxitin 2 g intravenously once daily plus doxycycline 100 mg twice daily for 10 days in an outpatient randomised comparative study in 249 women [67]. *N. gonorrhoeae* was found in 16% of patients and *C. trachomatis* in 12%, all of whom were treated effectively with ofloxacin [67]. Ciprofloxacin 250 mg orally twice daily plus clindamycin 300 mg orally three times daily for 14 days was comparable in efficacy to ceftriaxone plus doxycycline (97% *versus* 95% clinical cure rate) in a study from South America [68]. In this study, the most prevalent isolates were streptococci, staphylococci, *Escherichia coli*, and anaerobes. *N. gonorrhoeae* was isolated from only 2% of patients (3 of 131) and *C. trachomatis* was isolated from 11% (15 of 131). The addition of clindamycin to ciprofloxacin gives better streptococcal, staphylococcal and anaerobic cover, but will not reliably eradicate *C. trachomatis*. The importance of anaerobes in the pathogenesis of PID remains uncertain. Concern that tissue damage may continue when anaerobes are sub-optimally treated has prompted the CDC and others to recommend therapeutic regimens for PID which include comprehensive anaerobic cover [69]. American, British and European guidelines all recommend oral ofloxacin 400 mg twice daily plus oral metronidazole 500 mg twice daily for 14 days for outpatient management of pelvic inflammatory disease [12, 13, 70]. For patients with more severe clinical disease, ofloxacin 400 mg intravenously twice daily plus metronidazole 500 mg intravenously three times daily for 14 days, or ciprofloxacin 200 mg intravenously twice daily plus doxycycline 100 mg intravenously or orally twice daily plus metronidazole 500 mg intravenously three times daily for 14 days, are alternative treatment regimens which include a quinolone [12, 13, 70]. Once clinical improvement has been established, the 2-week antimicrobial therapy course may be completed using the equivalent oral preparations.

Quinolones and sexually transmitted infections in pregnancy and paediatrics

Fluoroquinolones are contra-indicated in pregnancy. Their use in paediatrics has been limited because of fear of arthropathy. Ciprofloxacin has been used successfully in children with cystic fibrosis to treat *Pseudomonas aeroginosa* infection [71], and in children with typhoid fever [72], with no adverse effects on growth or joint symptomatology. As yet recommendations for the treatment of gonococcal and chlamydial infection in children do not include the fluoroquinolones.

Conclusion

Quinolones play an important role in the management of sexually transmitted infection in adults. Table 4 summarises the use of quinolones for the treatment of gonorrhoea, non-gonococcal genital infection, chancroid, donovanosis, epididymo-orchitis and pelvic inflammatory disease as recommended in the current American, European and British guidelines [12–14, 45, 56, 59, 64, 69].

Increasing resistance of *N. gonorrhoeae* to quinolones is limiting their clinical effectiveness on a global scale. The highest levels of quinolone-resistant *N. gonorrhoeae* isolates are found in Southeast Asia [29, 31, 33]. Current recommendations are that gonococcal infection acquired in Southeast Asia should be treated with ceftriaxone or spectinomycin, and not with a quinolone [12–14]. Accurate and effective surveillance programmes need to be continued worldwide in order to monitor the incidence and the antimicrobial resistance of gonococcal isolates. The CDC will continue to recommend the use of fluoroquinolones for the treatment of gonococcal infection as long as quinolone-resistant strains comprise <1% of all *N. gonorrhoeae* strains isolated through surveillance [12]. As demonstrated by Tapsall et al. [36], phenotyping is a useful and important tool in the understanding and management of an outbreak and should compliment surveillance.

Quinolone-, doxycycline-, and macrolide-resistant isolates of *C. trachomatis* have been reported [54]. Quinolone-resistant strains of *C. trachomatis* have also been developed in the laboratory by sub-culturing the organism in sub-inhibitory concentrations of quinolones [52, 53]. The importance of these findings remains to be seen and may foretell an emerging infectious disease problem.

Finally, quinolones play an important role in the management of epididymo-orchitis in men and pelvic inflammatory disease in women [12, 13, 65, 70].

Table 4. Summary of the recommended use of quinolones in the treatment of sexually transmitted infections [12–14, 46, 60, 65, 70]

Uncomplicated gonorrhoea

One of the following:

i) Ciprofloxacin 500 mg orally as a single dose

ii) Ofloxacin 400 mg orally as a single dose

Disseminated gonorrhoea

One of the following:

i) Ciprofloxacin 500 mg intravenously every 12 h until symptoms have improved and continuing with ciprofloxacin 500 mg orally every 12 h to complete a treatment course of 7 days

ii) Ofloxacin 400 mg intravenously every 12 h until symptoms have improved and continuing with ofloxacin 400 mg orally twice daily to complete a treatment course of 7 days.

Non-gonococcal genital infection

One of the following:

i) Ofloxacin 300 mg orally twice daily for 7 days

ii) Ofloxacin 200 mg orally twice daily for 7 days

iii) Ofloxacin 400 mg orally once daily for 7 days.

If a single dose of ofloxacin 400 mg orally or a single dose of ciprofloxacin 500 mg orally is given then further treatment with a macrolide or doxycycline is required.

Chancroid

Ciprofloxacin 500 mg orally twice daily for 3 days.

Donovanosis

One of the following:

i) Ciprofloxacin 500 mg orally twice daily until ulceration is healed

ii) Ciprofloxacin 750 mg orally twice daily until ulceration is healed

iii) Norfloxacin 400 mg orally twice daily until ulceration is healed

Epididymo-orchitis

One of the following:

i) Ofloxacin 300 mg orally twice daily for 10 days

ii) Ofloxacin 200 mg orally twice daily for 14 days

Pelvic inflammatory disease

For outpatient management:

Ofloxacin 400 mg orally twice daily plus metronidazole 500 mg orally twice daily for 14 days.

For inpatient management, one of the following:

i) Ofloxacin 400 mg intravenously twice daily plus metronidazole 500 mg intravenously three times daily until symptoms have improved, and continuing with ofloxacin 400 mg orally twice daily and metronidazole 500 mg orally twice daily to complete a treatment course of 14 days.

ii) Ciprofloxacin 200 mg intravenously twice daily plus doxycycline 100 mg intravenously or orally twice daily plus metronidazole 500 mg intravenously three times daily until symptoms have improved, and continuing with ciprofloxacin 250 mg orally twice daily plus doxycycline 100 mg orally twice daily plus metronidazole 500 mg orally twice daily to complete a treatment course of 14 days.

References

1 Robinson AJ, Ridgway GL (2000) Concurrent gonococcal and chlamydial infection. How best to treat. *Drugs* 59: 801–813
2 Brunham RC, Embree JE (1992) Sexually transmitted diseases: Current and future dimensions of the problem in the third world. *In*: A Germain, KK Holmes, P Piot et al (eds): *Reproductive tract infections: Global impact and priorities for women's reproductive health*. Plenum, New York, 35–58
3 Division of STD/HIVPrevention (1996) Sexually Transmitted Disease Surveillance, 1995. U.S. Department of Health and Human Services, Public Health Service. Atlanta: Centers for Disease Control and Prevention
4 Diagnoses of gonorrhoea reach ten year high. *Commun Dis Rep CDR Wkly* 2001: 11
5 Fitzgerald M, Bedford C (1996) National Standards for the management of gonorrhoea. *Int J STD AIDS* 7: 298–300
6 Centers for Disease Control Prevention (1989) Sexually transmitted diseases treatment guidelines. *MMWR Morb Mortal Wkly Rep* 38: 58
7 Black JR, Long JM, Zwickl BE, Ray BS, Verdan MS, Wetherby S, Hook EWIII, Handsfield HH (1989) Multicenter randomised study of single dose ofloxacin *versus* amoxicillin-probenecid for the treatment of uncomplicated gonococcal infection. *Antimicrob Agents Chemother* 33: 167–170
8 Lassus A, Renkonen OV, Ellmen J (1988) Fleroxacin *versus* standard therapy in gonococcal urethritis. *J Antimicrob Chemother* 22 (Suppl. D): 223–225
9 Hook EWIII, Jones RB, Martin DH, Bolan GA, Mroczkowski TF, Neumann TM, Haag JJ, Echols R (1993) Comparison of ciprofloxacin and ceftriaxone as single-dose therapy for uncomplicated gonorrhoea in women. *Antimicrob Agents Chemother* 37: 1670–1673
10 Tegelberg-Stassen MJ, van der Hoek JC, Mooi L, Wagenvoort JH, van Joost T, Michel MF, Stolz E (1986) Treatment of uncomplicated gonococcal urethritis in men with two dosages of ciprofloxacin. *Eur J Clin Microbiol* 5: 244–246
11 Echols RM, Heyd A, O'Keefe BJ, Schacht P (1994) Single dose ciprofloxacin for the treatment of uncomplicated gonorrhoea: A worldwide summary. *Sex Transm Dis* 21: 345–352
12 Centers for Disease Control Prevention (1998) 1998 Guidelines for treatment of sexually transmitted diseases. *MMWR Morb Mortal Wkly Rep* 47: RR-1
13 UK National Guidelines on sexually transmitted infections (1994) *Sex Transm Infect* 75 (Suppl 1)
14 Bignell CJ (2001) European guideline for the management of gonorrhoea. *Int J STD AIDS* 12 (Suppl 3): 27–29
15 Moi H, Morel P, Gianotti B, Barlow D, Phillips I, Jean C (1996) Comparative efficacy of single oral doses of sparfloxacin *versus* ciprofloxacin in the treatment of acute gonococcal urethritis in men. *J Antimicrob Chemother* 37 (Suppl A): 115–122
16 Hook EWIII, McCormack WM, Martin D, Jones RB, Bean K, Mavoli AN (1997) Comparison of single dose oral grepafloxacin with cefixime for treatment of uncomplicated gonorrhoea in men. *Antimicrob Agents Chemother* 41: 1843–1845
17 Jones RB, Schwebke J, Thorpe EMJnr Dalu ZA, Leone P, Johnson RB (1998) Randomised trial of trovafloxacin and ofloxacin for single dose therapy of gonorrhoea. Trovafloxacin Study Group. *Am J Med* 104: 28–32
18 Jones RN, Deshpande LM, Erwin ME, Barrett MS, Beach ML (2000) Anti-gonococcal activity of gemifloxacin against fluoroquinolone-resistant strains and a comparison of agar dilution and Etest methods. *J Antimicrob Chemother* 45 (Suppl. S1): 67–70
19 Ridgway GL (1999) Quinolones in sexually transmitted diseases. *Drugs* 58 (Suppl. 2): 92–95
20 National Committee for Clinical Laboratory Standards (1998) Performance standards for antimicrobial susceptibility testing. M100-38. Wayne. PA: National Committee for Clinical Laboratory Standards
21 Kam KM, Wong PW, Cheung MM, Ho NKY (1996) Detection of quinolone-resistant *Neisseria gonorrhoeae. J Clin Micro* 34: 1462–1464
22 Knapp JS, Fox KK, Trees DL, Whittington WL (1997) Fluoroquinolone resistance in *Neisseria gonorrhoeae. Emerg Inf Dis* 3: 33–39
23 Tanaka M, Takahashi K, Saika T, Kobayashi I, Ueno T, Kumazawa J (1998) Development of fluoroquinolone resistance and mutations involving Gyr A and Par C proteins among *Neisseria gonorrhoeae* isolates in Japan. *J Urol* 159: 2215–2219
24 Schultz TR, Tapsall JW, White PA (2001) Correlation of *in vitro* susceptibilities to newer

quinolones of naturally occurring quinolone-resistant *Neisseria gonorrhoeae* strains with changes in GyrA and ParC. *Antimicrob Agents Chemother* 45: 734–738
25 Carlyn CJ, Doyle LJ, Knapp CC, Ludwig MD, Washington JA (1995) Activities of three investigational fluoroquinolones (BAY y 3118, DU 6859a, and clinafloxacin) against *Neisseria gonorrhoeae* with diminished susceptibilities to ciprofloxacin and ofloxacin. *Antimicrob Agents Chemother* 39: 1606–1608
26 Gransden WR, Warren CA, Phillips I, Hodges M, Barlow D (1990) Decreased susceptibility of *Neisseria gonorrhoeae* in the United Kingdom. *Lancet* 335: 51
27 Tapsall JW, Schultz TR, Lovett R, Munro R (1992) Failure of 500 mg ciprofloxacin therapy in male urethral gonorrhoea. *Med J Aust* 156: 143
28 Ringuette L, Trudeau T, Turcotte P, Yeung K, Remis R, Perron L, Le Corre I (1996) Emergence of *Neisseria gonorrhoeae* strains with decreased susceptibility to ciprofloxacin-Quebec, 1994–1995. *Can Commun Dis Rep* 22: 121–125
29 Ng PP, Chan RK, Ling AE (1998) Gonorrhoea treatment failure and ciprofloxacin resistance. *Int J STD AIDS* 9: 323–325
30 Gordon SM, Carlyn CJ, Doyle LJ, Knapp CC, Longworth DL, Hall GS, Washington JA (1996) The emergence of *Neisseria gonorrhoeae* with decreased susceptibility to ciprofloxacin in Cleveland, Ohio: epidemiology and risk factors. *Ann Intern Med* 125: 465–470
31 Aplasca de los Reyes MR, Pato-Mesola V, Klausner JD, Manalastas R, Wi T, Tuazon CU, Dellabetta G, Whittington WL, Holmes KK (2001) A randomised trial of ciprofloxacin *versus* cefixime for treatment of gonorrhoea after rapid emergence of gonococcal ciprofloxacin resistance in the Philippines. *Clin Infect Dis* 32: 1313–1318
32 Ivens D, Martin I, Ison C (2000) *Neisseria gonorrhoeae* in a London sexually transmitted infection clinic not fully sensitive to quinolones: are isolates imported and how effective is ciprofloxacin as a first-line therapy? *Int J STD and AIDS* 11: 774–776
33 Knapp JS (1998) *Neisseria gonorrhoeae* resistant to ciprofloxacin and ofloxacin. *Sex Transm Dis* 25: 425–426
34 Kam KM, Lo KK, Chong LY, Au WF, Wong PY, Cheung MM (1999) Correlation between *in vitro* quinolone susceptibility of *Neisseria gonorrhoeae* and outcome of treatment of gonococcal urethritis with single dose ofloxacin. *Clin Infect Dis* 28: 1165–1166
35 Trees DL, Sandul AL, Neal SW, Higa H, Knapp JS (2001) Molecular epidemiology of *Neisseria gonorrhoeae* exhibiting decreased susceptibility and resistance to ciprofloxacin in Hawaii, 1991–1999. *Sex Transm Dis* 28: 309–314
36 Tapsall JW, Limnios EA, Shultz TR (1998) Continuing evolution of the pattern of quinolone resistance in *Neisseria gonorrhoeae* isolated in Sydney, Australia. *Sex Transm Dis* 25: 415–417
37 Moodley P, Pillay C, Goga R, Kharsany ABM, Sturm AW (2001) Evolution in the trends of antimicrobial resistance in *Neisseria gonorrhoeae* isolated in Durban over a 5 year period: impact of the introduction of syndromic management. *J Antimicrob Chemother* 48: 853–859
38 Tapsall JW (2000) Surveillance of antibiotic resistance in *Neisseria gonorrhoeae* in the WHO Western Pacific Region, 1998. The WHO Western Pacific Gonococcal Antimicrobial Surveillance Programme. *Commun Dis Intell* 24: 1–4
39 GRASP steering group (2001) The Gonococcal Resistance to Antimicrobials Surveillance Programme (GRASP) year 2000 report. London: Public Health Laboratory service
40 Taylor-Robinson D, Horner PJ (2001) The role of *Mycoplasma genitalium* in non-gonococcal urethritis. *Sex Transm Inf* 77: 229–231
41 Bowie WR, Wang SP, Alexander ER, Floyd J, Forsyth PS, Pollock HM, Lin JS, Buchanan TM, Holmes KK (1977) Etiology of non-gonococcal urethritis. Evidence for *Chlamydia trachomatis* and *Ureaplasma urealyticum*. *J Clin Invest* 59: 735–742
42 Woolley PD (2000) Anaerobic bacteria and non-gonococcal urethritis. *Int J STD AIDS* 11: 347–348
43 Miyashita N, Niki Y, Matsushima T (2001) *In vitro* and *in vivo* activities of sitafloxacin against *Chlamydia* Spp *Antimicrob Agents Chemother* 45: 3270–3272
44 Bébéar CM, Renaudin H, Boudjadja A, Bébéar C (1998) *In vitro* activity of Bay 12-8039, a new fluoroquinolone against mycoplasmas. *Antimicrob Agents Chemother* 42: 703–704
45 Hooton TM, Batteiger BE, Judson FM, Spruance SL, Stamm WE (1992) Ofloxacin *versus* doxycycline for treatment of cervical infection with *Chlamydia trachomatis*. *Antimicrob Agents Chemother* 36: 1144–1146
46 Stary A (2001) European guideline for the management of chlamydial infection. *Int J STD and*

AIDS 12 (Suppl. 3): 30–33
47 Blomer R, Bruch K, Klose V (1988) Ofloxacin in the treatment of gonococcal and chlamydial urethritis. *Clin Ther* 10: 263–265
48 Dreses-Werringloer U, Padubrin I, Jurgens-Saathoff B, Hudson AP, Zeidler H, Kohler L (2000) Persistance of *Chlamydia trachomatis* is induced by ciprofloxacin and ofloxacin *in vitro*. *Antimicrob Agents Chemother* 44: 3288–3297
49 Phillips I, Dimian C, Barlow D, Moi H, Stolz E, Weidner W, Perea E (1996) A comparative study of two different regimens of sparfloxacin *versus* doxycycline in the treatment of non-gonococcal urethritis in men. *J Antimicrob Chemother* 37 (Suppl A): 123–134
50 McCormack WM, Martin DH, Hook EWIII, Jones RB (1998) Daily oral grepafloxacin *versus* twice daily oral doxycycline in the treatment of *Chlamydia trachomatis* endocervical infection. *Infect Dis Obstet Gynaecol* 6: 109–115
51 McCormack WM, Dalu ZA, Martin DH, Hook EWIII, Laisi R, Kell P, Pluck ND, Johnson RB (1999) Double-blind comparison of trovafloxacin and doxycycline in the treatment of uncomplicated chlamydial urethritis and cervicitis. *Sex Transm Dis* 26: 531–536
52 Dessus-Babus S, Bébéar C, Charron A, Bébéar CM, de Barbeyrac B (1998) Sequencing of gyrase and topoisomerase IV quinolone-resistance determining regions of *Chlamydia trachomatis* and characterisation of quinolone-resistant mutants obtained *in vitro*. *Antimicrob Agents Chemother* 42: 2474–2481
53 Morrissey I, Salman H, Bakker S, Farrell D, Bébéar CM, Ridgway GL (2002) Serial passage of *Chlamydia* spp in sub-inhibitory fluoroquinolone concentrations and assessment of resistance development. Submitted *J Antimicrob Chemother* 49: 757–761
54 Somani J, Bhullar VB, Workowski KA, Farshy CE, Black CM (2000) Multiple drug-resistant *Chlamydia trachomatis* associated with clinical treatment failure. *J Infect Dis* 181: 1421–1427
55 Rice RJ, Bhullar V, Mitchell SH, Bullard J, Knapp JS (1995) Susceptibilities of *Chlamydia trachomatis* isolates causing uncomplicated female genital tract infections and pelvic inflammatory disease. *Antimicrob Agents Chemother* 39: 760–762
56 Jones RB, Van der Pol B, Johnson RB (1997) Susceptibilities of *Chlamydia trachomatis* to trovafloxacin. *J Antimicrob Chemother* 39 (Suppl. B): 63–65
57 National Guidelines for the Management of Lymphogranuloma venereum: Clinical Effectiveness Group (Association of Genito-urinary medicine Physicians, the Medical Society for the Study of Venereal Disease) (1999) *Sex Transm Inf* 75 (Suppl. 1): 540–542
58 Wall RA, Mabey DCW, Bello CSS, Felmingham D (1985) The comparative *in vitro* activity of twelve 4-quinolone antimicrobials against *Haemophilus ducreyi*. *J Antimicrob Chemother* 16: 165–168
59 Ridgway GL (1995) Quinolones in sexually transmitted diseases: Global experience. *Drugs* 49 (Suppl. 2): 115–122
60 Roest RW, van der Meijden WI (2001) European guideline for the management of tropical genito-ulcerative diseases. *Int J STD and AIDS* 12 (Suppl.3): 78–83
61 Malonza IM, Tyndall MW, Ndinya-Achola JO, Maclean I, Omar S, MacDonald S, Perriens J, Orle K, Plummer FA, Ronald AR, Mosel S (1999) A randomised double-blind, placebo-controlled trial of single-dose ciprofloxacin *versus* erythromycin for the treatment of chancroid in Nairobi, Kenya. *J Infect Dis* 180: 1886–1893
62 D'Souza P, Pandho RK, Khanna N, Rattan A, Misra RS (1998) A comparative study of therapeutic response of patients with clinical chancroid to ciprofloxacin, erythromycin and cotrimoxazole. *Sex Transm Dis* 25: 293–295
63 Plourde PJ, D'Costa LJ, Agoki E, Ombette J, Ndinya-Achola JO, Slaney LA, Ronald AR, Plummer FA (1992) A randomised, double blind study of the efficacy of fleroxacin *versus* trimethoprim-sulfamethoxazole in men with culture-proven chancroid. *J Infect Dis* 165: 949–952
64 Ramanan C, Sarma PS, Ghorpade A, Das M (1990) Treatment of donovanosis with norfloxacin. *Int J Dermatol* 29: 298–299
65 Horner PJ (2001) European guidelines for the management of epididymo-orchitis and syndromic management of acute scrotal swelling. *Int J STD and AIDS* 12 (Suppl. 3): 88–93
66 Bevan CD, Johal BJ, Mumtaz G, Ridgway GL, Siddle NC (1995) Clinical, laparoscopic and microbiological findings in acute salpingitis. Report on a United Kingdom cohort. *Br J Obstet Gynaecol* 102: 407–414
67 Martens MG, Gordon S, Yarborough DR, Faro S, Binder D, Berkeley A (1993) Multicenter randomised trial of ofloxacin *versus* cefoxitin and doxycycline in outpatient treatment of pelvic

inflammatory disease. *South Med J* 86: 604–610
68 Arredondo JL, Diaz V, Gaitan H, Maradiegue E, Oyarzun E, Paz R, Reynal JL, Stamm W, Zambrano D (1997) Oral clindamycin and ciprofloxacin *versus* intramuscular ceftriaxone and oral doxycycline in the treatment of mild-to-moderate pelvic inflammatory disease in outpatients. *Clin Infect Dis* 24: 170–178
69 Walker CK, Workowski KA, Washington AE, Soper D, Sweet RL (1999) Anaerobes in pelvic inflammatory disease: Implications for the Centers for Disease Control and Prevention's guidelines for the treatment of sexually transmitted diseases. *Clin Infect Dis* 28 (Suppl. 1): S29–36
70 Ross JDC (2001) European guideline for the management of pelvic inflammatory disease and perihepatitis. *Int J STD and AIDS* 12 (Suppl. 3): 84–87
71 Jick S (1997) Ciprofloxacin safety in a paediatric population. *Paediatric Infectious Disease Journal* 16: 130–134
72 Doherty CP, Saha SK, Cutting WA (2000) Typhoid fever, ciprofloxacin and growth in young children. *Ann Trop Paediatr* 20: 297–303

Fluoroquinolone Antibiotics
ed. by A.R. Ronald and D.E. Low

Gastrointestinal and intraabdominal infections

Anthony W. Chow

Division of Infectious Diseases, Department of Medicine, University of British Columbia and Vancouver Hospital Health Sciences Centre, Vancouver, B.C., Canada V5Z 3J5

Introduction

The fluoroquinolones have excellent *in vitro* activity against a variety of gastrointestinal pathogens including enteropathogenic *Escherichia coli, Salmonella* spp., *Shigella* spp., *Yersinia enterocolitica, Aeromonas hydrophila, Plesiomonas shigelloides,* and *Helicobacter pylori* [1–4]. The newer fluoroquinolones (trovafloxacin, gatifloxacin, gemifloxacin) are also active against many obligate anaerobes [5, 6]. Coupled with favorable bioavailability after oral administration, and the ability to achieve high concentrations in the intestinal mucosa, hepatobiliary tree, and in feces, it is not surprising that this antibiotic class has been studied extensively for the treatment of gastrointestinal infections. This chapter will review the impact of fluoroquinolones on the fecal flora, and their major clinical applications in gastrointestinal and intraabdominal infections. Particular emphasis is directed to large randomized, double-blind and controlled clinical trials before and since 1995.

Impact on fecal microflora

Even though their routes of elimination may differ, all fluoroquinolones reach much higher concentrations in the gastrointestinal tract than in serum, making them particularly attractive agents for the treatment of enteric infections [7] (Tab. 1). For ciprofloxacin, norfloxacin and pefloxacin, the transintestinal route of elimination is particularly prominent, accounting for extraordinarily high concentrations both in the intestinal mucosa and in feces [8]. Trovafloxacin and moxifloxacin are both eliminated primarily by biliary excretion [9–11], with recovery of fecal trovafloxacin predominantly in the unchanged rather than metabolized form (43% *versus* 13% of administered dose), and moxifloxacin predominantly in the metabolized form (36% *versus* 25%). Ofloxacin, fleroxacin, levofloxacin and gatifloxacin are primarily excreted by the renal route (~80%), with relatively lower concentrations in feces [12].

The impact of selected fluoroquinolones on the normal intestinal flora is summarized in Table 2. The facultative Gram-negative bacteria, particularly

Table 1. Faecal concentrations of selected fluoroquinolones from representative studies

Authors (year)	Drug	Dose	No. and type of subjects	Faecal conc. (μg/g ± SD)	Ref.
Brismar et al. (1990)	Ciprofloxacin	750 mg PO q12h × 1 day, 400 mg IV q12 h × 1 day	21 colorectal surgery	<0.1–858	[24]
Krueger et al. (1997)		400 mg IV q12h × 4 days	16 healthy volunteers	251–811	[108]
Krueger et al. (1999)		200 mg IV q12h × 3 days	10 hospitalized patients	109 ± 77	[109]
		200 mg IV q12h × 3 days plus sucralfate 1 g PO tid × 3 days	10 hospitalized patients	185 ± 159	
Edlund et al. (1987)	Norfloxacin	400 mg PO single dose	12 healthy volunteers	207–2716	[110]
Pecquet et al. (1987)	Ofloxacin	400 mg PO od × 5 days	5 healthy volunteers	327 (274	[111]
Edlund et al. (1997)		400 mg PO od × 7 days	10 healthy volunteers	78 ± 34	[112]
Midtvedt (1987)		200 mg PO q12h × 6 days	7 healthy volunteers	44	[113]
Janin et al. (1987)	Pefloxacin	400 mg PO q12h × 7 days	10 healthy volunteers	645 ± 67	[114]
Nakashima et al. (1988)	Fleroxacin	400 mg PO q12h × 7 days	30 healthy volunteers	159 ± 64	[115]
Edlund et al. (1997)	Levofloxacin	500 mg PO od × 7 days	10 healthy volunteers	94 ± 57	[112]
Garcia-Calvo et al. (2001)	Trovafloxacin	200 mg PO single dose	12 healthy volunteers	18 ± 34	[116]

(Continued on next page)

Table 1. (Continued)

Authors (year)	Drug	Dose	No. and type of subjects	Faecal conc. (μg/g ± SD)	Ref.
Dalvie et al. (1997)		200 mg PO single dose	4 healthy volunteers	43% of dose*	[11]
Stass & Kubitza (1999)	Moxifloxacin	400 mg PO single dose	6 healthy volunteers	25% of dose	[117]
		400 mg IV single dos	5 healthy volunteers	26% of dose	
Nakashima et al. (1995)	Gatifloxacin	400 mg PO single dose	6 healthy volunteers	6% of dose	[115]
Garcia-Calvo et al. (2001)	Gemifloxacin	320 mg PO single dose	12 healthy volunteers	75 ± 77	[116]

* faecal excretion of unchanged drug expressed as percent of dose administered

Table 2. Effect of selected fluoroquinolones on the intestinal microflora

Authors (year)	Drug	Dose	No. & type of subjects	Effect on:					Ref.
				Entero-bacteria-ceae	Entero-cocci	Anaer-obes	Coloni-zation with yeast	Emerg. of resist.	
de Vries-Hospers et al. (1985)	Norfloxacin	400 mg PO bid × 5 days	10 volunteers	+++	+	-	-	-	[118]
Bergan et al. (1986)	Ciprofloxacin	500 mg PO bid × 5 days	12 volunteers	+++	++	+	-	-	[119]
Brumfitt et al. (1984)		500 mg PO bid × 7 days	12 volunteers	+++	++	-	-	+	[120]
Brismar et al. (1990)		750 mg PO bid × 1 day, 400 mg IV bid × 1 day	21 colorectal surgery	+++	++	+	-	-	[24]
Shah et al. (1987)	Ofloxacin	200 mg PO bid × 7 days	10 volunteers	+++	+	-	-	-	[121]
Edlund et al. (1997)		400 mg PO od × 7 days	10 volunteers	+++	+	-	-	-	[112]
Janin et al. (1987)	Pefloxacin	400 mg PO bid × 7 days	10 volunteers	+++	+	+	-	-	[114]
Shah et al. (1988)	Fleroxacin	800 mg PO od × 7 days	10 volunteers	+++	+	-	-	-	[122]
Edlund et al. (1997)	Levofloxacin	500 mg PO od × 7 days	10 volunteers	+++	+	-	-	-	[112]

(Continued on next page).

Table 2. (Continued)

Authors (year)	Drug	Dose	No. & type of subjects	Effect on: Entero-bacteria-ceae	Entero-cocci	Anaer-obes	Coloni-zation with yeast	Emerg. of resist.	Ref.
van Nispen et al. (1998)	Trovafloxacin	200 mg PO od × 10 days	12 volunteers	+++	++	-	-	-	[123]
	Placebo	PO od × 10 days	6 volunteers	-	-	-	-	-	
Garcia-Calvo et al. (2001)	Trovafloxacin	200 mg PO single dose	12 volunteers	-	-	-	-	+	[116]
Edlund et al. (2000)	Moxifloxacin	400 mg PO od × 7 days	12 volunteers	+++	++	+	-	-	[124]
Edlund & Nord (1999)	Gatifloxacin	400 mg PO od × 10 days	18 volunteers	+++	++	+	-	-	[13]
Garcia-Calvo et al. (2001)	Gemifloxacin	320 mg PO single dose	12 volunteers	++	+	+	-	+	[116]
Barker et al. (2001)	Gemifloxacin	320 mg PO od × 7 days	10 volunteers	++	+	+	-	-	[125]
	Placebo	PO od × 7 days	5 volunteers	-	-	-	-	-	

+++ = strong suppression (>4 log10/g faeces; ++ = moderate suppression (~3 log10/g faeces); + = mild suppression (<2 log10/g faeces; - = no significant effect

Enterobacteriaceae, are profoundly suppressed or eliminated during therapy [13]. Facultative Gram-positive cocci are strongly suppressed by moxifloxacin, and to minor degrees by the other fluoroquinolones. The fourth generation fluoroquinolones, trovafloxacin, moxifloxacin and gatifloxacin, all have potent *in vitro* activity against obligate anaerobes including *Bacteroides fragilis* [5, 4, 14], but have only limited effects on the intestinal anaerobic microflora similar to the first and second generation fluoroquinolones [15]. Edlund et al. [16] reported that the fluoroquinolones bind to the bacterial fraction of feces. This may explain the apparent paradox that despite high fecal concentrations, these fluoroquinolones have relatively limited effect on the normal intestinal microflora. None of the fluoroquinolones are very active against *Clostridium difficile* [17], and *C. difficile* associated diarrhea following quinolone therapy has been well documented [18–20]. Contrary to reports from earlier studies, emergence of resistant facultative Gram-negative bacteria from the gastrointestinal tract during or following fluoroquinolone therapy is not uncommon [12, 21]. For this reason, the prophylactic use of fluoroquinolones is strongly discouraged.

Major clinical applications studied prior to 1995

The fluoroquinolones prior to 1995 (e.g., nalidixic acid, ciprofloxacin, norfloxacin, ofloxacin, pefloxacin, fleroxacin, lomefloxacin) are mainly active against Gram-negative bacteria (particularly *Enterobacteriaceae*), but have limited or no activity against Gram-positive or anaerobic bacteria. Earlier studies clearly established the use of second generation fluoroquinolones (norfloxacin, ciprofloxacin, ofloxacin, fleroxacin) as the agents of choice for the treatment of infectious and traveler's diarrhea in adults [22]. Since these agents lack activity against intestinal anaerobes and enterococci, and may preserve "colonization resistance" in the GI tract, they have also been studied for selective gut decontamination in patients undergoing colorectal surgery [23, 24] or bone marrow transplantation [25, 26]. The second generation fluoroquinolones have also been evaluated for the treatment and prevention of bacterial peritonitis in patients undergoing chronic ambulatory peritoneal dialysis (CAPD) and for spontaneous bacterial peritonitis in patients with cirrhosis. Finally, these fluoroquinolones have been investigated for the treatment of acute biliary tract infections (cholecystitis or cholangitis), and for the treatment or prevention of cholangitis following endoscopic retrograde cholangiopancreatography (ERCP).

Treatment and prevention of traveler's diarrhea

Traveler's diarrhea is characterized by a diarrheal illness after traveling from an industrialized country to a developing area of the world [27]. The clinical syndrome is defined by the passing of ≥ 3 loose stools within a 24-h period, and is associated with at least one symptom of enteric disease such as nausea, vomiting, cramps, fever, fecal urgency, tenesmus, or the passage of bloody mucoid stools. Bacterial enteropathogens cause at least 80% of traveler's diarrhea [22]. Although somewhat variable depending on the region of travel, the predominant causes in decreasing order of frequency include: enterotoxigenic *Escherichia coli, Shigella* species, *Campylobacter jejuni, Aeromonas* species, *Plesiomonas shigelloides, Salmonella* species, and non-cholera vibrios. Although traveler's diarrhea is usually self-limited and may not require antimicrobial therapy, patients who have severe disease, an underlying medical illness, or are immunocompromised may be candidates for anti-infective treatment. Several double-blind placebo-controlled trials have demonstrated the efficacy of fluoroquinolones in the treatment of traveler's diarrhea (Tab. 3). Either ciprofloxacin (750 mg as a single dose or 500 mg twice a day for 3 days), norfloxacin (800 mg as a single dose or 400 mg twice a day for 3 days), or ofloxacin (600 mg as a single dose or 300 mg twice a day for 3 days) is effective, and treatment reduces the duration of loose stools by 1 to 3 days compared to placebo [27, 28]. The addition of loperamide (up to 16 mg/day) to these agents appears to reduce the mean cumulative number of liquid stools relative to fluoroquinolones alone by about 25–50% at 48 h [29–31]. Whereas trimethoprim-sulfamethoxazole (TMP-SMZ) was comparable to the fluoroquinolones in several controlled trials and has been the treatment of choice for traveler's diarrhea for many years in the past, development of resistance to TMP-SMZ by a number of enteropathogens worldwide has severely limited its clinical utility [28].

Although ciprofloxacin and norfloxacin have both been demonstrated in double-blind placebo-controlled trials to be effective in preventing against traveler's diarrhea (89–94% *versus* 64–66% for placebo; $p < 0.05$) [32, 33], routine use of these agents for chemoprophylaxis of traveler's diarrhea is not recommended because of the concern of emerging resistance [28, 34].

Empiric treatment of acute infectious diarrhea

In a study of 173 patients with domestically acquired diarrhea, ciprofloxacin 500 mg twice daily for 5 days shortened the duration of diarrhea compared to placebo (2.4 *versus* 3.4 days; $p < 0.0005$) [35] (Tab. 3). In the same study, ciprofloxacin was also more effective than TMP-SMZ 160/800 mg or placebo ($p < 0.001$). In a separate study, fleroxacin given either as a single dose or three daily doses significantly shortened the clinical duration of diarrhea and eradicated the causative enteropathogen from stool cultures more rapidly compared to placebo [36, 37]. Short courses of fluoroquinolone therapy, however, have been relatively ineffective in intestinal clearance of *Salmonella* spp. [37, 38]. In light of this, and with the increasing threat of TMP-SMZ-resistant shigellosis and quinolone-resistant campylobacteriosis, it is strongly recommended

Table 3. Clinical and bacteriologic responses to fluoroquinolones in the treatment of traveler's diarrhea and non-travel-related acute infectious diarrhea

Authors (year)	Country	Treatment regimen	Clinical cure rate by 48–72 h	Microbiological cure rate	Reference
Traveler's Diarrhea					
DuPont et al. (1987)	International	Norfloxacin 400 mg PO bid × 5 days	116/131 (89%)	98%	[126]
		Norfloxacin 400 mg PO tid × 5 days	115/126 (91%)	100%	
		TMP-SMZ 160/800 mg PO bid × 5 days	105/135 (78%)	95%	
Taylor et al. (1991)	Cairo	Ciprofloxacin 500 mg PO bid × 3 days plus loperamide	45/50 (90%)		[29]
		Ciprofloxacin 500 mg PO bid × 3 days plus placebo	49/54 (90%)		
DuPont et al. (1992)	Mexico	Ofloxacin 300 mg PO bid × 5 days	59/66 (89%)*	75/78 (96%)*	[127]
		Ofloxacin 300 mg PO bid × 3 days	77/81 (95%)*		
		Placebo	56/79 (71%)	37/46 (80%)	
Petrucelli et al. (1992)	Central Thailand	Ciprofloxacin 750 mg PO single dose plus placebo	48/50 (96%)		[30]
		Ciprofloxacin 750 mg PO single dose plus loperamide	39/47 (83%)		
		Ciprofloxacin 500 mg PO bid × 3 days plus loperamide	37/45 (82%)		
Mattila et al. (1993)	Morocco	Norfloxacin 400 mg PO bid × 3 days	84%*		[51]
		Placebo	47%		
Salam et al. (1994)	Belize	Ciprofloxacin 500 mg PO single dose	42/45 (93%)		[128]
		Placebo	30/38 (79%)		
Acute Infectious Diarrhea (Non-traveler-related)					
Goodman et al. (1990)	USA	Ciprofloxacin 500 mg PO bid × 5 days	(92%)		[35]
		TMP-SMZ 160/800 mg PO bid × 5 days	(77%)		
		Placebo	(60%)		

(Continued on next page).

Table 3. (Continued)

Authors (year)	Country	Treatment regimen	Clinical cure rate by 48–72 h	Microbiological cure rate	Reference
DuPont et al. (1987)	USA	Norfloxacin 400 mg PO bid × 5 days	116/131 (89%)	105/106 (99%)	[126]
		Norfloxacin 400 mg PO tid × 5 days	115/126 (91%)		
		TMP-SMZ 160/800 mg PO bid × 5 days	105/135 (78%)	49/52 (94%)	
Wistrom et al. (1992)	Sweden	Norfloxacin 400 mg PO bid × 5 days	(63%)*		[129]
		Placebo	(51%)		
Butler et al. (1993)	International (Indonesia, Thailand, Ivory Coast, Mexico, Israel, Italy)	Fleroxacin 400 mg PO single dose	93/110 (85%)*	94%*	36
		Fleroxacin 400 mg PO od × 3 days	92/112 (82%)*	93%*	
		Placebo	68/110 (62%)	57%	
Dryden et al. (1996)	United Kingdom	Ciprofloxacin 500 mg PO bid × 5 days	79/81 (97%)*	86%*	[52]
		Placebo	64/81 (79%)	34%	
Noguerado et al. (1995)	Spain	Ofloxacin 400 mg PO single dose	41/44 (93%)	31%* at day 2; 62% at day 15[Ψ]	[37]
		Placebo	40/46 (87%) 59% at day 15[Ψ]	3% at day 2;	
Halstensen et al. (1995)	Norway	Ofloxacin 400 mg PO od × 3 days	47/86 (55%)*	34%*	[38]
		Placebo	13/41 (32%)	11%	
Akalin (1995)	Turkey	Ofloxacin 400 mg PO single dose	74/74 (100%)	95%	[39]
		Ofloxacin 400 mg PO od × 3 days	74/75 (99%)	94%	

* Difference statistically significant ($p < 0.05$) compared to placebo.
[Ψ] Predominant stool isolates were *Salmonella* spp. in this study.

that fecal specimens be routinely obtained for culture and examined for evidence of an inflammatory process, particularly if invasive diarrhea is suspected and empiric antimicrobial therapy is contemplated [34]. A second generation fluoroquinolone (norfloxacin 400 mg, ciprofloxacin 500 mg, or ofloxacin 800 mg, each bid × 3 days) is recommended if enteropathogenic (enteroinvasive, enterohaemorrhagic or enteroaggregative) *Escherichia coli, Salmonella, Shigella* or *Aeromonas* infection is suspected in adults. TMP-SMZ plus a macrolide (e.g., azithromycin) is recommended if quinolone-resistant *Campylobacter* spp. is suspected, and metronidazole is advised if *Clostridium difficile* associated diarrhea is likely [34].

Treatment of specific enteric infections (Tab. 4)

Non-typhoidal Salmonella gastroenteritis

Antibiotic therapy in non-typhoidal salmonella gastroenteritis remains controversial since the illness is usually self-limited (resolving within 2–5 days), and treatment not only does not shorten the duration of symptoms but also may prolong the intestinal carrier state [39]. Both norfloxacin (400 mg twice daily) and ciprofloxacin (500 mg twice daily) for 5 days either delayed the elimination of salmonella from stool cultures or failed to prevent a high rate of bacteriological relapse [33, 40]. As well, the emergence of high-level quinolone resistance in *S. typhimurium* during or after therapy has been reported [39]. Thus, fluoroquinolones should be used with caution in patients with acute non-typhoidal salmonella gastroenteritis, and should be limited to patients with immune deficiency states such as AIDS or asplenia [39, 34].

Salmonella enteric fever

Fluoroquinolones are considered the treatment of choice for enteric fever caused by *S. typhi* or *S. paratyphi* primarily in light of increasing resistance to the betalactams, TMP-SMZ, and chloramphenicol. In noncomparative trials, all second generation fluoroquinolones (ciprofloxacin, norfloxacin, ofloxacin, pefloxacin, enoxacin) were equally effective when administered for 7–14 days, with clinical cure rates of 96–100% [41, 42]. Fluoroquinolones are highly active even against multi-resistant *S. typhi,* and is superior to short-course (3-day) ceftriaxone therapy in one study [43]. Although shorter courses of fluoroquinolones have been effective in patients with enteric fever, treatment for at least 7–10 days is generally advised [42].

Between 1–6% of patients with enteric fever become chronic fecal carriers of *S. typhi* [44]. In contrast to non-typhoidal *Salmonella* in which stool carriage may be prolonged following fluoroquinolone therapy, several studies have demonstrated that norfloxacin, ciprofloxacin or ofloxacin eradicated chronic carriage of *S. typhi* in 83–93% of patients [45]. In a double-blind, placebo-controlled trial, norfloxacin 400 mg twice a day for 28 days eradicated chronic carriage of *S. typhi* from stool and bile cultures in 11 of 12 (92%)

Table 4. Clinical and bacteriologic responses to fluoroquinolones in the treatment of acute diarrhea caused by specific pathogens

Authors (year)	Country	Treatment regimen	Clinical cure rate by 48–72 h	Microbiological cure rate	Reference
Escherichia coli gastroenteritis					
Butler (1993)	International	Fleroxacin 400 mg PO single dose Fleroxacin 400 mg PO od × 3 days Placebo	6/8 (75%) 10/10 (100%) 7/8 (88%)	88% 80% 100%	[36]
Non-typhoidal *Salmonella* gastroenteritis					
Butler (1993)	International	Fleroxacin 400 mg PO single dose Fleroxacin 400 mg PO od × 3 days Placebo	13/16 (81%) 11/16 (69%) 12/14 (86%)	88%* 88%* 43%	[36]
Sanchez et al. (1993)	Spain	Ciprofloxacin 500 mg PO bid × 5 days TMP-SMZ 160/800 mg PO bid × 5 days Placebo	No difference between groups in symptom resolution among 65 total patients	No difference between groups in stool clearance	[130]
Wistrom et al. (1992)	Sweden	Norfloxacin 400 mg PO bid × 5 days Placebo	No difference between groups in symptom resolution among 82 total patients	18%* 49%	[129]
Salmonella enteric fever					
Limson and Littaua (1989)	Phillippines	Ciprofloxacin 500 mg PO bid × 10 days TMP-SMZ 160/800 mg PO bid × 14 days	100% 90%		[131]
Unal et al. (1996)	Turkey	Pefloxacin 400 mg PO bid × 5 days Pefloxacin 400 mg PO bid × 7 days	21/22 (96%) 24/24 (100%)	96% 100%	[132]
Smith et al. (1994)	Vietnam	Ofloxacin 200 mg PO q12h × 5 days Ceftriaxone 3 g IV od × 3 days	22/22 (100%)* 18/25 (72%)		[43]
Tran et al. (1995)	Vietnam	Ofloxacin 15 mg/kg IV × 3 days Ofloxacin 10 mg/kg IV × 5 days	437/438 (99%) for total group		[133]
Uwaydah et al. (1992)	Arabian Gulf	Ciprofloxacin 500 mg PO bid × 7–10 days Ciprofloxacin 750 mg PO bid × 7–10 days	34/34 (100%) 27/28 (96%)		[134]

(Continued on next page)

Table 4. (Continued)

Authors (year)	Country	Treatment regimen	Clinical cure rate by 48–72 h	Microbiological cure rate	Reference
Shigella spp.					
Butler (1993)	International	Fleroxacin 400 mg PO single dose Fleroxacin 400 mg PO od × 3 days Placebo	10/14 (71%) 14/17 (82%) 9/16 (56%)	86%* 94%* 50%	[36]
Bennish et al. (1992)	Bangladesh	Ciprofloxacin 1 g PO single dose	S. dysenterie type 1: 6/10 (60%) Other: 30/30 (100%)		[48]
		Ciprofloxacin 1 g PO od × 2 days	S. dysenterie type 1: 13/15 (87%) Other: 28/28 (100%)		
		Ciprofloxacin 500 mg PO bid × 5 days	S. dysenterie type 1: 15/15 (100%) Other: 20/20 (100%)		
Bennish et al. (1990)	Bangladesh	Ciprofloxacin 500 mg PO bid × 5 days Ampicillin 500 mg PO qid × 5 days	57/60 (95%) Ampicillin sensitive: 23/26 (88%) Ampicillin resistant: 15/35 (43%)*	60/60 (100%)* 23/26 (88%) 30/35 (86%)	[135]
Salam and Bennish (1988)	Bangladesh	Nadilixic acid 55 mg/kg/day PO × 5 days Amipicillin 100 mg/kgday PO × 5 days	26/32 (81%) Ampicillin sensitive 17/22 (77%) Ampicillin resistant 3/14 (21%)*	32/32 (100%) 22/22 (100%) 10/13 (77%)*	[136]
Khan et al. (1997)	Bangladesh	Ciprofloxacin 500 mg PO bid × 5 days Azithromycin 500 mg PO, then 250 mg PO od × 4 days	32/36 (89%) 28/34 (82%)	36/36 (100%) 32/34 (94%)	[137]
Gotuzzo et al. (1989)	Peru	Norfloxacin 800 mg PO single dose TMP-SMZ 160/800 mg PO bid × 5 days	No difference in symptom resolution between groups	23/24 (96%) 25/25 (100%)	[138]

(Continued on next page)

Table 4. (Continued)

Authors (year)	Country	Treatment regimen	Clinical cure rate by 48–72 h	Microbiological cure rate	Reference
Vibrio cholerae					
Butler (1993)	International	Fleroxacin 400 mg PO single dose	40/48 (83%)*	96%*%	[36]
		Fleroxacin 400 mg PO od × 3 days	35/46 (76%)*	96%*	
		Placebo	24/51 (47%)	63%	
Khan et al. (1996)	Bangladesh	Ciprofloxacin 1 g PO single dose	*V. cholerae* O1: 62/66 (94%)*	95%*	
			V. cholerae O139 54/59 (92%)	98%*	[50]
		Doxycycline 300 mg PO single dose	*V. cholerae* O1 47/64 (73%)	69%	
			V. cholerae O139 65/71 (92%)	79%	
Gotuzzo et al. (1995)	Peru	Ciprofloxacin 250 mg PO od × 3 days	No difference in duration	99%	[139]
		Tetracycline 500 mg PO qid × 3 days	diarrhea between groups	95%	
Khan et al. (1995)	Bangladesh	Ciprofloxacin 500 mg PO bid × 3 days	14/15 (93%)	100%*	[140]
		Tetracycline 500 mg PO qid × 3 days	5/12 (42%)*	20%	
		Erythromycin 500 mg PO qid × 3 days	12/15 (80%)	8%	
Vibrio parahaemolyticus					
Butler (1993)	International	Fleroxacin 400 mg PO single dose	22/23 (96%)	100%*	[36]
		Fleroxacin 400 mg PO od × 3 days	17/18 (94%)	94%*	
		Placebo	10/13 (77%)	46%	

* Difference statistically significant ($p < 0.05$) compared to placebo or the comparison group.

individuals compared to 0 of 12 in the placebo group ($p < 0.005$) [46]. Overall, the eradication rate with norfloxacin for 23 individuals with chronic *S. typhi* carriage was 78%. In a separate study, ciprofloxacin 750 mg twice a day for 28 days eliminated chronic carriage of *S. typhi* in 11 of 12 (92%) patients [44]. The optimal duration required for the treatment of chronic *S. typhi* carriage remains undetermined, however.

Shigellosis

A 3–5 day course of ciprofloxacin, norfloxacin, ofloxacin or fleroxacin was highly effective in patients with shigellosis (Tab. 4). The addition of loperamide to ciprofloxacin may further shorten the duration of diarrhea compared to ciprofloxacin alone (median duration 19 h *versus* 42 h) [47]. Even a single dose can be effective in acute shigellosis except in those cases caused by *S. dysenteriae* type 1, for whom a 5–10 day course of treatment is required [48]. An increasing frequency of *Shigella* strains develop multidrug resistance to ampicillin, TMP-SMZ and nalidixic acid, and these agents are no longer useful for the treatment of shigellosis in Bangladesh and elsewhere [49].

Cholera

Antimicrobial therapy reduces the volume of diarrhea by approximately one half, and shortens the duration of fecal excretion of *V. cholerae* compared to placebo controls. Although tetracycline has been the treatment of choice, the emergence of resistant strains of *V. cholerae* O1 has prompted a search for alternative regimens. The fluoroquinolones are highly active against both *V. cholerae* O1 and O139 infections [41] (Tab. 4). A single-dose regimen of ciprofloxacin 1 g is superior to single-dose doxycycline 300 mg in *V. cholerae* O1 infection, both in reducing the volume of diarrhea and in bacteriological eradication [50].

Campylobacter enteritis

The value of antimicrobial therapy in *Campylobacter* enteritis is limited since most patients are already recovering by the time laboratory confirmation of the diagnosis is received. However, studies of placebo-controlled empiric treatment of community acquired gastroenteritis with norfloxacin or ciprofloxacin for 5 days have shown a shortening of the duration of diarrhea by an average of 3.2 days [51, 52]. Unfortunately, rapid emergence of resistant strains during treatment is relatively common [53–55]. An alarming trend is the rapid appearance of quinolone-resistant *Campylobacter* enteritis both in the United States and abroad, especially in Spain and Southeast Asia [56–58]. In the United States, surveillance of 4,953 *Campylobacter* isolates submitted to the Minnesota Department of Health revealed an increasing rate of quinolone resistance, rising from 1.3% in 1992 to 10.2% in 1998 [59]. This study also reported a high rate of *C. jejuni* recovery (74%) from retail chicken products, including ciprofloxacin resistant strains (14%). A direct link between human and poultry isolates was confirmed by molecular subtyping. Erythromycin remains the antibiotic of choice for the treatment of *Campylobacter* enteritis, with resistance rates seldom exceeding 5%. Treatment with azithromycin has been found to be superior to ciprofloxacin (each administered at 500 mg daily for 3 days), particularly for ciprofloxacin-resistant infections [60]. It has been recommended that a second generation fluoroquinolone be considered for the initial empiric treatment of acute infectious gastroenteritis if antimicrobial therapy is warranted. Once the diagnosis of *Campylobacter* infection is confirmed bacteriologically, a macrolide may be added or substituted for specific treatment [34].

Other enteric infections
Patients infected with *V. parahaemolyticus* responded promptly to either a single-dose or 3-day treatment with fleroxacin 400 mg [36] (Tab. 4). There was significant reduction in the number of liquid stools on day 3 compared with patients treated with placebo ($p < 0.05$), and in positive stool cultures by day 3–5 ($p < 0.0001$). In patients with gastroenteritis caused by less common enteropathogens, such as *Yersinia enterocolitica, Plesiomonas shigelloides,* or *Aeromonas* spp., treatment with a fluoroquinolone has resulted in successful eradication of the causative organisms from stool cultures, but there is insufficient data to document the effect of quinolone therapy on the duration or severity of clinical illness.

Selective gut decontamination and infection prevention

Since fluoroquinolones result in selective suppression of the facultative Gram-negative intestinal flora, particularly *Enterobacteriaceae*, there was considerable interest in the use of these agents for the prevention of postoperative wound infection following colorectal surgery, and Gram-negative sepsis in the neurtropenic host.

Colorectal surgery
Single-dose regimens of oral or intravenous ciprofloxacin with or without metronidazole [23, 61], and single-dose intravenous trovafloxacin [62] were evaluated in double-blind randomized trials for wound prophylaxis following colorectal surgery. The rates of postoperative infectious complications in these studies ranged from 7% to 28% and were not significantly different from comparator standard regimens. Since effective antimicrobial therapy for postoperative wound sepsis is readily available, and because fluoroquinolones are inactive against both methicillin-resistant *S. aureus* and enterococci, two relatively common causes of surgical wound infections, the risk of promoting widespread quinolone resistance appears to outweigh any potential benefit from quinolone prophylaxis for patients undergoing colorectal surgery at this time.

Neutropenic host

A meta-analysis of 2,112 patients suggested that fluoroquinolones (ciprofloxacin, norfloxacin, ofloxacin and pefloxacin) alone were more effective than control groups (TMP-SMZ, oral nonabsorbable antimicrobials, or placebo) in preventing microbiologically documented infections and Gram-negative bacteremia as well as febrile mortality in the neutropenic host, but not Gram-positive bacteremia [63]. In comparative studies with other fluoroquinolones, ciprofloxacin was more effective than norfloxacin, ofloxacin or pefloxacin in reducing the incidence of infections caused by Gram-negative bacteria [64, 65]. However, the rapid emergence of resistant microorganisms, including high-level quinolone-resistant *E. coli* bacteremia in neutropenic patients who had received fluoroquinolone prophylaxis [66, 67], has greatly dampened the enthusiasm for prophylactic use of this drug class in this patient population [41].

Treatment and prevention of bacterial peritonitis in cirrhotic patients or following CAPD

Patients with cirrhosis are at high risk for recurrent spontaneous bacterial peritonitis caused by enteric facultative Gram-negative organisms. Treatment with oral ofloxacin was as effective as intravenous cefotaxime in one randomized comparative study of 123 cirrhotics with spontaneous bacterial peritonitis (84% *versus* 85%) [68]. Although prophylaxis with oral ciprofloxacin (750 mg once weekly) or norfloxacin (400 mg once daily) has been shown to reduce recurrences of spontaneous peritonitis by three-fold [69, 70], prolonged treatment has resulted in the rapid emergence of resistant bacteria and is not recommended [71].

Use of fluoroquinolones in peritonitis has also been evaluated in patients undergoing chronic ambulatory peritoneal dialysis (CAPD). In noncomparative studies, clinical cure rates (defined as the absence of symptoms of peritonitis with clear dialysate effluent) ranged from 75 to 83% of episodes following treatment with intraperitoneal ciprofloxacin (25 or 50 mg/L in each bag of dialysate for 5 or 7 days) [41]. Not surprisingly, the clinical and microbiological cure rates were higher in Gram-negative (19 of 20; 95%) than in Gram-positive (39 of 58; 67%) infections. A cure rate of 83% was reported in a study which used sequential intraperitoneal ciprofloxacin (50 mg/L in each bag of dialysate for 5 days) followed by oral ciprofloxacin (500 mg bid for 10 days) [72]. In another comparative study, success rates with intraperitoneal ciprofloxacin (20 mg/L in each bag of dialysate) for 10 days was similar to the standard regimen of intraperitoneal vancomycin plus gentamicin (95% *versus* 80%) [73]. Compared to intraperitoneal ciprofloxacin (200 mg IP loading dose, then 25 mg/L in each bag of dialysate for 10 days), oral ciprofloxacin (750 mg bid for 10 days) produced lower cure rates (67% *versus* 42%) [74]. Resistant Gram-positive infections accounted for about half of the treatment failures in this study. Others also reported the high rate of treatment failures with oral ciprofloxacin or ofloxacin, primarily due to the emergence and spread of ciprofloxacin-resistant coagulase-negative staphylococci [75, 76].

Acute biliary tract infections

The fluoroquinolones can reach high concentrations in the hepatobiliary tract, either by direct excretion into bile or through tissue penetration [77, 78]. Concentrations of ciprofloxacin in bile may reach up to 10-fold higher than in serum. Remarkably, fluoroquinolone concentrations in bile remain high even in the presence of biliary tract obstruction [79]. Since acute biliary tract infections are primarily caused by enteric facultative Gram-negative bacteria and the role of enterococci is less certain, standard empiric treatment for such infections has been either with an aminoglycoside, a second or third generation cephalosporin, or a ureidopenicillin such as mezlocillin or piperacillin [80]. Coverage for anaerobic bacteria is generally not required, unless there is prior bile duct-bowel anastomosis, in the elderly, or in patients with serious clinical conditions. TMP-SMZ and fluoroquinolones are alternative agents, but there have been relatively few comparative studies that evaluated their efficacy.

Cholecystitis or cholangitis

Clinical cure or improvement with ciprofloxacin therapy by sequential intravenous (200 mg q12h) and oral (750 mg q12h) administration was observed in 28 of 32 (88%) patients with acute biliary tract infection (cholecystitis, cholangitis, or both) [81]. In a comparative study of 90 patients with acute suppurative cholangitis, the clinical cure rate following intravenous ciprofloxacin (200 mg q12h) was similar to combination therapy with intravenous ceftazidime (1 g q12h) plus ampicillin (500 mg q6h) and metronidazole (500 mg q8h) (85% *versus* 77%) [82]. However, the mean durations of fever (1.7 *versus* 2.4 days) and hospitalization (6.6 *versus* 7.7 days) were both significantly shorter in the ciprofloxacin group ($p < 0.05$).

ERCP

Cholangitis and septicemia are serious complications of endoscopic retrograde cholangiopancreatography (ERCP). Antibiotic prophylaxis with piperacillin was found to be effective in preventing cholangitis and bacteremia following ERCP in randomized, double-blind placebo-controlled trials [83]. Both ciprofloxacin, fleroxacin and moxifloxacin are actively excreted into bile [77, 79, 84]. However, there have been few well-controlled studies evaluating the efficacy of fluoroquinolones prior to ERCP. A recent meta-analysis of seven randomized, double-blind, placebo-controlled trials concluded that although antibiotic prophylaxis prior to ERCP may reduce the incidence of bacteremia, prophylaxis does not substantially reduce the incidence of sepsis/cholangitis and thus the routine use of antibiotic prophylaxis cannot be recommended

[85]. Subhani et al. [86] suggested that antibiotic prophylaxis prior to ERCP should be restricted to patients who require stenting due to incomplete draining of the biliary system. Such patients have a high risk of developing cholangitis and Gram-negative bacteremia. By restricting antibiotic prophylaxis to this patient group who are most likely to benefit from treatment, antibiotic use can be avoided in 90% of all patients having an ERCP. More comparative studies are warranted to examine the efficacy of an oral fluoroquinolone compared to intravenous regimens such as piperacillin, ceftriaxone or an aminoglycoside in this high risk population [87].

Major clinical applications studied since 1995

The fluoroquinolones developed since 1995 (e.g., levofloxacin, trovafloxacin, moxifloxacin, clinafloxacin, gatifloxacin, gemifloxacin, etc.) have retained much of the activity of ciprofloxacin and ofloxacin against enteric Gram-negative bacteria [12]. However, they have greater potency than ciprofloxacin against Gram-positive cocci including *S. pneumoniae,* viridans streptococci and some staphylococci, although activity against enterococci remains only marginal. Most methicillin sensitive *S. aureus* are sensitive, but many methicillin resistant *S. aureus* have acquired high-level cross-resistance to ciprofloxacin as well as the newer fluoroquinolones [12]. The fourth generation fluoroquinolones (trovafloxacin, moxifloxacin, gatifloxacin, clinafloxacin, gatifloxacin, gemifloxacin) also have excellent anti-anaerobe activity, including members of the *Bacteroides fragilis* group, *Peptostreptococcus* spp., and some *Clostridium* spp. but not *C. difficile* [5, 88, 89]. Furthermore, these fluoroquinolones have excellent penetration into abdominal tissues including colonic mucosa, bile and peritoneal fluid. Thus, these fourth generation fluoroquinolones show considerable promise as monotherapy for the treatment of intraabdominal infections which are usually polymicrobial and caused by a mixture of anaerobes and facultative Gram-negative aerobes. In addition, there has been a resurgence of interest in the use of fluoroquinolones for the eradication of *Helicobacter pylori* in patients with gastritis and peptic ulcer disease.

Intraabdominal sepsis

Among the fourth generation fluoroquinolones, only trovafloxacin, moxifloxacin and gatifloxacin are released for clinical use. Clinafloxacin has been withdrawn by the manufacturer because of concerns of severe adverse effects such as phototoxicity and hypoglycemia, while gemifloxacin is still under clinical investigation. Unfortunately, trovafloxacin has only limited clinical application because of the risk of liver failure, and its clinical use is restricted to patients with life- or limb-threatening infections for whom it is believed that the potential benefits of trovafloxacin therapy outweigh the risks. Thus at present, only moxifloxacin and gatifloxacin are widely available, but neither of these fourth generation fluoroquinolones are currently approved for the treatment of intra-abdominal infections. Nevertheless, a number of randomized, double-blind controlled clinical trials have documented the potential use of fluoroquinolones, either in combination with an anti-anaerobe agent (e.g., ciprofloxacin plus either metronidazole or clindamycin) or as monotherapy (e.g., trovafloxacin or clinafloxacin) for the treatment of intraabdominal infections (Tab. 5).

Ciprofloxacin in combination with an anti-anaerobe agent

Yoshioka et al. [90] compared prospectively the combination of ciprofloxacin plus metronidazole *versus* amoxicillin-clavulanate in 78 patients with established intraabdominal infection, two-thirds of whom had a prior surgical procedure. The rates for clinical cure or improvement at 5 days were similar (97% *versus* 90%). Hoogkamp-Korstanje [91] reported that ciprofloxacin plus metronidazole was more effective than triple therapy with cefotaxime plus gentamicin and metronidazole in 79 post-surgical patients with intraabdominal infection (clinical cure/improvement rates 77% *versus* 57%; $p < 0.05$). In a more recent double-blind multicentre trial, 691 patients with complicated intraabdominal infections (largely due to diseases of the colon, small bowel and appendix) were randomized to receive either ciprofloxacin 400 mg IV q12h plus metronidazole 500 mg IV q6h, or imipenem-cilastatin 500 mg IV q6h [92]. The study also evaluated whether ciprofloxacin/metronidazole therapy was effective when given PO once the patient was taking oral feedings. Clinical success rates were similar in all three arms of the study in both the intent-to-treat (82%, 84%, and 82%, respectively), and evaluable patients (84%, 86%, and 81%, respectively) (Tab. 5). In the subset of patients who were randomized to sequential IV/PO therapy, the success rate among those randomized to ciprofloxacin/metronidazole PO was 96%, compared to 89% for those treated with ciprofloxacin/metronidazole IV, and 89% for those treated with imipenem-cilastatin IV. Thus, for complicated intraabdominal infections, treatment with ciprofloxacin plus metronidazole was equivalent to imipenem-cilastatin. Furthermore, in patients able to receive oral therapy, sequential IV to oral treatment with ciprofloxacin plus metronidazole was more cost-effective compared with full IV courses of ciprofloxacin plus metronidazole or imipenem-cilastatin [93]. Importantly, patient outcomes correlated significantly with their APACHE (Acute Physiology and Chronic Health Evaluation) scores (9.2 in the ciprofloxacin/metronidazole groups; 10.5 in the imipenem-cilastatin group), but did not differ between treatment groups with different pathogens isolated. However, the failure rate was higher in all treatment groups among those from whom enterococci were isolated than if they were not present (28% *versus* 14%; $p = 0.006$). It is not clear whether these differences reflect limited efficacy of the antibiotics against enterococcal infection, or whether the presence of enterococci was simply a marker for patients with more severe infection.

Table 5. Clinical and bacteriologic responses to fluoroquinolones in the treatment of Intraabdominal Infections

Authors (year)	Treatment regimen	Clinical cure rate	Reference
Yoshioka et al. (1991)	Ciprofloxacin plus metronidazole Amoxicillin-clavulanate plus metronidazole	97% 90%	[90]
Hoogkamp-Karstanje (1995)	Ciprofloxacin plus metronidazole Cefotaxime plus gentamicin and metronidazole	77%* 57%	[91]
Solomkin et al. (1996)	Ciprofloxacin 400 mg IV q12h plus metronidazole 500 mg IV q6h	ITT: 182/222 (82%) Evaluable: 93/111 (84%) Evaluable for IV/PO: 48/54 (89%)	[92]
	Ciprofloxacin, 400 mg IV q12h then 500 mg PO bid, plus metronidazole, 500 mg IV q6h then 500 mg PO qid	ITT: 183/219 (84%) Evaluable: 91/106 (86%) Evaluable for IV/PO: 44/46 (96%)	
	Imipenem-cilastatin 500 mg IV q6h	ITT: 113/189 (82%) Evaluable: 91/113 (81%) Evaluable for IV/PO: 49/55 (89%)	
Donahue et al. (1998)	Trovafloxacin (alatrofloxacin) 300 mg IV daily followed by 200 mg PO daily Imipenem-cilastatin 1 g IV q8h followed by amoxicillin/clavulanate 500 mg PO tid	129/156 (83%) 127/152 (84%)	[95]
Roy et al. (1998)	Trovafloxacin (alatrofloxacin) 300 mg IV daily followed by 200 mg PO daily Cefotetan 2 g IV q6h followed by amoxicillin/clavulanate 500 mg PO tid	96/107 (90%) 102/119 (86%)	[96]
Solomkin et al. (2001)	Clinafloxacin 200 mg IV q12h	ITT: 219/250 (85%) Evaluable: 123/150 (82%)	[97]
	Imipenem-cilastatin 500 mg IV q6h	ITT: 219/270 (81%) Evaluable: 130/162 (80%)	

ITT, intent-to-treat;
* difference significant compared to the comparison group ($p < 0.05$).

Trovafloxacin monotherapy
In a similar study, 404 patients with complicated intraabdominal infection were randomized to receive either trovafloxacin IV/PO sequential therapy or imipenem-cilastatin IV 94 [95]. The clinical success rates, which again correlated with APACHE scores, were comparable in the two groups (83% *versus* 84%), including the subgroup of patients from whom *B. fragilis* was isolated (97% *versus* 82%). The results of this study suggest that trovafloxacin may be used as monotherapy for mixed aerobic and anaerobic intraabdominal infections. However, since the APACHE scores in the trovafloxacin and comparator groups were both relatively low (6.4 *versus* 7.0), reflecting the dominance of patients with appendicitis in the study population, the efficacy of trovafloxacin monotherapy in more severely ill patients remains to be determined.

A similar regimen of trovafloxacin IV/PO sequential therapy was compared to intravenous cefotetan followed by amoxicillin-clavulanate PO for women with acute gynecologic infections (primarily puerperal endomyometritis) [96]. The overall clinical response rates were again comparable for the two regimens (90% *versus* 86%), and did not differ in the smaller subgroups of patients from whom Gram-negative aerobes, Gram-positive aerobes, and anaerobes were isolated. However, because of reports of liver failure associated with the drug, the FDA has issued an advisory to limit the use of trovafloxacin to complicated intraabdominal infections that are serious or life-threatening and are treated in hospital.

Clinafloxacin monotherapy
Clinafloxacin is another fourth generation fluoroquinolone with activity against facultative Gram-negative bacilli as well as aerobic Gram-positive cocci and obligate anaerobes [88]. A prospective, randomized, double-blind and controlled trial was conducted in 529 patients with complicated intraabdominal infections, comparing clinafloxacin 200 mg IV q12h with imipenem-cilastatin IV 500 mg q6h [97]. Patients with a wide range of infections were enrolled, with perforated or abscessed appendicitis being the most common (approximately 50%). The clinical cure rate was similar for the two groups both in the intent-to-treat (85% *versus* 81%) and evaluable (82% *versus* 80%) study populations. There were substantially more Gram-negative organisms recovered from the patients with treatment failure who were initially treated with imipenem-cilastatin compared with those treated with clinafloxacin (14/18 *versus* 5/15; $p = 0.015$). However, due to concerns of serious adverse effects including phototoxicity and hypoglycemia, clinafloxacin has been withdrawn by the manufacturer.

Helicobacter pylori gastritis and peptic ulcer disease

Although fluoroquinolones are generally active against *Helicobacter pylori in vitro* [4, 98], studies prior to 1995 have consistently demonstrated treatment failure with ciprofloxacin, norfloxacin or ofloxacin in *H. pylori*-associated gastritis [99–101]. Furthermore, emergence of resistant strains during treatment has been reported [102]. Since the bactericidal activity of fluoroquinolones is markedly reduced at acidic pH, Dresner et al. [103] investigated the efficacy of ciprofloxacin in eradicating *H. pylori* when administered in combination with omeprazole, a proton pump inhibitor that alters the gastric pH. Forty-four consecutive patients infected with *H pylori* were prospectively studied in a randomized, double-blind, controlled trial comparing ciprofloxacin with a placebo for 2 weeks (Tab. 6). Both treatment groups received bismuth and omeprazole. In 36 patients, follow-up endoscopy was performed 4 weeks after the cessation of all study drugs. Concurrent administration of omeprazole with ciprofloxacin cleared the *H. pylori* infection in 13 of 17 patients (76%) compared to 5 of 19 (26%) in the placebo group ($p < 0.01$). Since then, a number of other studies have reported similar results when norfloxacin or levofloxacin was administered in combination with a proton pump inhibitor with or without amoxicillin or tinidazole [104, 105] (Tab. 6). More recent studies have also reported markedly enhanced *in vitro* activity of the fourth generation fluoroquinolones against gastric biopsy isolates of *H. pylori,* particularly sitafloxacin, clinafloxacin, gatifloxacin and gemifloxacin compared to moxifloxacin, ciprofloxacin or levofloxacin [98, 106]. Of particular interest is a new class of quinolones in which the fundamental C-6 fluorine atom has been replaced by an amino or nitro group. These C-6 substituted quinolones are highly active against *H. pylori* even at acid pH [107]. Their safety profile and *in vivo* efficacy for *H. pylori*-associated gastritis and peptic ulcer disease remains to be determined.

Research priorities over the next 5 years

Based on the critical review of the clinical application of fluoroquinolones in gastrointestinal and intraabdominal infections summarized above, a number of research priorities in the near future are identified. These include:

- The need for more comparative studies to evaluate the role of the fourth generation fluoroquinolones in the treatment of complicated intraabdominal infections is clearly evident and may represent an important new niche for this antibiotic class. Particular emphasis should be directed at elucidating the pharmacodynamic parameters which can predict clinical success of fluoroquinolone therapy in patients with severe underlying disease in spite of high APACHE scores. Fluoroquinolones with broad spectrum *in vitro* activity and *in vivo* efficacy similar to trovafloxacin and clinafloxacin, but with an improved safety profile, are greatly needed.
- The role of fluoroquinolones in the treatment of acute biliary tract infections, including acute cholangitis, should be further clarified. Host determinants that identify the high risk patient population who are most likely to benefit from antimicrobial therapy or prophylaxis should be elucidated. The

Table 6. Clinical and bacteriologic responses to fluoroquinolones in the treatment of *H. pylori* gastritis and peptic ulcer disease

Authors (year)	Country	Treatment regimen	Clinical cure rate	Microbiological cure rate	Reference
Dresner and Coyle (1996)	USA	Ciprofloxacin 500 mg PO bid × 14 days plus omeprazole 20 mg PO bid × 30 days plus bismuth subsalicyclate 2 tablets qid × 30 days	13/17 (76%)* by endoscopy and urease testing at 4 weeks after cessation of al study drugs	13/17 (76%)*	[103]
		Placebo plus omeprazole 20 mg PO bid × 30 days plus bismuth subsalicyclate 2 t ablets qid × 30 days	5/19 (26%)	5/19 (26%)	
Gupta et al. (1997)	India	Norfloxacin 400 mg PO bid plus omeprazole 20 mg PO bid × 14 days	Healing at 2 weeks: 21/22 (95%) Recurrence at 6 mo: 2/22 (9%)	Eradication at 4 wk: 14/22 (64%) Recurrence at 6 mo: 2/22 (9%)	[104]
		Norfloxacin 400 mg PO bid plus lansoprazole 30 mg PO od × 14 days	Healing at 2 weeks: 25/26 (96%) Recurrence at 6 mo: 1/26 (4%)	Eradication at 4 wk: 20/26 (77%) Recurrence at 6 mo: 1/26 (4%)	
Cammarota et al. (2000)	Italy	Levofloxacin 500 mg PO od plus rabeprazole 20 mg PO od plus amoxycillin 1 g PO bid × 7 days	not stated	Eradication at 8 wk: 46/50 (92%)	[105]
		Levofloxacin 500 mg PO od plus rabeprazole 20 mg PO od plus tinidazole 500 mg PO bid × 7 days	not stated	Eradication at 8 wk: 45/50 (90%)	

* difference significant compared to the comparator group ($p < 0.05$).

cost-effectiveness of single-dose oral fluoroquinolone prophylaxis for the prevention of Gram-negative sepsis and cholangitis following ERCP requires critical evaluation.

- The development of newer fluoroquinolones with chemical modifications that improve their *in vivo* efficacy in the treatment of more chronic conditions such as *H. pylori* gastritis or the chronic *S. typhi* carrier state is strongly recommended. *In vivo* efficacy of the newly developed, acid-resistant C-6 substituted quinolones, in which the fluorine atom is replaced by an amino or nitro group, in the treatment of enteric infections will be of particular interest.
- The development of newer fluoroquinolones effective in eradicating *C. jejuni* both in dairy animals and in human disease, including those with high level resistance to currently available fluoroquinolones, is to be strongly encouraged. Future development of new fluoroquinolones should focus on chemical modifications that retard the selection for resistance.
- The availability of newer fluoroquinolones with improved *in vitro* and *in vivo* activity against nosocomial Gram-positive bacteria, including methicillin-resistant and vancomycin resistant *S. aureus* or coagulase-negative staphylococci, and vancomycin-resistant enterococci (VRE) will be particularly welcomed.

References

1 Karlowsky JA, Kelly LJ, Thornsberry C, Jones ME, Evangelista AT, Critchley IA, Sahm DF (2002) Susceptibility to fluoroquinolones among commonly isolated Gram-negative bacilli in 2000: TRUST and TSN data for the United States. Tracking Resistance in the United States Today. The Surveillance Network. *Int J Antimicrob Agents* 19: 21–31

2 Goossens H, De Mol P, Coignau H, Levy J, Grados O, Ghysels G, Innocent H, Butzler JP (1985) Comparative *in vitro* activities of aztreonam, ciprofloxacin, norfloxacin, ofloxacin, HR810 (a new cephalosporin), RU28965 (a new macrokide), and other agents against enteropathogens. *Antimicrob Agents Chemother* 27: 388–392

3 Fernandez-Roblas R, Cabria F, Esteban J, Lopez JC, Gadea I, Soriano F (2000) *In vitro* activity of gemifloxacin (SB-265805) compared with 14 other antimicrobials against intestinal pathogens. *J Antimicrob Chemother* 46: 1023–1027

4 Rhomberg PR, Biedenbach DJ, Jones RN (2001) Activity of BMS284756 (T-3811) tested against anaerobic bacteria, *Campylobacter jejuni, Helicobacter pylori* and *Legionella* spp. *Diagn Microbiol Infect Dis* 40: 45–49

5 Ackermann G, Schaumann R, Pless B, Claros MC, Goldstein EJ, Rodloff AC (2000) Comparative activity of moxifloxacin *in vitro* against obligately anaerobic bacteria. *Eur J Clin Microbiol Infect Dis* 19: 228–232

6 Appelbaum PC (1999) Quinolone activity against anaerobes. *Drugs* 58 (Suppl 2): 60–64

7 Korten V, Murray BE (1993) Impact of the fluoroquinolones on gastrointestinal flora. *Drugs* 45 (Suppl 3): 125–133

8 Rohwedder RW, Bergan T, Thorsteinsson SB, Scholl H (1990) Transintestinal elimination of ciprofloxacin. *Diagn Microbiol Infect Dis* 13: 127–133

9 Melnik G, Schwesinger WH, Teng R, Dogolo LC, Vincent J (1998) Hepatobiliary elimination of trovafloxacin and metabolites following single oral doses in healthy volunteers. *Eur J Clin Microbiol Infect Dis* 17: 424–426

10 Wise R (1999) A review of the clinical pharmacology of moxifloxacin, a new

8-methoxyquinolone, and its potential relation to therapeutic efficacy. *Clin Drug Invest* 17: 365–387
11 Dalvie DK, Khosla N, Vincent J (1997) Excretion and metabolism of trovafloxacin in humans. *Drug Metab Dispos* 25: 423–427
12 Hooper DC (2000) New uses for new and old quinolones and the challenge of resistance. *Clin Infect Dis* 30: 243–254
13 Edlund C, Nord CE (1999) Ecological effect of gatifloxacin on the normal human intestinal microflora. *J Chemother* 11: 50–53
14 Schaumann R, Ackermann G, Pless B, Claros MC, Goldstein EJ, Rodloff AC (2000) *In vitro* activities of fourteen antimicrobial agents against obligately anaerobic bacteria. *Int J Antimicrob Agents* 16: 225–232
15 Edlund C, Nord CE (1999) Effect of quinolones on intestinal ecology. *Drugs* 58 (Suppl 2): 65–70
16 Edlund C, Lindqvist L, Nord CE (1988) Norfloxacin binds to human fecal material. *Antimicrob Agents Chemother* 32: 1869–1874
17 Alonso R, Pelaez T, Gonzalez-Abad MJ, Alcala L, Munoz P, Rodriguez-Creixems M, Bouza E (2001) *In vitro* activity of new quinolones against *Clostridium difficile*. *J Antimicrob Chemother* 47: 195–197
18 Ozawa TT, Valadez T (2002) *Clostridium difficile* infection associated with levofloxacin treatment. *Tenn Med* 95: 113–115
19 Yip C, Loeb M, Salama S, Moss L, Olde J (2001) Quinolone use as a risk factor for nosocomial *Clostridium difficile*-associated diarrhea. *Infect Control Hosp Epidemiol* 22: 572–575
20 McFarland LV, Bauwens JE, Melcher SA, Surawicz CM, Greenberg RN, Elmer GW (1995) Ciprofloxacin-associated *Clostridium difficile* disease. *Lancet* 346: 977–978
21 Richard P, Delangle MH, Raffi F, Espaze E, Richet H (2001) Impact of fluoroquinolone administration on the emergence of fluoroquinolone-resistant Gram-negative bacilli from gastrointestinal flora. *Clin Infect Dis* 32: 162–166
22 DuPont HL, Ericsson CD (1993) Prevention and treatment of traveler's diarrhea. *New Engl J Med* 328: 1821–1827
23 Gortz G, Boese-Landgraf J, Hopfenmuller W, Rodloff A, Kotwas J (1990) Ciprofloxacin as single-dose antibiotic prophylaxis in colorectal surgery: results of a randomized, double-blind trial. *Diag Micro Infect Dis* 13: 181–185
24 Brismar B, Edlund C, Malmborg AS, Nord CE (1990) ciprofloxacin concentrations and impact of the colon microflora in patients undergoing colorectal surgery. *Antimicrob Agents Chemother* 34: 481–483
25 Giuliano M, Pantosti A, Gentile G, Venditti M, Arcese W, Martino P (1989) Effects on oral and intestinal microfloras of norfloxacin and pefloxacin for selective decontamination in bone marrow transplant patients. *Antimicrob Agents Chemother* 33: 1709–1713
26 Rozenberg-Arska M, Dekker AW, Verhoef J (1985) Ciprofloxacin for selective decontamination of the alimentary tract in patients with acute leukemia during remission induction treatment: the effect on fecal flora. *J Infect Dis* 152: 104–107
27 Ericsson CD, DuPont HL (1993) Travelers' diarrhea: approaches to prevention and treatment. *Clin Infect Dis* 16: 616–626
28 Adachi JA, Ostrosky-Zeichner L, DuPont HL, Ericsson CD (2000) Empirical antimicrobial therapy for traveler's diarrhea. *Clin Infect Dis* 31: 1079–1083
29 Taylor DN, Sanchez JL, Candler W, Thornton S, McQueen C, Echeverria P (1991) Treatment of travelers' diarrhea: ciprofloxacin plus loperamide compared with ciprofloxacin alone. A placebo-controlled, randomized trial. *Ann Intern Med* 114: 731–734
30 Petruccelli BP, Murphy GS, Scnchez JL, Walz S, DeFraites R, Gelnett J, Laberberger RL, Echeverria P, Taylor DN (1992) Treatment of traveler's diarrhea with ciprofloxacin and loperamide. *J Infect Dis* 165: 557–560
31 Ericsson CD, DuPont HL, Mathewson JJ (1997) Single dose ofloxacin plus loperamide compared with single dose or three days of ofloxacin in the treatment of traveler's diarrhea. *J Travel Med* 4: 3–7
32 Rademaker CMA, Hoepelman IM, Wolfhagen MJHM et al (1989) Results of a double-blind placebo-controlled study using ciprofloxacin for prevention of traveler's diarrhea. *Eur J Clin Microbiol* 8: 690–694
33 Wistrom JNSR, Burman LG, Lundholm R, Jellheden B et al (1987) Norfloxacin *versus* placebo for prophylaxis against travellers' diarrhea. *J Antimicrob Chemother* 20: 563–574

34 Guerrant RL, Van Gilder T, Steiner TS, Thielman NM, Slutsker L, Tauxe RV, Hennessy T, Griffin PM, DuPont H, Sack RB et al (2001) Practice guidelines for the management of infectious diarrhea. *Clin Infect Dis* 32: 331–351
35 Goodman IJ, Trenholme GM, Kaplan RL et al (1990) Empiric antimicrobial therapy of domestically acquired acute diarrhea in urban adults. *Arch Intern Med* 150: 546
36 Butler T, Lolekha S, Rasidi C, Kadio A, Del Rosal PL, Iskandar H, Rubinstein E, Pastore G (1993) Treatment of acute bacterial diarrhea: a multicenter international trial comparing placebo with fleroxacin given as a single dose or once daily for 3 days. *Am J Med* 94 (suppl 3A): 187S-194S
37 Noguerado A, Garcia-Polo I, Isasia T, Jimenez ML, Bermudez P, Pita J, Gabriel R (1995) Early single dose therapy with ofloxacin for empirical treatment of acute gastroenteritis: a randomized placebo-controlled double-blind clinical trial. *J Antimicrob Chemother* 36: 665–672
38 Halstensen A, Voltersvik P, Gossius GDA, Peterson LE, Rolstad T, Solberg CO (1995) Double-blind comparison of ofloxacin for 3 days and placebo in acute bacterial enteritis. *Drugs* 49: 52–54
39 Akalin HE (1995) Role of quinolones in the treatment of diarrhoeal diseases. *Drugs* 49: 1–4
40 Neill MA, Opal SM, Heelan J et al (1991) Failure of ciprofloxacin to eradicate convalescent faecal excretion after acute salmonellosis: experience during an outbreak in health care workers. *Ann Intern Med* 114: 195–199
41 Davis R, Markham A, Balfour JA (1996) Ciprofloxacin: an updated review of its pharmacology, therapeutic efficacy and tolerability. *Drugs* 51: 1019–1074
42 Limson BM (1995) Short course quinolone therapy of typhoid fever in developing countries. *Drugs* 49: 27–29
43 Smith MD, Duong NM, Hoa NT, Wain J, Ha HD, Diep TS, Day NP, Hien TT, White NJ (1994) Comparison of ofloxacin and ceftriaxone for short-course treatment of enteric fever. *Antimicrob Agents Chemother* 38: 1716–1720
44 Ferreccio C, Morris JG Jr, Valdivieso C, Prenzel I, Sotomayor V, Drusano GL, Levine MM (1988) Efficacy of ciprofloxacin in the treatment of chronic typhoid carriers. *J Infect Dis* 157: 1235–1239
45 Zavala T, I, Quiroz C, Gutierrez MA, Arias J, Renteria M (1991) Fluoroquinolones in the treatment of typhoid fever and the carrier state. *Eur J Clin Microbiol Infect Dis* 10: 334–341
46 Gotuzzo E, Guerra JG, Benavente L, Palomino JC, Carrillo C, Lopera J, Delgado F, Nalin DR, Sabbaj J (1988) Use of norfloxacin to treat chronic typhoid carriers. *J Infect Dis* 157: 1221–1225
47 Murphy GS, Bodhidatta L, Echeverria P, Tansuphaswadikul S, Hoge CW, Imlarp S, Tamura K (1993) Ciprofloxacin and loperamide in the treatment of bacillary dysentery. *Ann Intern Med* 118: 582–586
48 Bennish ML, Salam MA, Khan WA, Khan AM (1992) Treatment of shigellosis: III. Comparison of one- or two-dose ciprofloxacin with standard 5-day therapy. A randomized, blinded trial. *Ann Intern Med* 117: 727–734
49 Bennish ML, Salam MA, Hossain MA, Myaux J, Khan EH, Chakraborty J, Henry F, Ronsmans C (1992) Antimicrobial resistance of *Shigella* isolates in Bangladesh, 1983–1990: increasing frequency of strains multiply resistant to ampicillin, trimethoprim-sulfamethoxazole, and nalidixic acid. *Clin Infect Dis* 14: 1055–1060
50 Khan WA, Bennish ML, Seas C, Khan EH, Ronan A, Dhar U, Busch W, Salam MA (1996) Randomised controlled comparison of single-dose ciprofloxacin and doxycycline for cholera caused by *Vibrio cholerae* 01 or 0139. *Lancet* 348: 296–300
51 Mattila L, Peltola H, Siitonen A, Kyronseppa H, Simula I, Kataja M (1993) Short-term treatment of traveler's diarrhea with norfloxacin: a double-blind, placebo-controlled study during two seasons. *Clin Infect Dis* 17: 779–782
52 Dryden MS, Gabb RJ, Wright SK (1996) Empirical treatment of severe acute community-acquired gastroenteritis with ciprofloxacin. *Clin Infect Dis* 22: 1019–1025
53 Adler-Mosca H, Luthy-Hottenstein J, Martinetti LG, Burnens A, Altwegg M (1991) Development of resistance to quinolones in five patients with campylobacteriosis treated with norfloxacin or ciprofloxacin. *Eur J Clin Microbiol Infect Dis* 10: 953–957
54 Obana M, Matsuoka Y, Irimajiri S, Tonooka H (1992) [Clinical studies on the treatment of *Campylobacter* enteritis – emergence of quinolone-resistant *Campylobacter jejuni* after treatment with new quinolones]. *Kansenshogaku Zasshi* 66: 923–929
55 Wretlind B, Stromberg A, Ostlund L, Sjogren E, Kaijser B (1992) Rapid emergence of quinolone resistance in *Campylobacter jejuni* in patients treated with norfloxacin. *Scand J Infect Dis* 24: 685–686
56 Engberg J, Aarestrup FM, Taylor DE, Gerner-Smidt P, Nachamkin I (2001) Quinolone and

macrolide resistance in *Campylobacter jejuni* and C. coli: resistance mechanisms and trends in human isolates. *Emerg Infect Dis* 7: 24–34
57 DuPont HL (1995) Antimicrobial-resistant *Campylobacter* species – a new threat to travelers to Thailand. *Clin Infect Dis* 21: 542–543
58 Sjogren E, Lindblom GB, Kaijser B (1997) Norfloxacin resistance in *Campylobacter jejuni* and *Campylobacter* coli isolates from Swedish patients. *J Antimicrob Chemother* 40: 257–261
59 Smith KE, Besser JM, Hedberg CW, Leano FT, Bender JB, Wicklund JH, Johnson BP, Moore KA, Osterholm MT, The Investigation Team (1999) Quinolone-Resistant *Campylobacter jejuni* Infections in Minnesota, 1992–1998. *N Engl J Med* 340: 1525–1532
60 Kuschner RA, Trofa AF, Thomas RJ, Hoge CW, Pitarangsi C, Amato S, Olafson RP, Echeverria P, Sadoff JC, Taylor DN (1995) Use of azithromycin for the treatment of *Campylobacter* enteritis in travelers to Thailand, an area where ciprofloxacin resistance is prevalent. *Clin Infect Dis* 21: 536–541
61 Rohwedder R, Bonadeo F, Benati M, Ojea QG, Schlecker H, Vaccaro C (1993) Single-dose oral ciprofloxacin plus parenteral metronidazole for perioperative antibiotic prophylaxis in colorectal surgery. *Chemotherapy* 39: 218–224
62 Milsom JW, Smith DL, Corman ML, Howerton RA, Yellin AE, Luke DR, Trovafloxacdin Surgical Group (1998) Double-blind comparison of single-dose alatroflaxacin and cefotetan as prophylaxis of infection following elective colorectal surgery. *Am J Surg* 176 (Suppl 6A): 46S–52S
63 Cruciani M, Rampazzo R, Malena M, Lazzarini L, Todeschini G, Messori A, Concia E (1996) Prophylaxis with fluoroquinolones for bacterial infections in neutropenic patients: a meta-analysis. *Clin Infect Dis* 23: 795–805
64 GIMEMAInfection Program (1991) Prevention of bacterial infection in neutropenic patients with hematologic malignancies. A randomized, multicenter trial comparing norfloxacin with ciprofloxacin. The GIMEMA Infection Program. Gruppo Italiano Malattie Ematologiche Maligne dell'Adulto. *Ann Intern Med* 115: 7–12
65 D'Antonio D, Piccolomini R, Iacone A, Fioritoni G, Parruti G, Betti S, Quaglietta AM, Accorsi P, Dell'Isola M, Favalli C (1994) Comparison of ciprofloxacin, ofloxacin and pefloxacin for the prevention of the bacterial infection in neutropenic patients with haematological malignancies. *J Antimicrob Chemother* 33: 837–844
66 Carratala J, Fernandez-Sevilla A, Tubau F, Callis M, Gudiol F (1995) Emergence of quinolone-resistant *Escherichia coli* bacteremia in neutropenic patients with cancer who have received prophylactic norfloxacin. *Clin Infect Dis* 20: 557–560
67 Oethinger M, Jellen-Ritter AS, Conrad S, Marre R, Kern WV (1998) Colonization and infection with fluoroquinolone-resistant *Escherichia coli* among cancer patients: clonal analysis. *Infection* 26: 379–384
68 Navasa M, Follo A, Llovet JM, Clemente G, Vargas V, Rimola A, Marco F, Guarner C, Forne M, Planas R et al (1996) Randomized, comparative study of oral ofloxacin *versus* intravenous cefotaxime in spontaneous bacterial peritonitis. *Gastroenterology* 111: 1011–1017
69 Hsieh WJ, Lin HC, Hwang SJ, Hou MC, Lee FY, Chang FY, Lee SD (1998) The effect of ciprofloxacin in the prevention of bacterial infection in patients with cirrhosis after upper gastrointestinal bleeding. *Am J Gastroenterol* 93: 962–966
70 Gines P, Rimola A, Planas R et al (1990) Norfloxacin prevents spontaneous bacterial peritonitis recurrence in dirrhosis: resultws of a double-blind, placebo-controlled trial. *Hepatology* 12: 716–724
71 Dupeyron C, Mangeney N, Sedrati L et al (1994) Rapid emergence of quinolone resistance in cirrhotic patients treated with norfloxacin to prevent spontaneous bacterial peritonitis. *Antimicrob Agents Chemother* 38: 340–344
72 Perez-Fontan M, Rosales M, Fernandez F et al (1993) Treatment of CAPD peritonitis with ciprofloxacin – long-term results. *Nefrologia* 13: 149–154
73 Friedlan JS, IvesonTJ, Frise AP et al (1990) A comparison between intraperitoneal ciprofloxacin and intraperitoneal vancomycin and gentamicin in the treatment of peritonitis associated with continuous ambulatory peritoneal dialysis (CAPD). *J Antimicrob Chemother* 26 (Suppl F): 77–81
74 Cheng IK, Chan CY, Wong WT et al (1993) A randomized prospective comparison of oral *versus* intraperitoneal ciprofloxacin as the primary treatment of peritonitis complicating continuous ambulatory peritoneal dialysis. *Perit Dial Int* 13 (Suppl 2): S351–S354
75 Chan MK, Chau PY, Chan WWN (1988) Oral treatment of peritonitis in CAPD patients with two dosage regimens of ofloxacin. *J Antimicrob Chemother* 22: 371–375

76 Dryden MS, Talsania H, McCann M et al (1992) The epidemiology of ciprofloxacin resistance in coagulase-negative staphylococci in CAPD patients. *Epdemiol Inf* 109: 97–112
77 Edmiston CE Jr, Suarez EC, Walker AP, Demeure MP, Frantzides CT, Schulte WJ, Wilson SD (1996) Penetration of ciprofloxacin and fleroxacin into biliary tract. *Antimicrob Agents Chemother* 40: 787–791
78 Hayton WL, Vlahov V, Bacracheva N, Viachki I, Portmann R, Muirhead G, Stoeckel K, Weidekamm E (1990) Pharmacokinetics and biliary concentrations of fleroxacin in cholecystectomized patients. *Antimicrob Agents Chemother* 34: 2375–2380
79 van den Hazel SJ, de Vries XH, Speelman P, Dankert J, Tytgat GN, Huibregtse K, van Leeuwen DJ (1996) Biliary excretion of ciprofloxacin and piperacillin in the obstructed biliary tract. *Antimicrob Agents Chemother* 40: 2658–2660
80 Westphal JF, Brogard JM (1999) Biliary tract infections: a guide to drug treatment. *Drugs* 57: 81–91
81 Karachalios GN, Zografos G, Patrikakos V (1993) Biliary tract infections treated with ciprofloxacin. *Infection* 21: 362–364
82 Sung JJ, Lyon DJ, Suen R, Chung SC, Co AL, Cheng AF, Leung JW, Li AK (1995) Intravenous ciprofloxacin as treatment for patients with acute suppurative cholangitis: a randomized, controlled clinical trial. *J Antimicrob Chemother* 35: 855–864
83 Byl B, Deviere J, Struelens MJ, Roucloux I, De Coninck A, Thys JP, Cremer M (1995) Antibiotic prophylaxis for infectious complications after therapeutic endoscopic retrograde cholangiopancreatography: a randomized, double-blind, placebo-controlled study. *Clin Infect Dis* 20: 1236–1240
84 Vincent J, Teng R, Dalvie DK, Friedman HL (1998) Pharmacokinetics and metabolism of single oral doses of trovafloxacin. *Am J Surg* 176: 8S–13S
85 Harris A, Chan AC, Torres-Viera C, Hammett R, Carr-Locke D (1999) Meta-analysis of antibiotic prophylaxis in endoscopic retrograde cholangiopancreatography (ERCP). *Endoscopy* 31: 718–724
86 Subhani JM, Kibbler C, Dooley JS (1999) Review article: antibiotic prophylaxis for endoscopic retrograde cholangiopancreatography (ERCP). *Aliment Pharmacol Ther* 13: 103–116
87 Rey JR, Axon A, Budzynska A, Kruse A, Nowak A (1998) Guidelines of the European Society of Gastrointestinal Endoscopy (E.S.G.E.) antibiotic prophylaxis for gastrointestinal endoscopy. European Society of Gastrointestinal Endoscopy. *Endoscopy* 30: 318–324
88 Deshpande LM, Diekema DJ, Jones RN (1999) Comparative activity of clinafloxacin and nine other compounds tested against 2000 contemporary clinical isolates from patients in United States hospitals. *Diagnostic Microbiology and Infectious Disease* 35: 81–88
89 Schaumann R, Ackermann G, Pless B, Claros MC, Rodloff AC (1999) *In vitro* activities of gatifloxacin, two other quinolones, and five nonquinolone antimicrobials against obligately anaerobic bacteria. *Antimicrob Agents Chemother* 43: 2783–2786
90 Yoshioka K, Youngs DJ, Keighley MRB (1991) A randomized prospective controlled study of ciprofloxacin with metronidazole *versus* amoxicillin/clavulanic acid with metronidazole in the treatment of intra-abdominal infection. *Infection* 19: 25–29
91 Hoogkamp-Korstanje JAA (1995) Ciprofloxacin *versus* cefotaxime regimens for the treatment of intra-abdominal infections. *Infection* 23: 278–282
92 Solomkin JS, Reinhart HH, Dellinger EP, Bohnen JM, Rotstein OD, Vogel SB, Simms HH, Hill CS, Bjornson HS, Haverstock DC et al (1996) Results of a randomized trial comparing sequential intravenous/oral treatment with ciprofloxacin plus metronidazole to imipenem/cilastatin for intra-abdominal infections. The Intra-Abdominal Infection Study Group. *Ann Surg* 223: 303–315
93 Walters DJ, Solomkin JS, Paladino JA (1999) Cost effectiveness of ciprofloxacin plus metronidazole *versus* imipenem-cilastatin in the treatment of intra-abdominal infections. *Pharmacoeconomics* 16: 551–561
94 Madrid AM, Hurtado C, Venegas M, Cumsille F, Defilippi C (2001) Long-Term treatment with cisapride and antibiotics in liver cirrhosis: effect on small intestinal motility, bacterial overgrowth, and liver function. *Am J Gastroenterol* 96: 1251–1255
95 Donahue PE, Smith DL, Yellin AE, Mintz SJ, Bur F, Luke DR, Trovafloxacin Surgical Group (1998) Trovafloxacin in the treatment of intra-abdominal infections: results of a double-blind, multicenter comparison with imipenem/cilastatin. *Am J Surg* 176 (Suppl 6A): 53S–61S
96 Roy S, Koltun W, Chatwani A, Martens MG, Dittrich R, Luke DR (1998) Treatment of acute gynecologic infections with trovafloxacin. Trovafloxacin Surgical Group. *Am J Surg* 176: 67S–73S

97 Solomkin JS, Wilson SE, Christou NV, Rotstein OD, Dellinger EP, Bennion RS, Pak R, Tack K (2001) Results of a clinical trial of clinafloxacin *versus* imipenem/cilastatin for intraabdominal infections. *Ann Surg* 233: 79–87
98 Minehart HW, Chalker AF (2001) *In vitro* activity of gemifloxacin against *Helicobacter pylori*. *J Antimicrob Chemother* 47: 360–361
99 Glupczynski Y, Labbe M, Burette A, Delmee M, Avesani V, Bruck C (1987) Treatment failure of ofloxacin in *Campylobacter* pylori infection. *Lancet* 1: 1096
100 Mertens JC, Dekker W, Ligtvoet EE, Blok P (1989) Treatment failure of norfloxacin against *Campylobacter* pylori and chronic gastritis in patients with nonulcerative dyspepsia. *Antimicrob Agents Chemother* 33: 256–257
101 Stone JW, Wise R, Donovan IA, Gearty J (1988) Failure of ciprofloxacin to eradicate *Campylobacter* pylori from the stomach. *J Antimicrob Chemother* 22: 92–93
102 Andriole VT (1993) The future of the quinolones. *Drugs* 45 (syook 3): 1–7
103 Dresner D, Coyle W, Nemec R, Peterson R, Duntemann T, Lawson JM (1996) Efficacy of ciprofloxacin in the eradication of *Helicobacter pylori*. *South Med J* 89: 775–778
104 Gupta VK, Dhar A, Srinivasan S, Rattan A, Sharma MP (1997) Eradication of *H. pylori* in a developing country: comparison of lansoprazole *versus* omeprazole with norfloxacin, in a dual-therapy study. *Am J Gastroenterol* 92: 1140–1142
105 Cammarota G, Cianci R, Cannizzaro O, Cuoco L, Pirozzi G, Gasbarrini A, Armuzzi A, Zocco MA, Santarelli L, Arancio F et al (2000) Efficacy of two one-week rabeprazole/levofloxacin-based triple therapies for *Helicobacter pylori* infection. *Aliment Pharmacol Ther* 14: 1339–1343
106 Sanchez JE, Saenz NG, Rincon MR, Martin IT, Sanchez EG, Martinez MJ (2000) Susceptibility of *Helicobacter pylori* to mupirocin, oxazolidinones, quinupristin/dalfopristin and new quinolones. *J Antimicrob Chemother* 46: 283–285
107 Carbone M, Fera MT, Cecchetti V, Tabarrini O, Losi E, Cusumano V, Teti G (1997) *In vitro* activities of new quinolones against *Helicobacter pylori*. *Antimicrob Agents Chemother* 41: 2790–2792
108 Krueger WA, Ruckdeschel G, Unertl K (1997) Influence of intravenously administered ciprofloxacin on aerobic intestinal microflora and fecal drug levels when administered simultaneously with sucralfate. *Antimicrob Agents Chemother* 41: 1725–1730
109 Krueger WA, Ruckdeschel G, Unertl K (1999) Elimination of fecal Enterobacteriaceae by intravenous ciprofloxacin is not inhibited by concomitant sucralfate – a microbiological and pharmacokinetic study in patients. *Infection* 27: 335–340
110 Cofsky RD, duBouchet L, Landesman SH (1984) Recovery of norfloxacin in feces after administration of a single oral dose to human volunteers. *Antimicrob Agents Chemother* 26: 110–111
111 Pecquet S, Andremont A, Tancrede C (1987) Effect of oral ofloxacin on fecal bacteria in human volunteers. *Antimicrob Agents Chemother* 31: 124–125
112 Edlund C, Sjostedt S, Nord CE (1997) Comparative effects of levofloxacin and ofloxacin on the normal oral and intestinal microflora. *Scand J Infect Dis* 29: 383–386
113 Midtvedt T (1987) Influence of ofloxacin on the faecal flora. *Drugs* 34 (Suppl 1): 154–158
114 Janin N, Meugnier H, Desnottes JF, Woehrle R, Fleurette J (1987) Recovery of pefloxacin in saliva and feces and its action on oral and fecal floras of healthy volunteers. *Antimicrob Agents Chemother* 31: 1665–1668
115 Nakashima M, Kanamaru M, Uematsu T, Takiguchi A, Mizuno A, Itaya T, Kawahara F, Ooie T, Saito S, Uchida H et al (1988) Clinical pharmacokinetics and tolerance of fleroxacin in healthy male volunteers. *J Antimicrob Chemother* 22 (Suppl D): 133–144
116 Garcia-Calvo G, Molleja A, Gimenez MJ, Parra A, Nieto E, Ponte C, Aguilar L, Soriano F (2001) Effects of single oral doses of gemifloxacin (320 milligrams) *versus* trovafloxacin (200 milligrams) on fecal flora in healthy volunteers. *Antimicrob Agents Chemother* 45: 608–611
117 Stass H, Kubitza D (1999) Pharmacokinetics and elimination of moxifloxacin after oral and intravenous administration in man. *J Antimicrob Chemother* 43 (Suppl B): 83–90
118 Vries-Hospers HG, Welling GW, van der WD (1987) Influence of quinolones on throat- and faecal flora of healthy volunteers. *Pharm Weekbl Sci* 9 (Suppl): S41–S44
119 Bergan T, Delin C, Johansen S, Kolstad IM, Nord CE, Thorsteinsson SB (1986) Pharmacokinetics of ciprofloxacin and effect of repeated dosage on salivary and fecal microflora. *Antimicrob Agents Chemother* 29: 298–302
120 Brumfitt W, Franklin I, Grady D, Hamilton-Miller JMT, Iliffe A (1984) Changes in the pharmacokinetics of ciprofloxacin and fecal flora during administration of a 7-day course to human vol-

unteers. *Antimicrob Agents Chemother* 26: 757–761
121 Shah PM, Enzensberger R, Glogau O, Knothe H (1987) Influence of oral ciprofloxacin or ofloxacin on fecal flora of healthy volunteers. *Am J Med* 82 (Suppl 4A): 333–335
122 Shah PM, Sammann A, Schafer V, Seczendi M, Knothe H (1988) Fleroxacin: safety, tolerance and effect on the faecal flora of healthy volunteers. *J Antimicrob Chemother* 22 (Suppl D): 209–213
123 van Nispen CH, Hoepelman AI, Rozenberg-Arska M, Verhoef J, Purkins L, Willavize SA (1998) A double-blind, placebo-controlled, parallel group study of oral trovafloxacin on bowel microflora in healthy male volunteers. *Am J Surg* 176: 27S-31S
124 Edlund C, Beyer G, Hiemer-Bau M, Ziege S, Lode H, Nord CE (2000) Comparative effects of moxifloxacin and clarithromycin on the normal intestinal microflora. *Scand J Infect Dis* 32: 81–85
125 Barker PJ, Sheehan R, Teillol-Foo M, Palmgren AC, Nord CE (2001) Impact of gemifloxacin on the normal human intestinal microflora. *J Chemother* 13: 47–51
126 DuPont H, Corrado ML, Subbaj J (1987) Use of norfloxacin in the treatment of acute diarrheal disease. *Am J Med* 82 (Suppl 6B): 79–83
127 DuPont H, Ericsson CD, Mathewson JJ et al (1992) Five *versus* three days of ofloxacin therapy for traveller's diarrhoea: a placebo-controlled study. *Antimicrob Agents Chemother* 36: 87–91
128 Salam I, Katelaris P, Leigh-Smith s Farthing MJG (1994) Randomised trial of single-dose ciprofloxacin for travellers' diarrhea. *Lancet* 344: 1537–1539
129 Wistrom J, Jertborn M, Ekwall E, Norlin K, Soderquist B, Stromberg A, Lundholm R, Hogevik H, Lagergren L, Englund G et al (1992) Empiric treatment of acute diarrheal disease with norfloxacin. A randomized, placebo-controlled study. Swedish Study Group. *Ann Intern Med* 117: 202–208
130 Sanchez C, Garcia-Restoy E, Garau J, Bella F, Freixas N, Simo M, Lite J, Sanchez P, Espejo E, Cobo E et al (1993) Ciprofloxacin and trimethoprim-sulfamethoxazole *versus* placebo in acute uncomplicated *Salmonella* enteritis: a double-blind trial. *J Infect Dis* 168: 1304–1307
131 Limson BM, Littaua RT (1989) Comparative study of ciprofloxacin *versus* co-trimoxazole in the treatment of *Salmonella* enteric fever. *Infection* 17: 105–106
132 Unal S, Hayran M, Tuncer S, Gur D, Uzun O, Akova M, Akalin HE (1996) Treatment of enteric fever with pefloxacin for 7 days *versus* 5 days: a randomized clinical trial. *Antimicrob Agents Chemother* 40: 2898–2900
133 Tran TH, Bethell DB, Nguyen TT, Wain J, To SD, Le TP, Bui MC, Nguyen MD, Pham TT, Walsh AL et al (1995) Short course of ofloxacin for treatment of multidrug-resistant typhoid. *Clin Infect Dis* 20: 917–923
134 Uwaydah AK, al Soub H, Matar I (1992) Randomized prospective study comparing two dosage regimens of ciprofloxacin for the treatment of typhoid fever. *J Antimicrob Chemother* 30: 707–711
135 Bennish ML, Salam MA, Haider R, Barza M (1990) Therapy for shigellosis. II. Randomized, double-blind comparison of ciprofloxacin and ampicillin. *J Infect Dis* 162: 711–716
136 Salam MA, Bennish ML (1988) Therapy for shigellosis. I. Randomized, double-blind trial of nalidixic acid in childhood shigellosis. *J Pediatr* 113: 901–907
137 Khan WA, Seas C, Dhar U, Salam MA, Bennish ML (1997) Treatment of shigellosis: V. Comparison of azithromycin and ciprofloxacin. A double-blind, randomized, controlled trial. *Ann Intern Med* 126: 697–703
138 Gotuzzo E, Obergelman RA, Maguina C, Berry SJ, Yi a Guzman M, Ruiz R, Leon-Barua R, Sack RB (1989) Comparison of single-dose treatment with norfloxacin and standard 5-day treatment with trimethoprim-sulfamethoxazole for acute shigellosis in adults. *Antimicrob Agents Chemother* 33: 1101–1104
139 Gotuzzo E, Seas C, Echevarria J, Carrillo C, Mostorino R, Ruiz R (1995) Ciprofloxacin for the treatment of cholera: a randomized, double-blind, controlled clinical trial of a single daily dose in Peruvian adults. *Clin Infect Dis* 20: 1485–1490
140 Khan WA, Begum M, Salam MA, Bardhan PK, Islam MR, Mahalanabis D (1995) Comparative trial of five antimicrobial compounds in the treatment of cholera in adults. *Trans R Soc Trop Med Hyg* 89: 103–106

Fluoroquinolone Antibiotics
ed. by A.R. Ronald and D.E. Low

The quinolones in otitis media and upper respiratory infections

Eugene Leibovitz and Ron Dagan

Pediatric Infectious Disease Unit, Soroka University Medical Center and the Faculty of Health Sciences, Ben-Gurion University of the Negev, Beer-Sheva 84101, Israel

Introduction

Upper respiratory tract infections are a frequent cause of illness. In children, acute otitis media (AOM) is the most common illness for which children receive medical attention. In adults, 20 million cases of bacterial sinusitis are reported yearly and the disease represents the fifth most common diagnosis for which an antibiotic is prescribed [1].

Pediatric acute otitis media and sinusitis and adult sinusitis share common etiological agents, the vast majority of bacterial infections being caused mainly by *Streptococcus pneumoniae*, *H. influenzae*, *Moraxella catarrhalis* and *Streptococcus pyogenes*. While penicillins and aminopenicillins remain the first-line therapy for the majority of cases of pediatric upper respiratory tract infections, the increasing prevalence of penicillin-resistant and β-lactamase-producing microorganisms required a re-evaluation of the traditional antimicrobial strategies used in the treatment of upper respiratory tract infections in children. Some cephalosporins (particularly the second generation cefuroxime-axetil and third generation ceftriaxone) represent valuable second-line or alternative first-line therapeutic options.

This article reviews the available literature pertaining to the use of another group of antibiotics, the fluoroquinolones, in the treatment of upper respiratory tract infections. While broadly accepted for the treatment of many infections, as a result of their favorable pharmacokinetic properties, high antimicrobial activity and low incidence of adverse effects, their limited activity against *S. pneumoniae* and methicillin-resistant *Staphylococcus aureus* has caused reluctance in using these compounds for the treatment of respiratory tract infections. The new fluoroquinolones, by exhibiting greater potency than the older ones (ciprofloxacin and ofloxacin) against Gram-positive cocci and particularly against *S. pneumoniae*, represent today a valuable choice for the treatment of respiratory tract infections.

There is only limited experience with the use of fluoroquinolones in the treatment of acute nonresponsive/recurrent AOM and in chronic suppurative otitis media but there is no pediatric experience with these compounds in sinusitis. A section in this chapter will review the experience accumulated with the use of fluoroquinolones in the treatment of sinusitis in adults.

Quinolones in pediatrics

Quinolone usage in children has been limited following the observation of arthrotoxicity in juvenile animals [2]. This phenomenon has been initially described with nalidixic acid [3]. The arthropathy evolves within days to weeks of drug administration and is characterized by typical histopathological lesions: fluid-filled blisters, fissures, erosions, and clusters of chondrocytes. These lesions are associated with noninflammatory joint effusions, and it is hypothesized that the effect of quinolones in some animal species may reflect inhibition of mitochondrial DNA replication in immature chondrocytes. Ironically, the drug with the greatest arthropathic effect in animals, nalidixic acid, is the only one approved for use in children and has proved to be well tolerated in this population [4].

While a clear-cut species and drug differences in quinolones effect on cartilage exists, the only evidence of any arthropathy in prepubertal humans was manifested by infrequent joint complaints occurring among pediatric patients (mainly-[60%]-in adolescent patients with cystic fibrosis, in whom arthropathy may also occur without administration of fluoroquinolones) who were followed after treatment with fluoroquinolones [5].

Overall, arthralgia occurred during 31/2030 (1.5%) ciprofloxacin oral or intravenous ciprofloxacin treatments of 1795 children, an adverse event pattern that was similar to that seen in adults; the majority were of mild to moderate intensity and resolved without intervention. A comprehensive review of 31 previous reports showed no quinolone-associated arthropathy in over 7,000 children and adolescents who received ciprofloxacin, ofloxacin or nalidixic acid [6].

Acute otitis media

More than 24 million cases of acute otitis media (AOM) are seen annually in the US and the number of cases has increased substantially during the last two decades [7]. The disease can be met already early in life and at 1 year of age about 75% of children will have developed at least one AOM episode [8]. The rate of recurrent AOM episodes has also increased from 18% of all AOM cases in 1981 to 26% in 1988 [9]. AOM represents today the main reason for antimicrobial therapy and for surgery in the pediatric population in the United States [7]. Although antibiotic therapy is required in only 20–30% of all cases of AOM, most of the patients are treated with antibiotics since this small proportion cannot be quickly and easily identified, and thus antibiotics are the standard of care for the treatment of AOM in the US and many other countries [9].

Antibiotic resistance

By using appropriate microbiologic detection techniques, pathogenic bacteria may be recovered from the MEF of up to 70–90% of patients with AOM [10]. The main bacterial causes of AOM are *Streptococcus pneumoniae*, non- typable *Haemophilus influenzae* and *Moraxella catarrhalis* [11]. *Streptococcus pneumoniae* causes 30–40% of all cases of AOM and is the least likely to resolve without treatment [12]. A dramatic emergence of multiple-drug resistant *S. pneumoniae* has been reported all over the world [11, 12]. A substantial amount of cross-resistance exists between macrolides, trimethoprim-sulfamethoxazole (TMP/SMX) and penicillin.

Most of the oral cephalosporins, with the exception of cefuroxime-axetil, cefpodoxime-proxetil and cefprozil are not active against penicillin-intermediate and resistant strains of *S. pneumoniae*. Among intravenous cephalosporins, ceftriaxone and cefotaxime have the lowest MICs, but high-level resistance of *S. pneumoniae* to these agents has been reported [11, 12]. *Streptococcus pneumoniae* is either very sensitive or highly resistant to macrolides (including erythromycin, azithromycin and clarithromycin) and TMP/SMX [11, 12].

Haemophilus influenzae causes 30–35% of all cases of AOM and only 5–10% belong to serotype b, the remaining usually being untypable. Between 15 to 50% of *H. influenzae* isolates produce β-lactamase. *Moraxella catarrhalis* is recovered in 5–10% of cases of AOM and >90% of the strains are β-lactamase producers.

In a recent multinational study on the prevalence of antimicrobial-resistant pathogens in MEF during 1994–1995 in the United States, Central and Eastern Europe and Israel, 30% of *S. pneumoniae* isolates were intermediately or fully resistant to penicillin while 31% and 100%, respectively, of the *H. influenzae* and *M. catarrhalis* isolates were β-lactamase producers [13].

In southern Israel, a major increase in antibiotic-resistance was observed among *S. pneumoniae* isolated from MEF of patients with AOM [10]. While 10% of *S. pneumoniae* strains were non- susceptible to penicillin (MIC > 0.1 μg/ml) in 1992, their number rose to 58% in 1998 and 71% in 1999. Forty-two percent of these pneumococcal isolates were also resistant to second generation cephalosporins. The resistance to macrolides rose from 3% to 14% and the resistance to TMP-SMX from 13% to around 50%. The resistance of *S. pneumoniae* to three antibiotic classes (multi-drug resistance) rose from 1% only in 1992 to 17% in 1999. The resistance of *H. influenzae* to TMP-SMX was around 30% during 1998 [10].

Current recommendations for the management of acute otitis media

In general, antibiotics have to be administered if AOM is diagnosed in infants and young children with recurrent AOM, in those with structural or immunologic abnormalities and in those patients who are severely ill. Older children

(>2 years age), patients without fever and those with minimal clinical signs may be managed without antibiotics, but a follow-up evaluation is required 24–72 h after initiation of treatment.

The Drug-resistant *S. pneumoniae* Therapeutic Working Group of the CDC has recently published new guidelines for the antibiotic treatment of AOM in the present era of pneumococcal resistance [14]. According to these guidelines, amoxicillin (40–50 mg/kg/day or the high dosage of 70–90 mg/kg/day) represents the first-line treatment of choice for AOM (Fig. 1).

The three second-line antibiotic drugs recommended at present time for clinical failures are: 1) amoxicillin/clavulanate (the 45 mg/kg/day amoxicillin dose or in the future the 90 mg/kg/day dose) for 10 days; 2) cefuroxime-axetil (30 mg/kg/day) for 10 days; 3) intramuscular ceftriaxone (50 mg/kg/day) for 3 days.

I. FIRST-LINE THERAPY

1) *Amoxicillin 50 mg/kg/day for 10 days:*
   - empiric treatment of first episode of AOM
   - empiric treatment of AOM in older children (>2 years of age)
   - empiric treatment of AOM areas with low prevalence of pneumococcal penicillin resistance

2) *Amoxicillin 80–90 mg/kg/day for 10 days:*
   - empiric treatment of AOM in areas with high prevalence of pneumococcal penicillin resistance
   - empiric treatment of AOM in young children (<2 years of age)

3) *β-lactam stable drugs for 10 days:*
   - empiric treatment of AOM in neonates
   - empiric treatment of AOM in immunocompromized patients
   - empiric treatment of AOM in area with high prevalence of β-lactamase producing organisms

II. SECOND –LINE THERAPY*

1) *Amoxicillin/clavulanate* (high dose) for 10 days
2) *Cefuroxime axetil* (30 mg/kg/day) for 10 days
3) *IM Ceftriaxone* (50 mg/kg/day) for 3 days

* therapeutic failure considered not before 72 h of first-line therapy; diagnostic and therapeutic tympanocentesis and MEF culture recommended before initiation of second-line therapy.

Figure 1. The antibiotic management of acute otitis media in the era of antibiotic-resistant *S. pneumoniae*

Non-responsive acute otitis media

Non-responsive AOM, defined as persistence of both clinical and otoscopic findings of tympanic membrane inflammation after 48–72 h of antibiotic therapy, occurs in >10% of children treated with antibiotics. Contributory factors to the development of this entity are low age of patients, presence of mixed bacterial and viral infection, a history of recurrent episodes of AOM, repeated previous courses of antibiotic therapy and daycare center attendance. *S. pneumoniae,* and particularly the resistant strains, are found significantly more frequently in the MEF of children with non-responsive AOM and/or having recurrent episodes of AOM [15].

Recent studies demonstrated a high correlation between antibiotic-resistant *S. pneumoniae* strains and the treatment failures: only 14–21% *S. pneumoniae* isolated from patients with non-responsive AOM were susceptible to the antibiotic drug previously prescribed [15].

Today, only three second-line drugs are considered as appropriate for the treatment of non-responsive AOM: amoxicillin/clavulanate, cefuroxime-axetil or intramuscular ceftriaxone [14]. Cefaclor, cefixime, loracarbef, ceftibuten, azithromycin and TMP/SMX can no longer be recommended for the empiric treatment of non-responsive AOM [14].

New fluoroquinolones in the treatment of acute otitis media

There is no place for fluoroquinolones in the therapy of simple uncomplicated AOM. However, the paucity of the therapeutic armamentarium in the treatment of persistent/non-responsive/recurrent AOM makes the search for alternative therapeutic options imperative. The only new fluoroquinolone studied at the present time in the treatment of complicated AOM is gatifloxacin. This new fluoroquinolone has an excellent activity against the three main pathogens causing AOM (MIC_{90} of 0.5, ≤ 0.03 and ≤ 0.03 μg/ml, respectively, against *S. pneumoniae*, *H. influenzae* and *M. catarrhalis*, respectively) [16]. In addition, susceptibility of *S. pneumoniae* for gatifloxacin was unchanged with penicillin-resistant strains and the drug was shown less frequently to select drug-resistant mutants from wild-type *S. pneumoniae* compared to other marketed quinolones [17, 18].

Leibovitz et al. [19] recently reported on the bacteriologic and clinical efficacy and safety of gatifloxacin oral suspension (10 mg/kg once daily for 10 days) in the treatment of 130 infants and young children aged 6–48 months (median age 11 months, 66 < 1 year age) with recurrent/non-responsive AOM. One hundred and seven (82%) patients completed the treatment with an overall bacteriologic and clinical efficacy of 97% and 98%, respectively. All *S. pneumoniae, H. influenzae and M. catarrhalis* isolates were sensitive to gatifloxacin. The adverse events rate was low (12%) and included mild and transient neutropenia (5%), vomiting (3%) impaired liver function tests (2%), and diarrhea, thrombocytopenia and rash (1% each), without any articular event during therapy and a 3-week follow-up period.

Dagan et al. [20] analyzed the dynamics of nasopharyngeal pneumococcal carriage in the same 130 infants and young children during and after gatifloxacin therapy. They reported that the gatifloxacin therapy reduced the nasopharyngeal pneumococcal carriage rate from 69% at enrollment (all sensitive to gatifloxacin, MIC < 0.5 μg/ml) to 33% on day 4–6 of therapy. However, the initial nasopharyngeal pneumococcal colonization rates were regained on day 12–14 (58%) and the rates peaked to above pre-treatment values (84%) on day 22–30 following initiation of therapy. The susceptibility patterns to gatifloxacin of the *S. pneumoniae* isolates before, during and after completion of therapy were similar. In contrast, non-susceptibility to penicillin (61%), TMP/SMX (48%) and erythromycin (13%) was lower on day 22–30 than before initiation of gatifloxacin therapy [20].

Arguedas et al. [21] enrolled 254 children with recurrent/non-responsive AOM (aged 6 months–7 years) with gatifoxacin oral suspension 10 mg/kg/once daily for 10 days and reported on clinical outcome of the 173 evaluable for analysis patients at 4–7 days after the last dose of the drug. The cure (defined as resolution of pain and tympanic membrane bulging and no additional prescription of antibiotics) rate in the evaluable patients was 87% (91% for those patients in whom *S. pneumoniae* was isolated at enrollment). The most frequent drug-related adverse events were vomiting (15%) and diarrhea (5%). There have been no reports of arthropathy.

These preliminary results showed that gatifloxacin was highly efficacious and safe in the therapy of recurrent/non-responsive AOM in children. However, this drug should be used with caution in the future in order to restrict the selection pressure on various bacterial populations. In addition, comparative studies with other antibiotic drugs in common use in the therapy of AOM are warranted.

Acute otitis media in adults

Otitis media is infrequent in adults, but the bacteriology and therapy are similar to those in children [22]. No information is available in the English medical literature regarding the use of fluoroquinolones in the treatment of AOM in adults.

Chronic suppurative otitis media

Chronic suppurative otitis media is defined as chronic inflammation of the middle ear and mastoid with a non-intact tympanic membrane and otorrhea. The yearly incidence of the disease is ~39/100,000 in children and 1.5% in adults [23, 24]. The most common organisms isolated from the middle ear fluid of children suffering from this condition include *P. aeruginosa*, *S. aureus*, *S. epidermidis*, viridans streptococci and *S. pneumoniae* [23–25].

The initial management of chronic suppurative otitis media includes thorough aural cleaning and administration of ototopical agents. The ototopical agents most commonly used are polymyxin B-neomycin-hydrocortisone and gentamycin ophthalmic drops [25]. The potential ototoxicity of these compounds created the need to look for alternative therapeutic options. Ofloxacin otic solution was found to be also efficacious in the treatment of this condition and is approved for use in children 12 years of age and older [25, 26]. Recently, the Cochrane systematic review of interventions in chronic otitis media showed that quinolone ear drops are more effective than non-quinolone ones both in reducing discharge and in eradicating bacteria [27].

Oral ciprofloxacin (30 mg/kg/day in two daily doses for 10 to 25 days) was used in 21 patients aged 22 months to 14 years who had failed conventional therapy for otitis; *P. aeruginosa* was isolated in 86% [28]. Suppuration disappeared in 86% of patients after a mean of 9.7 days, but three cases of failure with development of resistance to ciprofloxacin were documented. Relapse of disease occurred in 39% patients during a 16-month follow-up. Normal growth and no arthropathy were demonstrated during a follow-up period of 29 to 42 months.

Malignant external otitis

Although not an upper respiratory infection *per se*, this entity is often addressed when reporting on the therapeutic approach to these conditions. Invasive (malignant) otitis externa is a severe necrotizing infection caused exclusively by *P. aeruginosa* which spreads form the squamous epithelium of the ear canal to adjacent areas of soft tissue, blood vessels, cartilage and bone. Combination therapy consisting of an antipseudomonal agent (ceftazidime, ticarcillin of piperacillin) plus an aminoglycoside is the treatment of choice for this condition. Oral ciprofloxacin was also found efficacious when started early in the treatment of malignant external otitis [29].

Acute bacterial rhinosinusitis

Acute bacterial rhinosinusitis is a complication of viral upper respiratory infections in 0.5 to 2.0% of cases. In studies using antral sinus puncture or rhinoscopic middle meatal cultures, the bacterial species accounting for the majority of cases in both children and adults include *S. pneumoniae* (20–40%, of which up to 28–40% are nonsusceptible to penicillin), *H. influenzae* (20–30%) and *M. catarrhalis* (2–10%) and, to a lesser extent, *S. pyogenes*, other α-hemolytic streptococci, *S. aureus*, anerobic bacteria or fungi [30, 31]. Nosocomial sinusitis has been most often associated with *S. aureus*, *P. aerug-*

inosa, *Seratia marcescens*, *K. pneumoniae*, *Enterobacter* spp and *P. mirabilis* and is often polymicrobial [31].

The antimicrobial therapy for acute rhinosinusitis is usually empirical. There is no published experience with the use of fluoroquinolones in the treatment of rhinosinusitis in children.

While ciprofloxacin has already been proven as efficacious as cefuroxime axetil in the treatment of acute rhinosinusitis in the community [32], its inferior activity against Gram-positive pathogens and particularly against *S. pneumoniae* are limiting factors in considering its use in the treatment of the disease in adults. Present recommendations for initial therapy of mild-moderate disease in adults who did not receive antibiotics during the previous 4–6 weeks include the use of new fluoroquinolones as first-line option in those patients allergic or intolerant to β-lactams. Recommendations for initial therapy in adults with moderate disease who have received antibiotics in the previous 4–6 weeks include levofloxacin, gatifloxacin, moxifloxacin, amoxicillin/clavulanate or combination therapy [32]. Levofloxacin and gatifloxacin were proven in recent studies as identical to clarithromycin and amoxicillin/clavulanate in terms of bacteriological efficacy and clinical outcome in adult patients with acute rhinosinusitis and received FDA approval for this indication [33–37].

Approximately 5–10% of cases of acute sinusitis do not improve (bacteriologically and clinically) after a course of antimicrobial therapy and develop chronic sinusitis. Limited information is available on the etiology of this entity and it seems that the pathogens recovered from sinus aspirates in patients with chronic sinusitis and their susceptibility patterns to the antibiotics administered are not different than those isolated in the acute form of this disease [38]. The commonly used therapeutic approach in the management of chronic sinusitis relies on additional courses of antimicrobials, sinus aspirates, intranasal or oral steroids and consideration of sinus surgery. The only fluoroquinolone evaluated in the treatment of chronic sinusitis was ciprofloxacin. In a double-blind comparison between ciprofloxacin and amoxicillin/clavulanic acid in 215 adults with chronic sinusitis, the reported clinical and bacteriologocal cure rates were 58.6% *versus* 51.2% and 88.9% *versus* 90.5%, respectively, in addition to better tolerability rates (mainly related to a larger number of gastrointestinal adverse event in the amoxicillin/clavulanic acid group) for the ciprofloxacin-treated patients [39].

References

1 McCraig LF, Hughes JM (1995) Trends in antimicrobial drug prescription among office-based physicians in the United States. *JAMA* 273: 214–219

2 Hooper DC, Wolfson JS (1991) Fluoroquinolone antimicrobial agents. *New England J Med* 324: 384–394

3 Norrby SR (1991) Side-effects of quinolones: comparison between quinolones and other antibiotics. *Eur J Clin Microbiol Infect Dis* 10: 378–383

4 Nuutinen M, Turtinen J, Uhari M (1994) Growth and joint symptoms in children treated with

nalidixic acid. *Pediatr Infect Dis J* 13: 798–800
5 Hampel B, Hullmann R, Schmidt H (1977) Ciprofloxacin in pediatrics: worldwide clinical experience based on compassionate use-safety report. *Pediatr Infect Dis J* 16: 127–129
6 Burkhardt JE, Walterspiel JN, Schaad UB (1997) Quinolone arthropathy in animals *versus* children. *Clin Infect Dis* 25: 1196–1204
7 Faden H, Duffy L, Boeve M (1998) Otitis media: back to basics. *Pediatr Infect Dis J* 17: 1105–1113
8 Lanphear BP, Byrd RS, Awinger P, Hall CB (1997) Increasing prevalence of recurrent acute otitis media among children in the United States. *Pediatrics* 99(3): E1
9 Kaleida PH, Casselbrandt ML, Rockette HE et al (1991) Amoxicillin or miringotomy or both for acute otitis media: results of a randomized clinical trial. *Pediatrics* 87: 466–474
10 Dagan R (2000) Clinical significance of resistant organisms in otitis media. *Pediatr Infect Dis J* 19: 378–382
11 Appelbaum PC (1992) Antimicrobial resistance in *Streptococcus pneumoniae*: an overview. *Clin Infect Dis* 15: 77–83
12 Jacobs MR (1996) Increasing importance of antibiotic-resistant *Streptococcus pneumoniae* in acute otitis media. *Pediatr Infect Dis J* 15: 940–943
13 Jacobs MR, Dagan R, Appelbaum PC, Burch DJ (1998) Prevalence of antimicrobial-resistant pathogens in middle ear fluid: multinational study of 917 children with acute otitis media. *Antimicrob Agents Chemother* 42: 589–595
14 Dowell SF, Butler JC, Giebink SG et al (1999) Acute otitis media: management and surveillance in an era of pneumococcal resistance- a report from the Drug-resistant *Streptococcus pneumoniae* Therapeutic Working Group. *Pediatr Infect Dis J* 18: 1–9
15 Leibovitz E, Raiz S, Piglansky L et al (1998) Resistance pattern of middle ear fluid isolates in acute otitis media recently treated with antibiotics. *Pediatr Infect Dis J* 17: 463–469
16 Perry CM, Barman Balfour JA, Lamb HM (1999) Gatifloxacin. *Drugs* 58: 683–696
17 Hoelmann DB, Lin G, Jacobs MR, Appelbaum PC (1999) Antipneumococcal activity of gatifloxacin compared with other quinolone and non-quinolone agents. *J Antimicrob Chemother* 43: 645–649
18 Fukuda H, Hiramatsu K (1999) Primary targets of fluoroquinolones in *Streptococcus pneumoniae*. *Antimicrob Agents Chemother* 43: 410–412
19 Leibovitz E, Piglansky L, Raiz S et al (2001) Bacteriological efficacy of gatifloxacin in the treatment of recurrent/non-responsive acute otitis media. *In*: Program and abstracts of the 41st Interscience Conference on Antimicrobial Agents and Chemotherapy, December 16–19, 2001, Chicago, MI (abstract 1558a)
20 Dagan R, Piglansky L, Greenberg D et al (2001) Dynamics of nasopharyngeal pneumococcal carriage in children with recurrent and non-responsive acute otitis media treated with gatifloxacin. *In*: Program and abstracts of the 41st Interscience Conference on Antimicrobial Agents and Chemotherapy, December 16–19, 2001, Chicago, MI (abstract G-1825)
21 Arguedas A, Sher L, Lopez E, Saez-Llorens X, Skuba K, Pierce P (2001) Gatifloxacin treatment of recurrent/non-responsive acute otitis media. *In*: Program and abstracts of the 41st Interscience Conference on Antimicrobial Agents and Chemotherapy, December 16–19, 2001, Chicago, MI (abstract 1534)
22 Celin S, Bluestone C, Stephenson J et al (1991) Bacteriology of acute otitis media in adults. *JAMA* 266: 2249–2252
23 Fliss DM, Shoham I, Leiberman A, Dagan R (1991) Chronic suppurative otitis media without cholesteatoma in children in Southern Israel. *Pediatr Infect Dis J* 10: 895–899
24 Fliss DM, Dagn R, Meidan N, Leiberman A (1992) Aerobic bacteriology of chronic suppurative otitis media without cholesteatoma in children. *Ann Otol Rhinol Laryngol* 101: 866–869
25 Sabella C (2000) Mangement of otorrhea in infants and children. *Pediatr Infect Dis J* 19: 1007–1008
26 Ghosh S, Panarese A, Parker AJ, Bull PD (2000) Quinolone ear drops for chronic otitis media. They are safer and more effective than aminoglycosides. *BMJ* 321: 126–127
27 Acuin J, Smith A, Mc Kenzie I (1999) Interventions for chronic suppurative otitis media. *In*: Cochrane Collaboration. Cochrane Library. Issue 4. Oxford: Update Software
28 Lang R, Goshen S, Raas-Rothschild A, Raz A, Ophir D, Wollach B, Berger I (1992) Oral ciprofloxacin in the management of chronic suppurative otitis media without cholesteatoma in children: preliminary experience in 21 children. *Pediatr Infect Dis J* 11: 925–929

29 Gehanno P (1994) Ciprofloxacin in the treatment of malignant external otitis. *Chemotherapy* 40: 35–40 (suppl 1)

30 Wald ER (1998) Microbiology of acute and chronic sinusitis in children and adults. *Am J Med Sci* 316: 13–20

31 (2000) Sinus and Allergy Health Partnership. Antimicrobial treatment guidelines for acute bacterial rhinosinusitis. *Otolaryngol Head Neck Surg* 123: S4–32

32 Weiss M, Hendrick K, Tillotson G, Gravelle K, the Rhinosinusitis Investigation Group (1998) Multicenter comparative trial of ciprofloxacin *versus* cefuroxime axetil in the treatment of acute rhinosinusitis in a primary care setting. *Clin Therap* 20: 921–931

33 Syndor TA, Kopp EJ, Anthony KE, LoCoco JM, Kim SS, Fowler CL (1998) Open-label assessment of levofloxacin for the treatment of acute bacterial sinusitis in adults. *Ann Allergy Asthma Immunol* 80: 357–362

34 Adelgass J, Jones TM, Ruoff G et al (1998) A multicenter, investigator-blinded, randomized comparison of oral levofloxacin an oral clarithromycin in the treatment of acute bacterial sinusitis. *Pharmacotherapy* 18: 1255–1263

35 Adelglass J, DeAbate CA, McElvaine P, Fowler CL, LoCocco J, Campbell T (1999) Comparison of the effectiveness of levofloxacin and amoxicillin-clavulanate for the treatment of acute sinusitis in adults. *Otolaryngol Head Neck Surg* 120: 320–327

36 Sisniega J, Jones RW, Kaminszczik G et al (1999) Treating acute, uncomplicated bacterial sinusitis with gatifloxacin. *J Resp Dis* 20: S11–16

37 Fogarty C, McAdoo MA, Paster RZ, Martel AY, Macko AC, Breen J (1999) Gatifloxacin *versus* clarithromycin in the management of acute sinusitis. *J Resp Dis* 20: S23–29

38 Winther B, Vickery CL, Gross CW, Hendley JO (1996) Microbiology of the maxillary sinus in adults with chronic sinus disease. *Am J Rhinol* 10: 347–350

39 Legent F, Bordure P, Beauvillain C, Berche P (1994) A double-blind comparison of ciprofloxacin and amoxycillin/clavulanic acid in the treatment of chronic sinusitis. *Chemotherapy* 40 suppl 1: 8–15

Fluoroquinolone Antibiotics
ed. by A.R. Ronald and D.E. Low

Quinolones in pneumonia

Thomas J. Marrie

Department of Medicine University of Alberta, 2F1.30 Walter C. Mackenzie Health Sciences Center, 6440 112th Street, Edmonton, Alberta, Canada, T6H 2B7

Pneumonia is an infectious process involving the alveoli and distal airways. It can be divided into three entities based upon the site of acquisition of the pneumonia – community; nursing home; nosocomial.

Community-acquired pneumonia

In order to understand the role of quinolones in the treatment of community-acquired pneumonia (CAP) it is necessary to understand the entity of CAP. Pneumonia is a common and often a serious illness. It is the sixth leading cause of death in the United States. About 600,000 persons are hospitalized with pneumonia each year and there are 64 million days of restricted activity due to this illness [1, 2]. Pneumonia has a clinical spectrum that ranges from mild severity to critical illness. The overall mortality rate for patients with CAP who require admission to hospital is 8% [3]. About 80% of adults with CAP are treated on an ambulatory basis.

Etiology of community-acquired pneumonia

Streptococcus pneumoniae is the most common cause of community-acquired pneumonia [4], accounting for about 50% of all cases [4]. *Chlamydia pneumoniae, Haemophilus influenzae,* aerobic Gram-negative bacilli, *Staphylococcus aureus, Legionella pneumophila* as well as other *Legionella* species, and *Mycoplasma pneumoniae,* are other causes of pneumonia. Indeed, over 100 microbial agents cause pneumonia. Inspite of this the etiology of pneumonia is established in only 40% to 50% of patients in research studies and in even fewer in everyday practice. Most patients who are treated for pneumonia in a physician's office have no studies done to determine the etiology of the pneumonia. Thus most antibiotic therapy for CAP is empirical. To aid the practitioner in choosing such therapy guidelines have been issued from the Canadian Infectious Diseases Society [5], the Infectious Diseases Society of America [6] and the American Thoracic Society [7]. For the first time both the

CIDS and IDSA guidelines recommend a respiratory fluoroquinolone (levofloxacin, moxifloxacin, gatifloxacin) for the treatment of adults with CAP admitted to hospital for treatment. In addition the CIDS guidelines [5] recommend a respiratory fluoroquinolone for adults with complicated ambulatory pneumonia (those with chronic obstructive pulmonary disease who have had antibiotic therapy and or oral corticosteroid therapy within the past 3 months). It is worth noting that a panel of experts convened by the Centers for Disease Control recommended that the new fluoroquinolones be limited to adults for whom other regimens have failed; those who are allergic to alternative agents or who have a documented infection with highly drug resistant pneumococci, e.g., penicillin MIC ≥ 4 mg/L [8]. Another factor that has impacted on the choice of antibiotic therapy for ambulatory pneumonia is the prevalence of penicillin and macrolide resistant *S. pneumoniae* in the community.

Why are the respiratory fluoroquinolones appropriate agents for the treatment of CAP?

The respiratory fluoroquinolones are active against penicillin and macrolide resistant *S. pneumoniae* [9, 10]. They are also active against most of the other microbial agents that cause CAP including – *S. aureus, H. influenzae, M. catarrhalis, C. pneumoniae, L. pneumophila, Legionella* species, *M. pneumoniae,* and most aerobic Gram-negative bacilli [10]. Both moxifloxacin and gatifloxacin are active against anaerobic bacteria [11, 12]. Peptostreptococci and most *Prevotella* and *Fusobacterium* spp. were inhibited by gatifloxacin at ≤ 1 mg/L in a US study while higher values ≤ 25 mg/L were noted in a Japanese study [11]. This antibiotic is also active against *Bacteroides* spp. [11]. Moxifloxacin inhibited 90% of 410 clinically important anaerobic bacterial strains at 2 mg/L [12]. *Clostridium, Fusobacterium, Eubacterium, Prevotella* and *Peptostreptoccus* spp., *Propionibactrium acnes* and some *Bacteroides* spp. were susceptible (MIC 90 ≤ 2 mg/L [12]). Ciprofloxacin is still the quinolone of choice for the treatment of pneumonia due to *Pseudomonas aeruginosa.* As a group the new so-called respiratory fluoroquinolones agents (levofloxacin, moxifloxacin, gatifloxacin) are well absorbed, ranging from 72% to 99% [10] and achieve high concentrations in bronchial mucosa, epithelial lining fluid and alveolar macrophages [9].

Results of treatment of CAP with respiratory fluoroquinolones

Antibiotic therapy is only one aspect of the treatment of CAP. Prompt diagnosis and attention to comorbidities and complications of pneumonia are essential for the successful management of the patient with CAP. Meehan et al. [13] carried out a retrospective multicenter cohort study of those >65 years of age presenting to emergency rooms with CAP using Medicare National Claims

History File from October 1, 1994 through September 30, 1995. Just over 75% of patients received antibiotics within 8 h of presenting at the emergency room. A significantly lower 30-day mortality rate was observed for those who received antibiotic therapy within 8 h of presentation.

Gleason et al. [14] reviewed the hospital records of 12,945 Medicare patients hospitalized for treatment of CAP and found that initial therapy with a second or third-generation cephalosporin plus a macrolide or a fluoroquinolone alone (the fluoroquinolones used were ciprofloxacin or ofloxacin) was associated with a lower 30-day mortality when compared with a non-pseudomonal third – generation cephalosporin alone. The combination of a beta-lactam/beta-lactamase inhibitor plus a macrolide and an aminoglycoside plus another agent was associated with an increased 30-day mortality.

Ball [9] reviewed 14 trials of new fluoroquinolones in the management of CAP. In only two of these trials a statistically significant difference in favor of the quinolone over the comparator was demonstrated. In one of these trials, File et al. [15] compared intravenous with stepdown to oral levofloxacin (or oral levofloxacin alone) vs IV ceftriaxone and/or oral cefuroxime with or without erythromycin. Ninety-six percent (217/226) of the levofloxacin treated subjects vs 90% (207/230) of the comparator treated patients demonstrated clinical success; the bacteriologic efficacy or eradication rates were 98% (125/128) for the levofloxacin treated patients vs 85% (122/144) for the comparator treated patients. In the trovafloxacin vs amoxicillin trial, 125/138 (91%) of the trovafloxacin treated patients vs 119/147 (81%) of the amoxicillin treated patients demonstrated clinical success ($p = 0.01$) [16]. Because of data showing an association with serious liver damage trovafloxacin is recommended only for patients with serious and life- or limb-threatening infections [17]. Indeed, in the review by Ball, 10 of the 14 trials reviewed involved trovafloxacin and grepafloxacin (no longer available, and sparfloxacin, which is not available in Canada). Two of the trials cited in Ball's review involve moxifloxacin vs amoxicillin or clarithromycin. In the moxifloxacin vs amoxicillin trial 136/159 (86%) of the moxifloxacin treated patients demonstrated clinical success at the end of study vs 138/169 (82%). Bacteriologic eradication rates were 63/70 (90%) vs 65/78 (83%). In the moxifloxacin vs clarithromycin trial the clinical success rates were 97% (107/110) for moxifloxacin and 95% (105/110) for clarithromycin. The bacteriologic eradication rates were not stated. Gatifloxacin resulted in cure of 95% of 184 patients with mild, moderate or severe CAP compared with 93% of 188 clarithromycin treated patients [18] and similar results were obtained in a trial of gatifloxacin vs intravenous ceftriaxone with stepdown to oral clarithromycin in patients with CAP requiring hospitalization [19].

Marrie et al. [20] conducted a randomized trial of a critical pathway for the treatment of CAP vs conventional management. The critical pathway consisted of a clinical prediction rule to guide the admission decision, levofloxacin therapy, and practice guidelines for switch from intravenous to oral levofloxacin and a discharge guideline. Nine hospitals were randomized to the pathway and 10 to conventional management. An intention to treat analysis was used. In 6 months 1743 patients were enrolled in the study, 795 in the intervention arm and 948 in the conventional treatment arm. Pathway use was associated with a 1.7 day reduction in the bed days per patient managed (4.4 vs 6.1 days; $p = .04$). Although inpatients at critical pathway hospitals had more severe disease, they required 1.7 fewer days of intravenous therapy (4.6 vs 6.3 days; $p = 0.1$) and were more likely to receive treatment with a single class of antibiotic (64% vs 27%; $p < .001$). Patients from this study were followed up at 2 and 6 weeks to determine factors that predicted resolution of symptoms [21]. Logistic regression analysis identified younger age, absence of asthma or chronic obstructive pulmonary disease, and levofloxacin treatment as significant predictors of symptom resolution.

Better and bigger trials are needed

Why do so many of the studies cited in this chapter show similar but very good outcomes for the antibiotic under investigation and for the comparator agent? Most of the patients included in these trials are only mildly to moderately ill. The sample sizes are generally too small to show a difference in cure rates, i.e., they are designed to show equivalency. It is also likely that the incorrect outcomes are being measured. Time to return to work and time to return to usual activities as well as the time to resolution of symptoms are measures that should be incorporated into future studies of community-acquired pneumonia. Studies of patients with acute exacerbation of chronic bronchitis have begun to use time to resolution of symptoms as an outcome measure. In this setting 40% of the patients treated with a quinolone, moxifloxacin, reported symptom relief within 3 days of starting therapy compared with 24% of patients treated with azithromycin ($p = 0.03$) [22]. Another important consideration is that these trials do not allow us to evaluate the impact of resistance because patients with pneumonia due to a resistant microorganism to the study agent and its comparator are excluded.

Resistance to fluoroquinolones

The new fluoroquinolones have been a significant advancement in the treatment of CAP. To maintain this important therapeutic advance it is critical that we use these antibiotics wisely so that our patients do not lose an easy to administer safe treatment. Thus the macrolides or doxycycline should remain the drugs of choice for the treatment of patients with CAP that can be treated on an ambulatory basis. Indeed, we are beginning to see resistance of *S. pneumoniae* emerging to the fluoroquinolones [23, 24]. In a study from Hong Kong Ho et al. found that the presence of chronic obstructive lung disease, nosocomial origin of infection, nursing home residence, fluroquinolone use during the 12 months prior to admission were all factors independently associated with levofloxacin resistant *S. pneumoniae* lower respiratory tract infection or colonization [23]. Chen et al. [24] performed susceptibility testing on 7551 isolates of *S. pneumoniae* collected in Canada from 1988 to 1998. They found that resistance to ciprofloxacin increased from 0 in 1993 to 1.7% in 1997 and 1998. The prevalence of resistance was higher in older patients (2.6% for those 65 years of age or older vs 1% among those 15–64 years of age) and higher among those from Ontario compared with the rest of Canada. They also noted that fluoroquinolone prescriptions increased from 0.8 to 5.5/100 persons/year. More recent data from Montreal [25] indicate that 13/672 (1.9%) isolates of *S. pneumoniae* were resistant to ciprofloxacin. The MICs increased over time – thus for the seven isolates from 1994–1997 the MIC was 4 mg/L while for the six isolates from 1998–2000 two had an MIC of 8 mg/L; one 16 mg/L and four had MICs of 32 mg/L. Fluoroquinolone resistant *S. pneumoniae* were clonal in Hong Kong [26] and exhibited considerable genetic variablility in Canada [27]. Data from these studies raise concerns about one of the recommendations in the Canadian Infectious Diseases Society guideline for the empiric treatment of CAP, namely use of a fluoroquinolone to treat patients with pneumonia who have COPD and have received antibiotic therapy or oral corticosteroid therapy in the previous 3 months [5].

Nursing home acquired pneumonia

With successful treatment of many diseases there has been a marked increase in the number of persons living to an old age. Twenty-one percent of those older than 85 years of age need help with bathing and 10% need help in using the toilet and transferring [28]. As a result facilities have evolved to care for these individuals. It has been estimated that 4.1% of those >65 years of age reside in nursing homes and 15% of those older than age 85 live in such facilities [29]. Individuals residing in these facilities exhibit a spectrum of health states, from healthy, self sufficient individuals to those who are frail and others who are bedridden. One of the most serious illnesses that can affect elderly residents of nursing homes is pneumonia.

Epidemiology

The attack rate for pneumonia is highest among those in nursing homes. Loeb et al. [30] studied 475 residents of five nursing homes and found that there were 1.2 episodes of pneumonia per 1,000 resident days. Pneumonia is the leading cause of infection requiring transfer of nursing home patients to hospital accounting for 10% to 18% of all pneumonia admissions [31].

Risk factors for pneumonia among residents of a nursing home

Profound disability (Karnofsky score of <10), bedfast state, urinary incontinence or deteriorating health status are risk factors for pneumonia in this setting [31]. In another study, old age, male gender, swallowing difficulty, and inability to take oral medications were risk factors for pneumonia while receipt of influenza vaccination was protective [30]. Factors that increase the risk of aspiration are likely to result in pneumonia. These are malnutrition, tube feedings, hyperextended neck, contractures, use of benzodiazepines and anticholinergic medications [28].

Etiology of nursing home-acquired pneumonia

El-Solh et al. [32] studied all patients >75 years of age admitted to intensive care with a diagnosis of CAP and requiring mechanical ventilation. Fifty-seven patients were admitted from home and 47 from a nursing home. Among the nursing home patients *Staphylococcus aureus* was the most common etiological agent at 35% (6% of the cases overall were due to methicillin resistant *S. aureus).* Aerobic Gram-negative bacilli as a group accounted for 18% of the cases (*Pseudomonas aeruginosa* accounted for 4% of the cases). *Streptococcus pneumoniae* was implicated in 9% of the cases and *Mycobacterium tuberculosis* in 2%. Outbreaks of influenza [33], respiratory syncytial virus [34], *Streptococcus pneumoniae* [35], and *Chlamydia pneumoniae* [36] may occur in nursing homes. Outbreaks of pneumonia due to *Legionella spp* in this setting seem to be uncommon but have occurred [37]. In addition colonization with methicillin resistant *Staphylococcus aureus* [38] and gentamicin and or ceftriaxone resistant Gram-negative bacilli are common among residents of some nursing homes [39]. Quinolone resistance among Gram-negative organisms isolated from nursing home residents ranged from 1% of *Escherichia coli* isolates to 72% of *Acinetobacter calcoaceticus* subspecies *anitratus* [40]. In six studies reporting on 471 patients with NHAP *S. pneumoniae* accounted for 12.9% of the cases, followed by *H. influenzae –6.4%;Staphylococcus aureus* –6.4% *Moraxella catarrhalis* –4.4%; aerobic Gram-negative bacilli –13.1% [41–46].

Treatment of nursing home acquired pneumonia

Naughton and Mylotte [47] performed a retrospective chart review of 239 episodes of NHAP and found that 72% were initially treated in nursing homes. 105/171 (61%) of these were treated only with an oral regime, while 66 (39%) were treated with an intramuscular antibiotic and subsequently with an oral regimen. There was no difference in the 30-day mortality rates between those initially treated in nursing homes (22%) and those initially treated in hospitals (31%). The most commonly used oral agent was cephalexin, followed by ciprofloxacin, and amoxicillin-clavulinic acid. A parenteral (intramuscular) antibiotic was prescribed for 39% of the episodes treated in a nursing home.

The major problem is that there is a paucity of randomized trials of antibiotic treatment of pneumonia in the nursing home.

Peterson et al. [48] carried out a trial of oral ciprofloxacin vs intramuscular cefamandole in patients with pneumonia and patients with acute bronchitis in a nursing home. The cure rates were high – 93% of the 30 patients treated with ciprofloxacin and 100% of the patients treated with cefamandole. In another study the same group of investigators [49] randomized 24 patients to receive ciprofloxacin IV and then P0 and 26 patients to receive ceftriaxone IV followed by IM. Fifty percent of the ciprofloxacin treated patients and 54% of the ceftriaxone treated patients had a favorable outcome. Recurrent oropharyngeal aspiration was the reason for treatment failure in most patients refractory to either antibiotic. The mortality rate was 8% in each group.

The Canadian Infectious Diseases Society and the Canadian Thoracic Society [5] guidelines recommend a respiratory fluoroquinolone or amoxicillin-clavulinic acid plus a macrolide for patients with NHAP who can be treated in the nursing home. A second generation cephalosporin plus a macrolide is an alternative. For those patients who require admission to hospital a respiratory fluorquinolone is recommended as the first choice. An alternative is a second, third, or fourth generation cephalosporin plus a macrolide. The Infectious Diseases Society of America guidelines for the treatment of community-acquired pneumonia do not deal at all with nursing home-acquired pneumonia [6]. The Society of Hospital Epidemiologists of America recommend trimethoprim – sulfamethoxazole, amoxicillin, cefuroxime axetil, macrolide, doxycycline; as second line antibiotics for the treatment of NHAP they recommend amoxicillin-clavulinic acid, quinolone, clindamycin (for aspiration pneumonia) [50].

Nosocomial pneumonia

Nosocomial pneumonia is pneumonia that develops after admission to hospital and was not incubating at the time of admission. Pneumonia is the third most common type of nosocomial infection (0.6% to 1.1% of hospitalized patients are affected) and one with a mortality rate of 28% to 37% [51]. Most patients who develop nosocomial pneumonia are receiving mechanical ventilation. The microbiology of nosocomial pneumonia is dominated by aerobic Gram-negative bacteria. Enterobacteriaceae account for almost half of all the isolates; *Staphylococcus aureus* 26%; *Pseudomonas aeruginosa* 9%; *Streptococcus pneumoniae* 31%; anaerobic bacteria 35%; and *Haemophilus influenzae* 17% [52]. Multi-drug resistant Enterobacteriaceae, *Pseudomonas aeruginosa* and methicillin resistant *Staphylococcus aureus* are common among patients with nosocomial pneumonia.

Prevention of nosocomial pneumonia is very important. The Centers for Disease Control have issued a comprehensive document that details the programs that hospitals should have to reduce occurrence of nosocomial pneumonia [53].

Correct empirical treatment of nosocomial pneumonia is vitally important. Celis and colleagues [54] found that 92% of patients with ventilator associated pneumonia died when treated with inappropriate antibiotics compared with a 31% mortality rate among those receiving appropriate antibiotics. Torres et al. [55] noted a 55% mortality among those receiving inappropriate antibiotics vs 23% for those with appropriate antibiotics.

There are very few good trials of treatment of nosocomial pneumonia. Fink et al. [56] carried out a randomized double blind trials of imipenem vs ciprofloxacin in severe pneumonia in hospitalized patients (78% of whom had nosocomial pneumonia). The dose of ciprofloxacin was 400 mg q 8 h and imipenem 1 gm q 8 h. There were 205 patients in the ciprofloxacin group and 200 in the imipenem group. One hundred and four and 85 in each group met the criteria for assessment of efficacy. Clinical resolution and bacterial eradication rates were significantly higher in the ciprofloxacin group than in the imipenem group both in the efficacy and intention to treat analyses. Emergence of resistance among *Pseudomonas aeruginosa* was common – 33% for the patients treated with ciprofloxacin who had this organism isolated vs 42% for the imipenem treated patients. These results suggest that neither of these agents should be used alone to treat nosocomial pneumonia because of the high rate of emergence of antimicrobial resistance. Zhanel et al. [10] carried out a comprehensive review of the literature on new fluoroquinolones between 1994 and 1998. They present in tabular form the results of 53 clinical trials in which these agents were used – only two of these trials included patients with nosocomial pneumonia. One trial compared clinafloxacin to ceftazidime and the other trovafloxacin with ciprofloxacin. A MEDLINE search of the literature since then failed to reveal any new clinical trials of these agents in the treatment of nosocomial pneumonia.

Concluding remarks

Most of the clinical trials of fluoroquinolones in the treatment of pneumonia involve patients with community-acquired pneumonia. The evidence suggests that they are effective. Currently there are no data to suggest that one fluoroquinolone is clinically superior to another, however this may be due to design of the trials which are powered to show equivalence and lack of trials comparing one fluoroquinolone to another. Because of emerging resistance to fluoroquinolones among isolates of *S. pneumoniae* these agents should be reserved for patients who require admission to hospital for the treatment of community-acquired pneumonia.

There are no data to allow conclusions as to the utility of new fluoroquinolones for the treatment of nursing home acquired pneumonia. Ciprofloxacin seems to be effective for the treatment of nursing home acquired pneumonia.

The newer fluoroquinolones lack activity against *P. aeruginosa* and hence should not be first line agents for the empiric treatment of nosocomial pneumonia, especially ventilator associated pneumonia.

If advances are to be made in the treatment of pneumonia we can no longer rely on pharmaceutical industry sponsored trials. Instead granting agencies should be prepared to fund multicenter clinical trials that are designed to answer key clinical questions.

Restriction of fluoroquinolone use for the treatment of patients with acute exacerbation of chronic bronchitis is likely to be the most important measure in controlling *S. pneumoniae* resistance to these agents.

References

1 Dixon RE (1985) Economic costs of respiratory tract infections in the United States. *Am J Med* 78: 45–51

2 National Centre for Health Statistics (1992) National hospital discharge survey: annual summary 1990. *Vital Health Statistics* 13: 1–225

3 Fine MJ, Stone RA, Singer DE et al (1999) Processes and outcomes of care for patients with community-acquired pneumonia. Results from the pneumonia patient outcomes research team (PORT) cohort. *Arch Intern Med* 159: 970–980 (*This study presents the results of a comprehensive observation study of community-acquired pneumonia. Data are given on both ambulatory and hospitalized patients with pneumonia.*)

4 Marrie TJ, Durant H, Yates L (1989) Community-acquired pneumonia requiring hospitalization: 5-year prospective study. *Rev Infect Dis* 11: 586–599 (*A longitudinal study of patients with community-acquired pneumonia requiring hospitalization for treatment. A major effort was made to define etiology of pneumonia. Patients with nursing home acquired pneumonia were included in the study and they are compared to patients from the community. All patients presenting with pneumonia were included in the study so it presents a comprehensive picture of CAP.*)

5 Mandell LA, Marrie TJ, Grossman RF, Chow AW, Hyland RH, the Canadian Community-Acquired Pneumonia Working Group (2000) Canadian guidelines for the initial management of community-acquired pneumonia: An evidence-based update by the Canadian Infectious Diseases Society and the Canadian Thoracic Society. *Clin Infect Dis* 31: 383–421 (*A comprehensive review of the literature on pneumonia with the objective of applying evidence based approach to guidelines for empiric treatment of community-acquired pneumonia.*)

6 Bartlett JG, Dowell SF, Mandell LA, File TMJr Musher DM, Fine MJ (2000) Practice guidelines for the management of community-acquired pneumonia in adults. *Clin Infect Dis* 31: 347–382 (*Also a comprehensive approach to guidelines for the empiric treatment of CAP. There are some differences between the Canadian and American approaches to this common problem especially in the management of ambulatory pneumonia.*)

7 Niederman MS, Mandell LA, Anzueto A et al (2001) Guidelines for the management of adults with community-acquired pneumonia. Diagnosis, assessment of severity, antimicrobial therapy and prevention. *Am J Respir Crit Care Med* 163: 1730–1754 (*The most recent of the guidelines trinity. There are subtle differences in the recommendations among the three sets of guidelines. It is useful to read all three. Both the Canadian and this guideline have separate recommendations for ambulatory patients who have chronic obstructive lung disease. These recommendations are based on expert opinion.*)

8 Heffelfinger JD, Dowell SF, Jorgensen JH et al (2000) Management of community-acquired pneumonia in the era of pneumococcal resistance. A report from the drug-resistant *Streptococcus pneumoniae* therapeutic working group. *Arch Intern Med* 160: 1339–1408 (*An admonition to reserve fluoroquinolones for the treatment of drug resistant* S. pneumoniae *and not to use them as first line agents in the empiric management of community-acquired pneumonia.*)

9 Ball P (1999) New Fluoroquinolones: real and potential roles. *Current Infect Dis Reports* 1: 470–479 (*A short but very good review of the new fluoroquinolones. A considerable portion of the*

paper deals with quinolones that are no longer in use.)

10 Zhanel GG, Waltky A, Vercaigne L, Karlowsky JA, Embil J, Gin AS et al (1999) The new fluoroquinolones: a critical review. *Can J Infect Dis* 10: 207–238 (*A comprehensive review of fluoroquinolones; unfortunately it too devotes a lot of space to the quinolones that are no longer in use. The extensive biliography* (*257 references*) *is helpful.*)

11 Perry CM, Barman Balfour JA, Lamb HM (1999) Gatifloxacin. *Drugs* 58: 683–696

12 Barman Balfour JA, Wiseman LR (1999) Moxifloxacin. *Drugs* 57: 363–373

13 Meehan TP, Fine MJ, Krumholz HM, Scinto JD, Galusha DH, Mockalis JT et al (1997) Quality of care, process and outcomes in elderly patients with pneumonia. *JAMA* 278: 2080 (*A study that proves that timely administration of antibiotics to elderly patients with community-acquired pneumonia saves lives.*)

14 Gleason PP, Meehan TP, Fine JM, Galusha DH, Fine MJ (1999) Associations between initial antimicrobial therapy and medical outcomes for hospitalized elderly patients with pneumonia. *Arch Intern Med* 159: 2562–2572 (*A retrospective chart review which indicates that there are differences in outcomes for elderly patients with community-acquired pneumonia according to the antibiotic therapy that is chosen. The study design weakens the conclusions.*)

15 File TM, Segreti J, Dunbar L et al (1997) A multicenter, randomised study comparing the efficacy and safety of intravenous and/or oral levofloxacin *versus* ceftriaxone and/or cefuroxime axetil in treatment of adults with community-acquired pneumonia. *Antimicrob Agents Chemother* 41: 1965–1972 (*A well designed study which indicates that levofloxacin is better than the cephalosporin comparators.*)

16 Tremolieres F, de Kock F, Pluck Daniel R (1998) Trovafloxacin *versus* high dose amoxicillin (1 g three times daily) in the treatment of community-acquired pneumonia. *Eur J Clin Microbiol Infect Dis* 17: 447–453 (*This study is now of historic interest only.*)

17 USDepartment of Health Human Services Food Drug Administration (1999) FDA issues public health advisory on liver toxicity associate with the antibiotic Trovan [FDA talk paper]. Rockville, MD

18 Ramirez J, Nguyen T-H, Tellier G et al (1999) Treating community-acquired pneumonia with once-daily gatifloxacin vs twice-daily clarithromycin. *J Respir Dis* 20: S40–S48

19 Dowell M, Mayer H, Anderson A et al (1999) A randomised, double-blind, multicenter, comparative study of gatifloxacin (GAT) 400 mg IV and PO vs ceftriaxone +/– erythromycin (CTX +/– ERY) in treatment of community-acquired pneumonia requiring hospitalisation [abstract]. 39th Interscience Conference on Antimicrobial Agents and Chemotherapy, 1999, Sep 26–29, San Francisco

20 Marrie TJ, Lau Cy Wheeler SL, Wong CJ, Vandervoort MK, Feagan BG for the CAPITALStudy Investigators (2000) A controlled trial of a critical pathway for treatment of community-acquired pneumonia. *JAMA* 283: 749–755 (*A trial that show that a critical pathway* (*practice guidelines for admission, switch from intravenous to oral antibiotic therapy and discharge*) *is equivalent to standard therapy for community acquired pneumonia in terms of mortality, intensive care admission rate, failure of outpatient therapy, and complications but is associated with a significant decrease in the number of bed days per patient managed and fewer days on intravenous therapy.*)

21 Marrie TJ, Lau CY, Wheeler SL, Wong CJ, Feagan BG (2000) Predictors of symptom resolution in patients with community-acquired pneumonia. *Clin Infect Dis* 31: 1362–1367 (*The antibiotic chosen to treat pneumonia is one of the factors associated with persistent symptoms at follow-up.*)

22 Kreis S, the Therapeutic Circle Investigators (2000) Moxifloxacin compared to azithromycin in the treatment of acute exacerbations of acute bronchitis: an interim analysis of the Therapeutics Circles Program. *Chest* 118: S243

23 Ho Pl Tse Ws Tsan KW, Kwok Tk NTk Cheung VCC, Chan RMT (2001) Risk factors for acquistion of lefofloxacin-resistant *Streptococcus pneumoniae*: A case-control study. *Clin Infect Dis* 32: 701–707

24 Chen DK, McGeer A, de Azavedo JC, Low DE, The Canadian Bacterial Surveillance Network (1999) Decreased susceptibility of *Streptococcus pneumoniae* to fluoroquinolones in Canada. *N Engl J Med* 341: 233–239

25 Robson HG, Lavallee J (2001) Rapidly increasing resistance of *Streptococcus pneumoniae* to penicillin, macrolides and fluoroquinolones in a Canadian teaching hospital. Abstract C2-704; 41 Interscience Conference on Antimicrobial Agents and Chemotherapy, page 133, American Society for Microbiology, Chicago, Illinois, December 2001

26 Morrissey I, Farrell DJ, Enright MC, Felmingham D. Molecular characterization of fluoroquinolone-resistant *Streptococcus pneumoniae* PROTEK 2000 isolates from Hong Kong. Abstract

C2-703. 41 Interscience Conference on Antimicrobial Agents and Chemotherapy, page 133, American Society for Microbiology, Chicago, Illinois, December 2001
27 Nichol KA, Smith Hj Hoban DJ, Zhanel GG (2001) Genetic relationship of fluoroquinolone (FQ)-resistant *Streptococcus pneumoniae* in Canada. Abstrac C2-701. 41 Interscience Conference on Antimicrobial Agents and Chemotherapy, American Society for Microbiology, Chicago, Illinois, 132
28 Palmer RM (1995) Acute care of the elderly: minimizing the risk of functional decline. *Cleveland Cl J Med* 62: 117–128
29 Medina-Walpole AM, Katz PR (1999) Nursing home-acquired pneumonia. *J Am Geriatric Soc* 47: 1005–1015
30 Loeb M, McGeer A, McArthur M, Walter S, Simor AS (1999) Risk factors for pneumonia and other lower respiratory tract infections in elderly residents of long – term care facilities. *Arch Intern Med* 159: 2058–2064
31 Muder RR (1998) Pneumonia in residents of long-term care facilities: epidemiology, etiology, management and prevention. *Am J Med* 105: 319–330
32 El-Solh AA, Sikka P, Ramadan F, Davies J (2001) Etiology of severe pneumonia in the very elderly. *Am J Respir Crit Care Med* 163: 645–651
33 Patriarca PA, Weber JA, Parker SA et al (1986) Risk factors for outbreaks of influenza in nursing homes. *Am J Epidemiol* 124: 114–119
34 Sorvillo FJ, Huie SF, Strassburg MA, Butsumyo A, Shandera WX, Fannin SL (1984) An outbreak of respiratory syncytial virus pneumonia in a nursing home for the elderly. *J Infect* 9: 252–256
35 Kludt P, Lett SM, De Maria A et al (1997) Outbreaks of pneumococcal pneumonia among unvaccinated residents in chronic care facilites – Massachusetts, October 1995, Oklahama, February 1996 and Maryland, May-June 1996. *Morbid Mortal Wkly Rpt* 46: 60–62
36 Troy CJ, Peeling RW, Ellis AG et al (1997) *Chlamydia pneumoniae* as a new source of infectious outbreaks in nursing homes. *JAMA* 277: 1214–1218
37 Loeb M, Simor AE, Mandell L et al (1999) Two nursing home outbreaks of respiratory infection with *Legionella sainthelensi*. *J Am Geriatr Soc* 47: 547–552
38 Kotilaninen P, Routamaa M, Peltonen R, Evesti P, Eerola E, Salmenlinna S et al (2001) Eradication of methicillin-resistant *Staphylococcus aureus* from a health center ward and associated nursing home. *Arch Intern Med* 161: 859–863
39 Terpenning MS, Bradley SF, Wan JY, Chenoweth CE, Jorgensen KA, Kauffman CA (1994) Colonization and infection with antibiotic resistant bacteria in a long-term care facility. *J Am Geriatr Soc* 42: 1062–1069
40 Flournoy DJ (1994) Antimicrobial susceptibilities of bacteria from nursing home residents in Oklahoma. *Gerontology* 40: 53–56
41 Marrie TJ, Durant H, Yates L (1989) Community-acquired pneumonia requiring hospitalization: 5-year prosepctive study. *Rev Infect Dis* 11: 586–599
42 Garb JL, Brown RB et al (1978) Differences in etiology of pneumonias in nursing home and community patients. *J Am Med Assoc* 240: 2169–2172
43 Orr PH, Peeling RW, Fast M et al (1996) Serological study of responses to selected pathogens causing respiratory tract infection in the institutionalized elderly. *Clinical Infect Dis* 23: 1240
44 Phillips SL, Branaman-Phillips J (1993) The use of intramuscular cefoperazone *versus* intramuscular ceftriaxone in patients with nursing home acquired pneumonia. *J Am Geriatr Soc* 41: 1071–1074
45 Drinka PJ, Gauerke C, Voeks S, Miller J, Schultz S, Krause P et al (1994) Pneumonia in a nursing home. *J Gen Intern Med* 9: 650–652
46 Chow CW, Senathiragah N, Rawji M et al (1994) Interim report on drug utilization review of community-acquired and nosocomial pneumonia: clinical bacteriological and radiological spectrum. *Can J Infect Dis* 5 Suppl C: 20C–27C
47 Naughton BJ, Mylotte JM (2000) Treatment guideline for nursing home-acquired pneumonia based on community practice. *J Am Geriatr Soc* 48: 82–88
48 Peterson PK, Stein D, Guay DRP et al (1988) Prospective study of lower respiratory tract infections in an extended-care nursing home program: Potential role of oral ciprofloxacin. *Am J Med* 85: 164–171
49 Hirta-Dulas CAI, Stein DJ, Guay DRP et al (1991) A randomized study of ciprofloxacin *versus* ceftriaxone in the treatment of nursing home-acquired lower respiratory tract infections. *J Am Geriatr Soc* 39: 979–985
50 Nicolle LE, Bentley DW, Garibaldi R, Neuhaus EG, Smith PW, the SHEALong Term-Care com-

mittee (2000) Antimicrobial use in long-term-care facilities. SHEA Long-Term-Care Committee. *Infect Control Hosp Epidemiol* 21: 537–545
51 Dal Nogare AR (1994) Nosocomial pneumonia in the medical and surgical patient. Risk factors and primary management. *Med Clin N Am* 78: 1081–1090
52 Bartlett JG, O'Keefe P, Tally FP et al (1986) Bacteriology of hospital-acquired pneumonia. *Arch Intern Med* 146: 868–871
53 Centers for Disease Control (1997) Guidelines for prevention of nosocomial pneumonia. *MMWR* 46: RR1: 1–85
54 Celis R, Torres A, Gatell JM et al (1988) Nosocomial pneumonia: a multivariate analysis of risk and prognosis. *Chest* 93: 318–324
55 Torres A, Aznar R, Gatell JM et al (1990) Incidence, risk, and prognosis factors of nosocomial pneumonia in mechanically ventilated patients. *Am Rev Respir Dis* 142: 523–528
56 Fink MP, Snydman DR, Niederman MS et al (1994) Treatment of severe pneumonia in hospitalizaed patients: Results of a multicenter, randomized, double-blind trial comparing intravenous ciprofloxacin with imipenem-cilastatin. *Antimicrobial Agents Chemother* 38: 547–557

Fluoroquinolone Antibiotics
ed. by A.R. Ronald and D.E. Low

Fluoroquinolones for the treatment of respiratory tract infections other than pneumonia

Donald E. Low

Department of Microbiology, Toronto Medical Laboratories/Mount Sinai Hospital, University of Toronto and Canadian Bacterial Diseases Network, 600 University Ave., Rm. 1487, Toronto, Ontario, Canada M5G 1X5

Introduction

A variety of bacterial species are associated with acute respiratory tract infections, including Gram-positive, Gram-negative, and atypical pathogens. The most common pathogens include *Streptococcus pneumoniae, Mycoplasma pneumoniae, Chlamydia pneumoniae, Legionella* species, *Haemophilus influenzae,* and *Moraxella catarrhalis.* Because of cost considerations and specimen collection difficulties, primary care physicians seldom attempt to identify the causative pathogen. As a result treatment is necessarily empiric with agents including: the β-lactams, macrolides, tetracyclines, and trimethoprim-sulfamethoxazole (TMP-SMX). However, antimicrobial resistance among the most common respiratory tract pathogens to these agents is increasing [1–5]. Specifically, the growing problem of multidrug resistant pneumococci has been the catalyst for the development of fluoroquinolones such as levofloxacin, gatifloxacin, which are effective against this resistant organism. However, there are reports of fluoroquinolone resistance emerging among pneumococci from a number of countries including: Canada, Spain, Hong Kong, Eastern and Central Europe, and Northern Ireland (Fig. 1). In Canada, Chen et al. [6] found that the prevalence of ciprofloxacin-resistant pneumococci (MIC ≥ 4 μg/ml) increased from 0% in 1993 to 1.7% in 1997–1998 ($p = 0.01$). In adults, the prevalence increased from 0% in 1993 to 3.7% in 1998. In addition to the increase in prevalence of pneumococci with reduced susceptibility to fluoroquinolones, the degree of resistance also increased. From 1994 to 1998, there was a statistically significant increase in the proportion of isolates with a MIC for ciprofloxacin of ≥ 32 μg/ml ($p = 0.04$). Linares et al. [7] found that in Spain an increase of ciprofloxacin-resistant pneumococci from 0.9% in 1991–1992 to 3% in 1997–1998. Ho and colleagues [8, 9] documented a marked increase in the overall prevalence of non-susceptibility to the fluoroquinolones when comparing results of surveillance studies carried out in 1998 and 2000. Over a 2-year period, the prevalence of levofloxacin non-susceptibility (MIC ≥ 4 μg/ml) increased from 5.5% to 13.3% among all

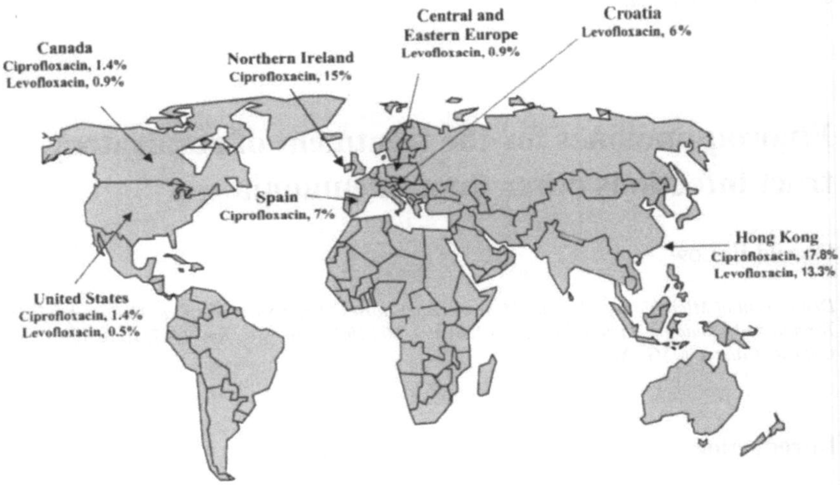

Figure 1. The prevalence of ciprofloxacin (MIC ≥ 4 μg/ml) and levofloxacin (MIC ≥ 4 μg/ml) resistance in *S. pneumoniae* worldwide. Adapted from references [2, 9, 10, 98, 99].

isolates and from 9.2% to 28.4% among the penicillin-resistant strains. Nagai and colleagues [10] carried out surveillance in 10 Central and Eastern European countries between 1999 and 2000. Overall, levofloxacin resistance was 0.9%, however, in Croatia, 6 (5.9%) of 101 isolates were levofloxacin resistant. In Northern Ireland, ciprofloxacin resistance was linked to penicillin resistance. Eighteen (42.9%) of 42 penicillin-resistant pneumococci were resistant to ciprofloxacin [11]. Rates of resistance in the United States are <2% [2, 12–15]. Doern et al. [2] reported ciprofloxacin resistance rates of 1.4%. The Centers for Disease Control's Active Bacterial Core Surveillance program carried out during 1995–1999 reported levofloxacin non-susceptible rates of 0.2% [15]. The CDC has not included ciprofloxacin as one of the agents they test.

In most countries reporting increasing ciprofloxacin resistance, it has been the result of the emergence of *de novo* resistance in many different serotypes [6, 16, 17]. However, in Hong Kong, the emergence of resistance has been due to the dissemination of a multiply resistant clone that shares an identical multilocus sequence typing allelic profile with the globally distributed strain Spain^{23F}-1 [9]. In Croatia, all six strains of levofloxacin resistant pneumococci had the same pulsed-field gel electrophoresis pattern and were serotype 23F [10]. McGee et al. [18] characterized a collection of 29 fluoroquinolone-resistant (ofloxacin MIC ≥ 4 mg/L) isolates of *S. pneumoniae* that were obtained from a study in Northern Ireland and from the Alexander Project, an international network that was established in 1992 to monitor the development of antimicrobial resistance to major lower respiratory tract bacterial pathogens over time. Of the 29 fluoroquinolone-resistant strains, eight (28%) belonged to serotype 23F, eight (28%) to serotype 9V and five (17%) to serogroup 6. Serotypes 35, 22, 34, 14 and 20 accounted for the remaining eight isolates.

Although treatment failures due to β-lactams, macrolides, and trimethoprim/sulphamethoxazole resistance in pneumococci have been reported with meningitis and otitis media; the relation between drug resistance and treatment failures among patients with other pneumococcal infections is less clear [19, 20]. However, ciprofloxacin and levofloxacin treatment failures of pneumococcal pneumonia when caused by fluoroquinolone resistant strains has been well described [21–28]. Reports of the development of resistance and clinical failures appeared shortly after the introduction of the ciprofloxacin in 1987 [24, 29–32]. Davidson et al. [26] report four cases of pneumococcal pneumonia, treated empirically with oral levofloxacin, that failed therapy. All cases were associated with the isolation of an organism that was either resistant to levofloxacin prior to therapy or which had acquired resistance during therapy. Two patients had previously been on ciprofloxacin. One of the four patients died after 6 days of monotherapy with levofloxacin. Kays et al. [28] reported a levofloxacin treatment failure in a patient who had pneumococcal pneumonia and had received three previous courses of levofloxacin therapy. Susceptibility testing revealed high-level resistance to levofloxacin, with MICs of >32 μg/ml and cross-resistance to moxifloxacin (MIC 4 μg/ml) and gatifloxacin (MIC 12 μg/ml). The patient was treated successfully with intravenous ceftriaxone followed by oral cefprozil.

These findings underscore the need to curtail the use of these drugs for infections that can be treated with other agents including the β-lactam or macrolide antimicrobials.

Ear infections

Otitis externa

Otitis externa is an inflammation of the external auditory canal, which can spread to the pinna, periauricular soft tissues, or even the temporal bone. Diffuse otitis externa is typically a bacterial infection, the most common pathogens being pseudomonas, staphylococci, and proteus, but fungi may also be involved (most commonly *Aspergillus* and *Candida*). Malignant (necrotizing) external otitis is a subset of osteomyelitis and is caused by *Pseudomonas aeruginosa* infection with involvement of the temporal bone and skull base [33–36]. The most important predisposing factor is the combination of advanced age (older than 60 years) and diabetes mellitus. Classic signs of infection (fever, leukocytosis, and systemic toxicity) are notably absent, making diagnosis difficult. Otalgia followed by severe and often excruciating headache is the most common presenting symptom. Cranial nerve dysfunction, especially facial nerve palsy, is a late complication [37]. On physical examination, the external auditory canal is abnormal in almost all patients. It usually appears inflamed, swollen or erythematous, and a purulent discharge is present. In most cases, granulation tissue is seen at the junction of the bony and cartilaginous canal. Diagnosis rests on abnormal findings of the temporal bone and skull by computed tomographic scan, an elevated erythrocyte sedimentation rate (ESR) (often exceeding 100 mm/h), and isolation of *P. aeruginosa* from the external auditory canal [38]. Because mortality has been reduced substantially with the advent of effective antipseudomonal therapy, recurrence is the major complication [39]. Interestingly, oral ciprofloxacin therapy (750 mg twice a day) appears to be as effective as parenteral combination antipseudomonal therapy [35, 39–43]. Treatment should be continued for 4 to 10 weeks, depending on the severity of infection at initiation of therapy. Normalization of the ESR has been useful in monitoring therapy. Surgery is rarely necessary except for local debridement or excision of accessible foci of infection *via* polypectomy or removal of sequestrum.

Early recognition and improved treatment have improved the outcome. However, patients who present with neurologic deficits have a worse prognosis [33]. Treatment failures can occur despite optimal therapy, and relapses are observed as long as 4 to 12 months after treatment.

Chronic suppurative otitis media

Chronic suppurative otitis media (CSOM) is defined by chronic infection in the middle ear and mastoid and a nonintact tympanic membrane (chronic perforation or tympanostomy tube). Otorrhea may or may not be present; infection can be present in the middle ear and mastoid, but otorrhea is not evident through the perforation or tympanostomy tube or in the external auditory canal. There is no consensus regarding the duration of otitis media to be designated CSOM. Even though 3 or more months appears to be an acceptable criterion, some clinicians consider a shorter duration, such as 3 or more weeks, of otitis media as being chronic, especially when the causative organism is pseudomonas [44].

CSOM is a major health problem in many populations around the world, affecting diverse racial and cultural groups not only in developing nations but also in highly industrialized countries [44]. Populations that are at highest risk for CSOM associated with chronic perforations are the Inuit of Alaska, Canada, and Greenland; Australian Aborigines; and certain Native Americans, e.g., Apache and Navajo tribes. Populations with moderately high rates include certain natives of the South Pacific islands, such as the Solomon Islands, and the Maori of New Zealand. Not only is CSOM common in these special populations, but with the widespread use of tympanostomy tube placement in the developed nations of the world, CSOM is also a potentially common complication in all infants and children in these countries [44].

CSOM can develop when the tympanic membrane is either intact or not intact. When the tympanic membrane is intact and an attack of acute otitis media occurs, a spontaneous perforation can develop with subsequent acute otorrhea. If the otorrhea persists into the chronic stage, the infection is then CSOM [45]. CSOM can also occur when there is a preexisting chronic perforation of the tympanic membrane or a tympanostomy tube is in place in which otitis media-mastoiditis is absent. The most common organism isolated from around the world when the diagnosis is CSOM is *P. aeruginosa* [46].

Currently the only United States Food and Drug Administration (FDA)-approved ototopical agent is ofloxacin, which is indicated for use when AOM with otorrhea occurs in children with a tympanostomy tube in place; it is the only topical antimicrobial agent that has been demonstrated to be safe and effective [47, 48] and approved for this indication in children; it is also indicated in children and adults when external otitis is the diagnosis. This ototopical agent is also approved for adults who have CSOM [49], but it is currently not approved for this indication in children, even though it has been reported to be effective in this age group [50]. Topical ofloxacin is more effective than the combination of neomycin-polymyxin B-hydrocortisone otic drops in adults with CSOM [51]. Ciprofloxacin with hydrocortisone has also been approved by the FDA, but only for treatment of external otitis in both children and adults. Orally administered ciprofloxacin has been shown to be effective in adults and children who had CSOM, but this agent currently is not approved in the United States for use in patients younger than 18 years of age [44].

Sinus infections

Acute sinusitis

The term sinusitis refers to inflammation of the mucosa of the paranasal sinuses. Because sinusitis is invariably accompanied by inflammation of the contiguous nasal mucosa, rhinosinusitis has become the preferred term. Primary care physicians tend to think of sinusitis as an acute bacterial infection and prescribe an antibiotic in 85% to 98% of cases. However, sinusitis is frequently caused by viral infection. It will often resolve in most patients without antibiotic treatment, even if it is bacterial in origin [52]. Acute rhinosinusitis is defined by symptom duration of less than 4 weeks. Acute bacterial sinusitis is usually a secondary infection resulting from sinus ostia obstruction, impaired mucus clearance mechanisms caused by an acute viral upper respiratory tract infection, or both. According to epidemiologic estimates, only 0.2% to 2% of viral upper respiratory tract infections in adults are complicated by bacterial rhinosinusitis. The gold standard for diagnosis of bacterial sinusitis is sinus puncture, and *S. pneumoniae* and *H. influenzae* are the bacteria most commonly isolated from infected maxillary sinuses [53]. Because no simple and accurate office-based test for acute bacterial sinusitis exists, clinicians rely on clinical findings to make the diagnosis. However, signs and symptoms of acute bacterial sinusitis and those of prolonged viral upper respiratory tract infections are very similar, resulting in frequent misclassification of viral cases. Antibiotics have potential value in treating acute rhinosinusitis only when true bacterial infection is present.

For acute bacterial rhinosinusitis, randomized, double-blind, placebo-controlled trials of antibiotic treatment using pretreatment and post-treatment culture of sinus aspirates have not been performed [52]. Five randomized, double-blind clinical trials with good methods have compared antibiotic treatment with placebo for acute rhinosinusitis in adults [54–58]. These studies basically concluded that although antibiotics are statistically more efficacious than placebo in reducing or eliminating symptoms at 10 and 14 days, the degree of benefit is relatively small.

The clinical diagnosis of acute bacterial rhinosinusitis should be reserved for patients with rhinosinusitis symptoms lasting 7 days or more who have purulent nasal secretions and maxillary facial or tooth pain or tenderness. Patients who have symptoms of rhinosinusitis for less than 7 days are unlikely to have bacterial infection. Antibiotic therapy should be reserved for patients with severe symptoms who meet the criteria for the clinical diagnosis of acute bacterial rhinosinusitis, regardless of duration of illness. Initial antibiotic treatment should be with narrow-spectrum agents that are active against the likely pathogens, *S. pneumoniae* and *H. influenzae* [52]. According to many authorities, amoxicillin continues to be the favored drug, although higher than customary doses may be required for suspected or proven penicillin-resistant pneumococci [52, 59, 60].

Several fluoroquinolones including: ciprofloxacin, levofloxacin, moxifloxacin, and gatifloxacin have approval for the treatment of acute sinusitis due to *S. pneumoniae* and *H. influenzae* [61] [62–70] (Tab. 1). A clinical trial was reported by Sher et al. [67] that compared the clinical efficacy of short-course (5-day) gatifloxacin with standard 10-day regimens of amoxicillin/clavulanate or gatifloxacin in patients with a diagnosis of acute, uncomplicated maxillary sinusitis. This was a multicenter, investigator-blinded study in patients with physical findings, signs and symptoms (for at least 7 days), and radiographic findings indicating acute, uncomplicated maxillary sinusitis. In this population of patients with acute, uncomplicated sinusitis of presumed bacterial origin, a short 5-day course of gatifloxacin therapy was associated with comparable

Table 1. Fluoroquinolones approved for the treatment of acute sinusitis

Fluoroquinolone	Adult dosage	Duration
Ciprofloxacin	500 mg bid	10 days
Levofloxacin	500 mg qd	10–14 days
Gatifloxacin	400 mg qd	5–10 days
Moxifloxacin	400 mg qd	10 days

clinical cure rates and tolerability to those of standard 10-day therapy with gatifloxacin or amoxicillin/clavulanate.

Throat infections

Acute pharyngitis

Acute pharyngitis is one of the most common illnesses for which patients visit primary care physicians. According to the National Ambulatory Medical Care Survey, upper respiratory tract infections, including acute pharyngitis, are responsible for 200 visits to a physician per 1000 population annually in the United States; a rate more than double that for any other category of infectious disease. Group A streptococcus is by far the most common bacterial cause of acute pharyngitis, accounting for approximately 15 to 30% of cases in children and 5 to 10% of cases in adults. Moreover, group A streptococcal pharyngitis is the only common form of the disease for which antimicrobial therapy is definitely indicated. Penicillin, to which the organism is uniformly susceptible, remains the treatment of choice for group A streptococcal pharyngitis because of its proven efficacy, narrow spectrum, safety, and low cost. Although there is no known reason as to why fluoroquinolones would be used to treat pharyngitis, there are anecdotal reports that in fact they are being used for such an indication. Ciprofloxacin and levofloxacin have only moderate activity against group A streptococci, with MIC_{90}s of 0.5 µg/ml. Despite this, reports of resistance of group A streptococci to the fluoroquinolones has been rare [71, 72]. However, in a nationwide multicenter susceptibility surveillance study in Spain by Pérez-Trallero et al. [17], 70 (3.4%) of 2,039 isolates of *S. pyogenes* had a ciprofloxacin MIC $\geq$ 4 µg/ml and were found equally in children and adults. Ciprofloxacin resistance was more prevalent among erythromycin-nonsusceptible group A streptococci than among erythromycin-susceptible ones.

Pulmonary infections

Acute exacerbations of chronic bronchitis

Patients with chronic obstructive lung disease often have a component of chronic bronchitis contributing to their airway obstruction and chronic symptoms. Chronic bronchitis is recognized clinically when a patient has cough and sputum production for 3 months of the year over at least 2 consecutive years. An acute exacerbation of chronic bronchitis (AECB) is characterized by symptoms of increased dyspnea, increased sputum volume, and increased sputum purulence [73]. Other symptoms may also be present, but these three represent the "cardinal symptoms" of an exacerbation, and the severity of the acute process can be graded by how many of these symptoms are present.

Anthonisen and colleagues graded exacerbations as Type I if all three symptoms were present; Type II if only two symptoms were present; and Type III if only one symptom was present [73]. The efficacy of antibiotic therapy in AECB varies with the severity of the acute episode.

When sputum is cultured from a patient with chronic bronchitis, bacteria often are present, with nontypable *H. influenzae*, *S. pneumoniae*, and *M. catarrhalis* being the most commonly recovered pathogens. The role of bacteria in actually causing an acute exacerbation is uncertain because the same organisms may be present when the patient is clinically stable or when the patient is having an acute exacerbation, reflecting the fact that these patients have chronic tracheobronchial colonization. Thus, the role of bacteria in patients with AECB is controversial, making the necessity of antibiotic therapy equally uncertain [74].

Despite many decades of therapeutic trials, the role for antimicrobial therapy in AECB treatment remains controversial. There have been a number of randomized trials examining the role of antibiotics in chronic bronchitis, and they have shown some benefit during acute exacerbations, but no benefit if used to prevent exacerbations [75, 76]. Saint et al. [76] carried out a meta-analysis of nine trials that were randomized and placebo-controlled evaluations of antibiotic therapy in AECB, conducted between 1957 and 1992. That analysis showed a small beneficial effect of antibiotic therapy when the end points were overall benefit and change in peak flow rate. Another analysis of placebo-controlled trials for AECB, conducted by Ball, reached similar conclusions [77].

The most common organisms leading to AECB are nontypable *H influenzae, M catarrhalis,* and *S pneumoniae*. When patients have multiple episodes of recurrent infection, either as a consequence of antibiotic therapy or as a result of ongoing bronchial injury, Gram-negatives, including *P. aeruginosa* can be found [78, 79]. When considering the target organisms of a selected antibiotic, it is important to profile the patient in order to define a likely spectrum of etiologic pathogens. This concept has been incorporated into the recently published Canadian chronic bronchitis guidelines and implies that the ideal antibiotic will vary for different individuals [80]. For patients with uncomplicated chronic bronchitis, characterized by individuals ≤ 65 years of age with fewer than four exacerbations per year, therapy should be directed at *H. influenzae*, *M. catarrhalis*, pneumococcus, and possibly atypical pathogens. Patients with more complicated disease, characterized by >65 years of age, four or more exacerbations per year, FEV1 <50% of predicted, or underlying comorbidity, antibiotic spectrum should include Gram-negatives. In addition, if the patient has recently received antibiotic therapy or had a nonresponse to an agent, then a resistant organism is possible and an agent from another class should be chosen.

Studies done in the early 1980s showed no differences in the outcome among the usual first-line antibiotics that included: amoxicillin/ampicillin, trimethoprim-sulfamethoxazole, and erythromycin. With the changing resistance patterns notably for *H. influenzae*, *M. catarrhalis*, and *S. pneumoniae*, it would not be surprising to expect some antibiotics to do better than others. A number of fluoroquinolones have been approved for their use in the treatment of AECB. To date, however, no randomized, placebo-controlled trial has proved the superiority of any one of the fluoroquinolones to standard first-line therapy [81–92].

There have been several advances proposed with the use of the fluoroquinolones. Several of these agents including moxifloxacin, gatifloxacin, and levofloxacin have been shown that when administered for 5 days to be as effective and a more convenient treatment than a standard course of antimicrobials for patients with AECB [83–86]. There is mounting evidence that fluoroquinolone treatment of AECB is associated with a longer infection-free interval: the length of time in days between the end of therapy and the beginning of the next AECB [93]. Chodosh and colleagues [90] performed a double-blind study comparing ciprofloxacin and clarithromycin to determine clinical and bacteriologic efficacy and safety of the two therapies. They also sought to compare the length of the infection-free interval between one AECB and the next exacerbation. Patients were randomized to receive two 250 mg tablets of either ciprofloxacin or clarithromycin. The antibiotics were administered twice daily for 14 days. The effectiveness of the antimicrobial agents was assessed by patient clinical response and laboratory measurements, with a physical examination at 2, 12, 24 and 36 weeks post-treatment, or when a treatment failure or a new exacerbation occurred. Throughout the 36-week follow-up period, 55% of the ciprofloxacin patients and 59% of the clarithromycin patients experienced a relapse or a new exacerbation. The median length of infection-free interval was 142 days in the ciprofloxacin group and 51 days in the clarithromycin group. Bacterial eradication at the end of therapy was 91% in the ciprofloxacin group but only 77% in the clarithromycin patients. The authors conclude from this study that patients taking ciprofloxacin showed a longer infection-free interval than did those treated with clarithromycin. Grossman et al. [94] studied the use of ciprofloxacin in a prospective 1-year study and demonstrated improved clinical outcome in patients with moderate to severe chronic bronchitis and at least four AECB in the previous year when compared to the usual antibiotic treatment. Treatment with ciprofloxacin tended to accelerate the resolution of all AECBs compared to usual care (relative risk = 1.20; 95% confidence interval [CI], 0.91 to 1.58; $p = 0.19$). Treatment assignment did not affect the interexacerbation period but a history of severe bronchitis, prolonged chronic bronchitis, and an increased number of AECBs in the past year were associated with shorter exacerbations-free periods. There was a slight, but not statistically significant, improvement in all quality of life measures with ciprofloxacin over usual care. The only factors predictive of hospitalization were duration of chronic bronchitis (odds ratio = 4.6; 95% CI, 1.6, 13.0) and severity of chronic bronchitis (odds ratio = 4.3; 95% CI, 0.8, 24.6). When the simple base case analysis was expanded to examine the effect of risk stratification, the presence of moderate or severe bronchitis and at least four AECBs in the previous year changed the economic and clinical analysis to one favorable to ciprofloxacin with the ciprofloxacin-treated group having a better clinical outcome at lower cost.

Finally, Nouira et al. [95] assessed the effects of ofloxacin in patients with AECB who required mechanical ventilation. A prospective, randomised, double-blind, placebo-controlled trial in 93 patients with AECB who required mechanical ventilation was carried out. Patients were randomly assigned to receive oral ofloxacin 400 mg once daily ($n = 47$) or placebo ($n = 46$) for 10 days. Primary endpoints were death in hospital or need for an additional course of antibiotics, both separately and in combination. Treatment with ofloxacin significantly reduced the need for additional courses of antibiotics (28.4%, 12.9–43.9, $p = 0.0006$). The combined frequency of death in hospital and need for additional antibiotics was significantly lower in patients assigned to ofloxacin than in those receiving placebo (45.9%, 29.1–62.7, $p < 0.0001$). The duration of mechanical ventilation and hospital stay was significantly shorter in the ofloxacin group than in the placebo group (absolute difference 4.2 days, 95% CI 2.5–5.9; and 9.6 days, 3.4–12.8, respectively).

A cautionary note regarding the use of the fluoroquinolones for the treatment of AECB has been the emergence of fluoroquinolone resistance to pneumococci and the association of resistance with clinical failures when a fluoroquinolone is used [6, 9, 25]. A number of risk factors have been recognized that identify patients that are likely to be colonized or infected with a ciprofloxacin or levofloxacin-resistant pneumococci: patients who are >64 years of age, have a history of chronic obstructive lung disease and/or prior fluoroquinolone exposure [6, 9, 13, 15, 96]. Weiss and colleagues [25] described a nosocomial outbreak of fluoroquinolone-resistant pneumococci. Over the course of a 20-month period, in a hospital respiratory ward where ciprofloxacin was often used as empirical antimicrobial therapy for lower respiratory tract infections, 16 patients with chronic bronchitis developed lower respiratory tract infections caused by a strain of penicillin- and ciprofloxacin-resistant *S. pneumoniae* (serotype 23F). The MIC of ciprofloxacin for all isolates was ≥ 4 μg/ml. All five patients with AECB treated with ciprofloxacin, failed therapy.

Whether or not the newer fluoroquinolones including moxifloxacin and gatifloxacin with enhanced pneumococcal activity and more favourable pharmacokinetic/pharmacodynamic parameters will slow or prevent the emergence of resistance and/or will be more effective for the treatment of AECB due to pneumococci with reduced susceptibilities to the fluoroquinolones is yet to be determined [97].

References

1 Low DE (2000) Trends and significance of antimicrobial resistance in respiratory pathogens. *Curr*

Opin Infect Dis 13: 145–153
2 Doern GV, Heilmann KP, Huynh HK, Rhomberg PR, Coffman SL, Brueggemann AB (2001) Antimicrobial resistance among clinical isolates of *Streptococcus pneumoniae* in the United States during 1999–2000, including a comparison of resistance rates since 1994–1995. *Antimicrob Agents Chemother* 45(6): 1721–1729
3 Doern GV, Jones RN, Pfaller MA, Kugler K (1999) *Haemophilus influenzae* and *Moraxella catarrhalis* from patients with community-acquired respiratory tract infections: antimicrobial susceptibility patterns from the SENTRY antimicrobial Surveillance Program (United States and Canada, 1997). *Antimicrob Agents Chemother* 43(2): 385–389
4 Zhanel GG, Karlowsky JA, Low DE, Hoban DJ (2000) Antibiotic resistance in respiratory tract isolates of *Haemophilus influenzae* and *Moraxella catarrhalis* collected from across Canada in 1997–1998. *J Antimicrob Chemother* 45(5): 655–662
5 Pfaller MA, Ehrhardt AF, Jones RN (2001) Frequency of pathogen occurrence and antimicrobial susceptibility among community-acquired respiratory tract infections in the respiratory surveillance program study: microbiology from the medical office practice environment. *Am J Med* 111 Suppl 9A: 4S–12S
6 Chen D, McGeer A, de Azavedo JC, Low DE, The Canadian Bacterial Surveillance Network (1999) Decreased susceptibility of *Streptococcus pneumoniae* to fluoroquinolones in Canada. *N Eng J Med* 341(4): 233–239
7 Linares J, De La Campa AG, Pallares R (1999) Fluoroquinolone resistance in *Streptococcus pneumoniae* [letter]. *N Engl J Med* 341(20): 1546–1547
8 Ho PL, Que TL, Tsang DN, Ng TK, Chow KH, Seto WH (1999) Emergence of fluoroquinolone resistance among multiply resistant strains of *Streptococcus pneumoniae* in Hong Kong. *Antimicrob Agents Chemother* 43(5): 1310–1313
9 Ho PL, Yung RW, Tsang DN, Que TL, Ho M, Seto WH, Ng TK, Yam WC, Ng WW (2001) Increasing resistance of *Streptococcus pneumoniae* to fluoroquinolones: results of a Hong Kong multicentre study in 2000. *J Antimicrob Chemother* 48(5): 659–665
10 Nagai K, Appelbaum PC, Davies TA, Kelly LM, Hoellman DB, Andrasevic AT, Drukalska L, Hryniewicz W, Jacobs MR, Kolman J et al (2002) Susceptibilities to telithromycin and six other agents and prevalence of macrolide resistance due to L4 ribosomal protein mutation among 992 pneumococci from 10 Central and Eastern European countries. *Antimicrob Agents Chemother* 46(2): 371–377
11 Goldsmith CE, Moore JE, Murphy PG, Ambler JE (1998) Increased incidence of ciprofloxacin resistance in penicillin-resistant pneumococci in Northern Ireland [letter; comment]. *J Antimicrob Chemother* 41(3): 420–421
12 Brueggemann AB, Coffman SL, Rhomberg P, Huynh H, Almer L, Nilius A, Flamm R, Doern GV (2002) Fluoroquinolone Resistance in *Streptococcus pneumoniae* in United States since 1994–1995. *Antimicrob Agents Chemother* 46(3): 680–688
13 Sahm DF, Peterson DE, Critchley IA, Thornsberry C (2000) Analysis of ciprofloxacin activity against *Streptococcus pneumoniae* after 10 years of use in the United States. *Antimicrob Agents Chemother* 44(9): 2521–2524
14 Sahm DF, Karlowsky JA, Kelly LJ, Critchley IA, Jones ME, Thornsberry C, Mauriz Y, Kahn J (2001) Need for annual surveillance of antimicrobial resistance in *Streptococcus pneumoniae* in the United States: 2-year longitudinal analysis. *Antimicrob Agents Chemother* 45(4): 1037–1042
15 Centers for Disease Control (2001) Resistance of *Streptococcus pneumoniae* to fluoroquinolones-United States, 1995–1999. *Morbid Mortal Weekly Rep* 50(37): 800–804
16 Alou L, Ramirez M, Garcia-Rey C, Prieto J, de Lencastre H (2001) *Streptococcus pneumoniae* isolates with reduced susceptibility to ciprofloxacin in Spain: clonal diversity and appearance of ciprofloxacin-resistant epidemic clones. *Antimicrob Agents Chemother* 45(10): 2955–2957
17 Perez-Trallero E, Fernandez-Mazarrasa C, Garcia-Rey C, Bouza E, Aguilar L, Garcia-de-Lomas J, Baquero F (2001) Antimicrobial susceptibilities of 1,684 *Streptococcus pneumoniae* and 2,039 *Streptococcus pyogenes* isolates and their ecological relationships: results of a 1-year (1998–1999) multicenter surveillance study in Spain. *Antimicrob Agents Chemother* 45(12): 3334–3340
18 McGee L, Goldsmith CE, Klugman KP (2002) Fluoroquinolone resistance among clinical isolates of *Streptococcus pneumoniae* belonging to international multiresistant clones. *J Antimicrob Chemother* 49(1): 173–176
19 Deeks SL, Palacio R, Ruvinsky R, Kertesz DA, Hortal M, Rossi A, Spika JS, Di Fabio JL (1999) Risk factors and course of illness among children with invasive penicillin-resistant *Streptococcus*

pneumoniae. The Streptococcus pneumoniae Working Group. *Pediatrics* 103(2): 409–413
20 Straus WL, Qazi SA, Kundi Z, Nomani NK, Schwartz B (1998) Antimicrobial resistance and clinical effectiveness of co-trimoxazole *versus* amoxycillin for pneumonia among children in Pakistan: randomised controlled trial. Pakistan Co-trimoxazole Study Group. *Lancet* 352(9124): 270–274
21 Davies BI, Maesen FP, Baur C (1986) Ciprofloxacin in the treatment of acute exacerbations of chronic bronchitis. *Eur J Clin Microbiol* 5(2): 226–231
22 Hoogkamp-Korstanje JA, Klein SJ (1986) Ciprofloxacin in acute exacerbations of chronic bronchitis. *J Antimicrob Chemother* 18(3): 407–413
23 Maesen FP, Davies BI, Geraedts WH, Baur C (1987) The use of quinolones in respiratory tract infections. *Drugs* 34 Suppl 1: 74–79
24 Thys JP (1988) Quinolones in the treatment of bronchopulmonary infections. *Rev Infect Dis* 10 Suppl 1: S212–S217
25 Weiss K, Restieri C, Laverdiere M, McGeer A, Davidson RJ, Kilburn L, Bast DJ, de Azavedo J, Low DE (2001) A nosocomial outbreak of fluoroquinolone-resistant *Streptococcus pneumoniae*. *Clin Inf Dis* 33(4): 517–522
26 Davidson R, Cavalcanti R, Brunton JL, Bast DJ, de Azavedo JC, Kibsey P, Fleming C, Low DE (2002) Resistance to levofloxacin and failure of treatment of pneumococcal pneumonia. *N Engl J Med* 346(10): 747–750
27 Empey PE, Jennings HR, Thornton AC, Rapp RP, Evans ME (2001) Levofloxacin failure in a patient with pneumococcal pneumonia. *Ann Pharmacother* 35(6): 687–690
28 Kays MB, Smith DW, Wack ME, Denys GA (2002) Levofloxacin treatment failure in a patient with fluoroquinolone- resistant *Streptococcus pneumoniae* pneumonia. *Pharmacotherapy* 22(3): 395–399
29 Lee BL, Kimbrough RC, Jones SR, Mills J, Sande MA (1991) Infectious complications with respiratory pathogens despite ciprofloxacin therapy. *N Engl J Med* 325(7): 520–521
30 Cooper B, Lawlor M (1989) Pneumococcal bacteremia during ciprofloxacin therapy for pneumococcal pneumonia [see comments]. *Am J Med* 87(4): 475
31 Perez-Trallero E, Garcia-Arenzana JM, Jimenez JA, Peris A (1990) Therapeutic failure and selection of resistance to quinolones in a case of pneumococcal pneumonia treated with ciprofloxacin. *Eur J Clin Microbiol Infect Dis* 9(12): 905–906
32 Gordon JJ, Kauffman CA (1990) Superinfection with *Streptococcus pneumoniae* during therapy with ciprofloxacin. *Am J Med* 89(3): 383–384
33. Pollack M (2000) *Pseudomona aeruginosa*. *In*: GL Mandell, JE Bennett, R Dolin (eds): *Mandell, Douglas, and Bennett's principles and practise of infectious diseases*. Toronto: Churchill Livingstone, 2310–2335
34 Chandler JR (1968) Malignant external otitis. *Laryngoscope* 78(8): 1257–1294
35 Rubin J, Yu VL (1988) Malignant external otitis: insights into pathogenesis, clinical manifestations, diagnosis, and therapy. *Am J Med* 85(3): 391–398
36 Zaky DA, Bentley DW, Lowy K, Betts RF, Douglas RG Jr (1976) Malignant external otitis: a severe form of otitis in diabetic patients. *Am J Med* 61(2): 298–302
37 Damiani JM, Damiani KK, Kinney SE (1979) Malignant external otitis with multiple cranial nerve involvement. *Am J Otol* 1(2): 115–120
38 Rubin J, Curtin HD, Yu VL, Kamerer DB (1990) Malignant external otitis: utility of CT in diagnosis and follow-up. *Radiology* 174(2): 391–394
39 Giamarellou H (1992) Malignant otitis externa: the therapeutic evolution of a lethal infection. *J Antimicrob Chemother* 30(6): 745–751
40 Morrison GA, Bailey CM (1988) Relapsing malignant otitis externa successfully treated with ciprofloxacin. *J Laryngol Otol* 102(10): 872–876
41 Lang R, Goshen S, Kitzes-Cohen R, Sade J (1990) Successful treatment of malignant external otitis with oral ciprofloxacin: report of experience with 23 patients. *J Infect Dis* 161(3): 537–540
42 Sade J, Lang R, Goshen S, Kitzes-Cohen R (1989) Ciprofloxacin treatment of malignant external otitis. *Am J Med* 87(5A): 138S-141S
43 Rubin J, Stoehr G, Yu VL, Muder RR, Matador A, Kamerer DB (1989) Efficacy of oral ciprofloxacin plus rifampin for treatment of malignant external otitis. *Arch Otolaryngol Head Neck Surg* 115(9): 1063–1069
44 Bluestone CD (2001) Efficacy of ofloxacin and other ototopical preparations for chronic suppurative otitis media in children. *Pediatr Infect Dis J* 20(1): 111–115

45 Bluestone CD (2000) Clinical course, complications and sequelae of acute otitis media. *Pediatr Infect Dis J* 19(5 Suppl): S37–S46
46 Kenna MA, Bluestone CD (1986) Microbiology of chronic suppurative otitis media in children. *Pediatr Infect Dis* 5(2): 223–225
47 Goldblatt EL, Dohar J, Nozza RJ, Nielsen RW, Goldberg T, Sidman JD, Seidlin M (1998) Topical ofloxacin *versus* systemic amoxicillin/clavulanate in purulent otorrhea in children with tympanostomy tubes. *Int J Pediatr Otorhinolaryngol* 46(1–2): 91–101
48 Dohar JE, Garner ET, Nielsen RW, Biel MA, Seidlin M (1999) Topical ofloxacin treatment of otorrhea in children with tympanostomy tubes. *Arch Otolaryngol Head Neck Surg* 125(5): 537–545
49 Agro AS, Garner ET, Wright JW, III, Caballeros dE, I, Villeda B, Seidlin M (1998) Clinical trial of ototopical ofloxacin for treatment of chronic suppurative otitis media. *Clin Ther* 20(4): 744–759
50 Kaga K, Ichimura K (1998) A preliminary report: clinical effects of otic solution of ofloxacin in infantile myringitis and chronic otitis media. *Int J Pediatr Otorhinolaryngol* 42(3): 199–205
51 Tong MC, Woo JK, van Hasselt CA (1996) A double-blind comparative study of ofloxacin otic drops *versus* neomycin-polymyxin B-hydrocortisone otic drops in the medical treatment of chronic suppurative otitis media. *J Laryngol Otol* 110(4): 309–314
52 Hickner JM, Bartlett JG, Besser RE, Gonzales R, Hoffman JR, Sande MA (2001) Principles of appropriate antibiotic use for acute rhinosinusitis in adults: background. *Ann Emerg Med* 37(6): 703–710
53 Gwaltney JM Jr (1996) Acute community-acquired sinusitis. *Clin Infect Dis* 23(6): 1209–1223
54 Lindbaek M, Hjortdahl P, Johnsen UL (1996) Randomised, double blind, placebo controlled trial of penicillin V and amoxycillin in treatment of acute sinus infections in adults. *BMJ* 313(7053): 325–329
55 Axelsson A, Chidekel N, Grebelius N, Jensen C (1970) Treatment of acute maxillary sinusitis. A comparison of four different methods. *Acta Otolaryngol* 70(1): 71–76
56 Gananca M, Trabulsi LR (1973) The therapeutic effects of cyclacillin in acute sinusitis: *in vitro* and *in vivo* correlations in a placebo-controlled study. *Curr Med Res Opin* 1(6): 362–368
57 Stalman W, van Essen GA, van der GY, de Melker RA (1997) The end of antibiotic treatment in adults with acute sinusitis-like complaints in general practice? A placebo-controlled double-blind randomized doxycycline trial. *Br J Gen Pract* 47(425): 794–799
58 van Buchem FL, Knottnerus JA, Schrijnemaekers VJ, Peeters MF (1997) Primary-care-based randomised placebo-controlled trial of antibiotic treatment in acute maxillary sinusitis [see comments]. *Lancet* 349(9053): 683–687
59 Antimicrobial treatment guidelines for acute bacterial rhinosinusitis Sinus, Allergy Health Partnership (2000) *Otolaryngol Head Neck Surg* 123(1 Pt 2): 5–31
60 Brook I, Gooch WM, III, Jenkins SG, Pichichero ME, Reiner SA, Sher L, Yamauchi T (2000) Medical management of acute bacterial sinusitis. Recommendations of a clinical advisory committee on pediatric and adult sinusitis. *Ann Otol Rhinol Laryngol Suppl* 182: 2–20
61 Clifford K, Huck W, Shan M, Tosiello R, Echols RM, Heyd A (1999) Double-blind comparative trial of ciprofloxacin *versus* clarithromycin in the treatment of acute bacterial sinusitis. Sinusitis Infection Study Group. *Ann Otol Rhinol Laryngol* 108(4): 360–367
62 Johnson PA, Rodriguez HP, Wazen JJ, Huck W, Shan M, Tosiello R, Heyd A, Echols RM (1999) Ciprofloxacin *versus* cefuroxime axetil in the treatment of acute bacterial sinusitis. Sinusitis Infection Study Group. *J Otolaryngol* 28(1): 3–12
63 Weis M, Hendrick K, Tillotson G, Gravelle K (1998) Multicenter comparative trial of ciprofloxacin *versus* cefuroxime axetil in the treatment of acute rhinosinusitis in a primary care setting. Rhinosinusitis Investigation Group. *Clin Ther* 20(5): 921–932
64 Klein GL, Whalen E, Echols RM, Heyd A (1998) Ciprofloxacin *versus* cefuroxime axetil in the treatment of adult patients with acute bacterial sinusitis. *J Otolaryngol* 27(1): 10–16
65 Rakkar S, Roberts K, Towe BF, Flores SM, Heyd A, Warner J (2001) Moxifloxacin *versus* amoxicillin clavulanate in the treatment of acute maxillary sinusitis: a primary care experience. *Int J Clin Pract* 55(5): 309–315
66 Burke T, Villanueva C, Mariano H Jr, Huck W, Orchard D, Haverstock D, Heyd A, Church D (1999) Comparison of moxifloxacin and cefuroxime axetil in the treatment of acute maxillary sinusitis. Sinusitis Infection Study Group. *Clin Ther* 21(10): 1664–1677
67 Sher LD, McAdoo MA, Bettis RB, Turner MA, Li NF, Pierce PF (2002) A multicenter, random-

ized, investigator-blinded study of 5- and 10-day gatifloxacin *versus* 10-day amoxicillin/clavulanate in patients with acute bacterial sinusitis. *Clin Ther* 24(2): 269–281
68 Lasko B, Lau CY, Saint-Pierre C, Reddington JL, Martel A, Anstey RJ (1998) Efficacy and safety of oral levofloxacin compared with clarithromycin in the treatment of acute sinusitis in adults: a multicentre, double- blind, randomized study. The Canadian Sinusitis Study Group. *J Int Med Res* 26(6): 281–291
69 Adelglass J, DeAbate CA, McElvaine P, Fowler CL, LoCocco J, Campbell T (1999) Comparison of the effectiveness of levofloxacin and amoxicillin- clavulanate for the treatment of acute sinusitis in adults. *Otolaryngol Head Neck Surg* 120(3): 320–327
70 Adelglass J, Jones TM, Ruoff G, Kahn JB, Wiesinger BA, Rielly-Gauvin K, Siu CO (1998) A multicenter, investigator-blinded, randomized comparison of oral levofloxacin and oral clarithromycin in the treatment of acute bacterial sinusitis. *Pharmacotherapy* 18(6): 1255–1263
71 Barry AL, Fuchs PC, Brown SD (2001) *In vitro* activities of three nonfluorinated quinolones against representative bacterial isolates. *Antimicrob Agents Chemother* 45(6): 1923–1927
72 Yan SS, Fox ML, Holland SM, Stock F, Gill VJ, Fedorko DP (2000) Resistance to multiple fluoroquinolones in a clinical isolate of *Streptococcus pyogenes*: identification of *gyrA* and *parC* and specification of point mutations associated with resistance. *Antimicrob Agents Chemother* 44(11): 3196–3198
73 Anthonisen NR, Manfreda J, Warren CP, Hershfield ES, Harding GK, Nelson NA (1987) Antibiotic therapy in exacerbations of chronic obstructive pulmonary disease. *Ann Intern Med* 106(2): 196–204
74 Murphy TF, Sethi S, Niederman MS (2000) The role of bacteria in exacerbations of COPD. A constructive view. *Chest* 118(1): 204–209
75 Murphy TF, Sethi S (1992) Bacterial infection in chronic obstructive pulmonary disease. *Am Rev Respir Dis* 146(4): 1067–1083
76 Saint S, Bent S, Vittinghoff E, Grady D (1995) Antibiotics in chronic obstructive pulmonary disease exacerbations. A meta-analysis [see comments]. *JAMA* 273(12): 957–960
77 Ball P (1995) Epidemiology and treatment of chronic bronchitis and its exacerbations. *Chest* 108(2 Suppl): 43S-52S
78 Fagon JY, Chastre J, Trouillet JL, Domart Y, Dombret MC, Bornet M, Gibert C (1990) Characterization of distal bronchial microflora during acute exacerbation of chronic bronchitis. Use of the protected specimen brush technique in 54 mechanically ventilated patients. *Am Rev Respir Dis* 142(5): 1004–1008
79 Monso E, Ruiz J, Rosell A, Manterola J, Fiz J, Morera J, Ausina V (1995) Bacterial infection in chronic obstructive pulmonary disease. A study of stable and exacerbated outpatients using the protected specimen brush. *Am J Respir Crit Care Med* 152(4 Pt 1): 1316–1320
80 Balter MS, Hyland RH, Low DE, Renzi PM (1994) Recommendations on the management of chronic bronchitis. *CMAJ* 151(Suppl 10): 7–23
81 Schaberg T, Ballin I, Huchon G, Bassaris H, Hampel B, Reimnitz P (2001) A multinational, multicentre, non-blinded, randomized study of moxifloxacin oral tablets compared with co-amoxiclav oral tablets in the treatment of acute exacerbation of chronic bronchitis. *J Int Med Res* 29(4): 314–328
82 DeAbate CA, Mathew CP, Warner JH, Heyd A, Church D (2000) The safety and efficacy of short course (5-day) moxifloxacin *versus* azithromycin in the treatment of patients with acute exacerbation of chronic bronchitis. *Respir Med* 94(11): 1029–1037
83 Chodosh S, DeAbate CA, Haverstock D, Aneiro L, Church D (2000) Short-course moxifloxacin therapy for treatment of acute bacterial exacerbations of chronic bronchitis. The Bronchitis Study Group. *Respir Med* 94(1): 18–27
84 Wilson R, Kubin R, Ballin I, Deppermann KM, Bassaris HP, Leophonte P, Schreurs AJ, Torres A, Sommerauer B (1999) Five day moxifloxacin therapy compared with 7 day clarithromycin therapy for the treatment of acute exacerbations of chronic bronchitis. *J Antimicrob Chemother* 44(4): 501–513
85 Gotfried MH, DeAbate CA, Fogarty C, Mathew CP, Sokol WN (2001) Comparison of 5-day, short-course gatifloxacin therapy with 7-day gatifloxacin therapy and 10-day clarithromycin therapy for acute exacerbation of chronic bronchitis. *Clin Ther* 23(1): 97–107
86 Masterton RG, Burley CJ (2001) Randomized, double-blind study comparing 5- and 7-day regimens of oral levofloxacin in patients with acute exacerbation of chronic bronchitis. *Int J Antimicrob Agents* 18(6): 503–512

87 Norrby SR (2001) Optimal treatment strategies for acute exacerbations of chronic bronchitis: high-risk patients. *Chemotherapy* 47 Suppl 4: 47–52
88 Read RC, Kuss A, Berrisoul F, Kearsley N, Torres A, Kubin R (1999) The efficacy and safety of a new ciprofloxacin suspension compared with co-amoxiclav tablets in the treatment of acute exacerbations of chronic bronchitis. *Respir Med* 93(4): 252–261
89 Anzueto A, Niederman MS, Tillotson GS (1998) Etiology, susceptibility, and treatment of acute bacterial exacerbations of complicated chronic bronchitis in the primary care setting: ciprofloxacin 750 mg b.i.d. *versus* clarithromycin 500 mg b.i.d. Bronchitis Study Group. *Clin Ther* 20(5): 885–900
90 Chodosh S, Schreurs A, Siami G, Barkman HW, Anzueto A, Shan Moesker H, Stack T, Kowalsky S, the Bronchitis Study Group (1998) Efficacy of oral ciprofloxacin *versus* clarithromycin for treatment of acute bacterial exacerbations of chronic bronchitis. *Clin Infect Dis* 27: 730–738
91 Chodosh S, McCarty J, Farkas S, Drehobl M, Tosiello R, Shan M, Aneiro L, Kowalsky S (1998) Randomized, double-blind study of ciprofloxacin and cefuroxime axetil for treatment of acute bacterial exacerbations of chronic bronchitis. The Bronchitis Study Group. *Clin Infect Dis* 27(4): 722–729
92 DeAbate CA, Henry D, Bensch G, Jubran A, Chodosh S, Harper L, Tipping D, Talbot GH (1998) Sparfloxacin vs ofloxacin in the treatment of acute bacterial exacerbations of chronic bronchitis: a multicenter, double-blind, randomized, comparative study. Sparfloxacin Multicenter ABECB Study Group. *Chest* 114(1): 120–130
93 Anzueto A, Rizzo JA, Grossman RF (1999) The infection-free interval: its use in evaluating antimicrobial treatment of acute exacerbation of chronic bronchitis. *Clin Infect Dis* 28(6): 1344–1345
94 Grossman RF (1998) The value of antibiotics and the outcomes of antibiotic therapy in exacerbations of COPD. *Chest* 113(4 Suppl): 249S-255S
95 Nouira S, Marghli S, Belghith M, Besbes L, Elatrous S, Abroug F (2001) Once daily oral ofloxacin in chronic obstructive pulmonary disease exacerbation requiring mechanical ventilation: a randomised placebo- controlled trial. *Lancet* 358(9298): 2020–2025
96 Ho PL, Tse WS, Tsang KW, Kwok TK, Ng TK, Cheng VC, Chan RM (2001) Risk factors for acquisition of levofloxacin-resistant *Streptococcus pneumoniae*: a case-control study. *Clin Infect Dis* 32(5): 701–707
97 Nicolau DP, Ambrose PG (2001) Pharmacodynamic profiling of levofloxacin and gatifloxacin using Monte Carlo simulation for community-acquired isolates of *Streptococcus pneumoniae*. *Am J Med* 111 Suppl 9A: 13S-18S
98 Low DE, de Azavedo J, Weiss CA, Mazzulli T, Kuhn M, Church D et al (2002) Antimicrobial resistance among clinical isolates of *Streptococcus pneumoniae* in Canada during 2000. *Antimicrob Agents Chemother* 46(5): 1295–1301
99 Thornsberry C, Sahm DF, Kelly LJ, Critchley IA, Jones ME, Evangelista AT, Karlowsky JA (2002) Regional trends in antimicrobial resistance among clinical isolates of *Streptococcus pneumoniae, Haemophilus influenzae*, and *Moraxella catarrhalis* in the United States: Results from the TRUST Surveillance Program, 1999–2000. *Clin Infect Dis* 34 Suppl 1: S4–S16

Fluoroquinolone Antibiotics
ed. by A.R. Ronald and D.E. Low

Quinolones for the treatment of skin, soft tissue, bone and prosthetic joint infections

John M. Embil

Infection Control Unit, Health Sciences Centre, MS 673–820 Sherbrook Street, Winnipeg, MB R3A 1R9, Canada

Introduction

The antimicrobial spectrum of activity of the early quinolones (i.e., norfloxacin, ofloxacin, ciprofloxacin) favor potency against Gram-negative microorganisms [1, 2]. The newer agents (levofloxacin, gatifloxacin, moxifloxacin) have expanded activity against the Gram-positive microorganisms [3, 4] and some of these newer agents which are currently available or in clinical trial (moxifloxacin, gatifloxacin, garenoxacin) also demonstrate excellent *in vitro* activity against the Gram-negative, Gram-positive, anaerobic, and atypical microorganisms [5–7]. Ciprofloxacin and levofloxacin have only moderate activity against the group A streptococci, with MIC_{90}s of 0.5 µg/ml, however, reports of resistance to these agents have been rare [8, 9]. In a nationwide multicenter susceptibility surveillance study in Spain [10], 70 (3.4%) of 2,039 isolates of *Streptococcus pyogenes* had a ciprofloxacin MIC ≥ 4 µg/ml. These microorganisms were found to be equally distributed between children and adults [10]. The early investigations with the then new fluoroquinolones, particularly ciprofloxacin, demonstrated *in vitro* activity against both methicillin-susceptible *Staphylococcus aureus* (MSSA) and methicillin-resistant *Staphylococcus aureus* (MRSA), although the activity was marginal with MIC_{90}s of 0.5 µg/ml [11, 12]. A single mutation in the primary target would increase the MIC of ciprofloxacin four- to 16-fold, a level of resistance at or above peak drug concentrations achievable in serum, providing an opportunity for such first-step mutants to survive and emerge when a patient was exposed to fluoroquinolones [13]. Fluoroquinolone resistance in MRSA and the coagulase-negative staphylococci is now >50% worldwide [14–16]. Fluoroquinolone resistance in methicillin-susceptible staphylococci vary from <5% to 22%, depending on the location of the study [17, 18]. An international study with isolates provided from countries in Europe, Asia, and Latin America demonstrated ciprofloxacin resistant rates in MRSA, MSSA, methicillin-resistant and -susceptible coagulase-negative staphylococci of 90%, 21%, 50% and 22% respectively [15]. Susceptibility testing was carried out on 602 geographically and genetically diverse *S. aureus* isolates from across North America. Initial investigations reported the successful use of oral ciprofloxacin in the eradication of MRSA colonization and in the treatment of MRSA and MSSA infections [19–21]. However, it was soon recognized that when a fluoroquinolone, such as ciprofloxacin, was used alone that resistance frequently developed and was often associated with clinical failures [20–23].

The quinolones have a rapid mechanism of antibacterial action by inhibiting DNA synthesis by interfering with DNA gyrase and type IV topoisomerase [1]. This rapid antibacterial activity coupled with excellent oral bioavailability [24, 25], broad tissue distribution and penetration [25–27] including intracellular concentration in neutrophils and macrophages, as well as infrequent dosing make the quinolones convenient and desirable agents for the management of infections. Favorable pharmacokinetics, and the availability of both oral and parenteral formulations of most quinolone agents allows a direct parenteral to oral stepdown once the patient is clinically stable or a suitable duration of therapy has been delivered parenterally. The oral administration of the quinolones with their excellent oral bioavailability offers a realistic alternative to parenteral therapy [25]. The quinolones may either be used as an initial oral first line therapy as an alternative to parenteral therapy, or, alternatively, as a rapid stepdown therapy to the parenteral agents. The quinolones are also a potential alternative in those individuals with β-lactam allergies. This chapter will provide an overview of the current data supporting the role of ciprofloxacin, levofloxacin, gatifloxacin, and moxifloxacin for the management of skin, soft tissue, and bone infections.

Skin and soft tissue infections

Bacterial skin and soft tissue infections are classified as uncomplicated where the infections are caused primarily by *S. aureus* or *S. pyogenes* and are not associated with necrotic soft tissue, and/or bone, deep abscesses, or underlying vascular insufficiency impairing delivery of antimicrobials to the infected area, impaired host immunity, and underlying host comorbidities which impede or delay healing [28]; and complicated where the infection involves ulcers, wounds, major abscesses, or there are significant underlying comorbidities such as diabetes, and/or peripheral vascular disease [29]. Although a multitude of quinolones have come to clinical trial, only a limited number of peer reviewed publications have arisen.

Ciprofloxacin and ofloxacin have been extensively evaluated [30–34] for skin, and soft tissue infections. Although the spectrum of activity of ciprofloxacin is primarily aerobic Gram-negative bacilli, with particular activity against *Pseudomonas auriginosa*, patients enrolled in randomized clinical trials treated with either ciprofloxacin or its comparator have had satisfactory clinical outcomes [30–32]. It is important to note that even patients from whose wounds *S. aureus* was recovered had a comparable outcome to those treated with the comparator agent with potentially superior anti-Gram-positive activity. In these studies, oral ciprofloxacin was compared to parenteral cefotaxime. Similar therapeutic outcomes have been observed in patients treated with oral ofloxacin *versus* intravenous cefotaxime [33] or with intravenous ofloxacin followed by oral ofloxacin compared to those receiving parenteral ampicillin/sulbactam followed by oral amoxicillin-clavulinic acid [34]. The overall cure rates were comparable for the quinolone and β-lactam regimens. A small study evaluating patients treated with cefazolin, imipenem-cilastatin, ciprofloxacin and ofloxacin for complicated skin and soft tissue infections revealed that all patients were cured or improved with the regimens provided, however, cefazolin demonstrated limited *in vitro* activity against the Gram-negative microorganisms recovered from open wounds when compared to imipenem-cilastatin, ciprofloxacin or ofloxacin [29]. These early clinical studies established ofloxacin and more so, ciprofloxacin, as antimicrobial agents suitable for both uncomplicated and complicated skin and soft tissue infections, however, these studies were only powered to show equivalence. These studies serve to further substantiate the disparity between *in vitro* susceptibility testing and the clinical effectiveness of certain antimicrobial agents as based upon the *in vitro* susceptibilities, these quinolones may have been regarded as suboptimal agents for the management of staphylococcal and streptococcal infections.

With the development of the new generation quinolones with their improved spectrum of activity against Gram-positive microorganisms such as *S. pyogenes* and *S. aureus*, it is anticipated that an expanded role for the quinolone will be observed in the management of community and nosocomial acquired skin and soft tissue infections [4]. Some of the new quinolones have the added advantage of possessing significant activity against the anaerobes making these agents ideal for the management of the polymicrobial animal or human bite wound and the diabetic foot infection, however, the newer agents possess suboptimal anti-pseudomonal activity [5–7].

In comparison to the number of published clinical trials for the management of upper and lower respiratory tract infections utilizing the new quinolones, there are remarkably few controlled clinical trials evaluating the new quinolones for the management of complicated or uncomplicated skin and soft tissue infections. Levofloxacin (500 mg po od for 7–10 days) has been compared to ciprofloxacin (500 mg po bid for 7–10 days) in patients with uncomplicated skin and soft tissue infections [35, 36]. In both studies, the overall clinical success rates (96 and 98% for the two levofloxacin groups, 94% for the two ciprofloxacin groups) and bacteriological eradication rates were similar. One can therefore conclude that levofloxacin had a comparable overall efficacy to ciprofloxacin in this study population, however, it is important to note that ciprofloxacin is not traditionally considered a first-line therapy for the management of skin or soft tissue infections. It would have, however, been anticipated that a potential therapeutic advantage may have been observed with levofloxacin in light of its improved *in vitro* activity against the Gram-positive microorganisms compared to that of ciprofloxacin. In a randomized, open-label clinical trial for complicated skin and skin structure infections, levofloxacin administered either 750 mg parenterally once a day or intravenously followed by oral step-down therapy was compared to ticarcillin-clavulanate followed by amoxicillin-clavulanate oral step-down therapy [37]. Therapeutic equivalence was demonstrated between levofloxacin and the ticarcillin-clavulanate and amoxicillin-clavulanate regimens (success rates of 84.1% and 80.3% respectively). For microbiologically evaluable subjects, the overall eradication rate was 83.7% in the levofloxacin arm compared to 71.4% for the ticarcillin-clavulanate and amoxicillin-clavulanate treatment group. These data suggest that levofloxacin 750 mg once per day is comparable to ticarcillin-clavulanate and amoxicillin-clavulanate for complicated skin and skin structure infections [37]. Oral gatifloxacin (400 mg od) has been compared to oral levofloxacin (500 mg od) for the treatment of uncomplicated skin and soft tissue infections in a double-blind multicentre study [28]. In this study, it was noted that the cure rates for gatifloxacin (91%) were numerically higher, albeit not statistically significantly different from those of levofloxacin (83%). Bacterial eradication rates were comparable in both groups [28]. It may, therefore, be concluded that gatifloxacin with its expanded spectrum of activity which includes anaerobes is comparable to levofloxacin for the management of uncomplicated skin and soft tissue infections. Moxifloxacin (400 mg po od) has been found to be as effective as cephalexin (500 mg po tid) in the clinical management of uncomplicated skin infections and in bacteriologically eradicating the most frequently recovered pathogen, *S. aureus* [38]. Cure rates of 90% and 91% were observed with moxifloxacin and cephalexin respectively in this study [38]. Garenoxacin, the des-fluoro [6] quinolone is currently undergoing phase III clinical trials. Based upon its *in vitro* activity against aerobic and anaerobic pathogens isolated from skin and soft tissue animal and human bite wound infections [7], it is anticipated that this agent will also be effective in the routine management of skin and soft tissue infections, particularly those which are complicated. The MIC for this agent are comparable or lower than other quinolone agents and other classes of antimicrobials such as the β-lactams traditionally used for the management of skin and soft tissue infections [7].

The β-lactam agents have served as the mainstay for the management of skin and soft tissue infections since their introduction into the therapeutic arena. Narrow spectrum agents such as cloxacillin and cephalexin are ideal for the management of infections presumed to be caused by *S. aureus*, where the endemic rates of MRSA are not excessive. Penicillin is the agent of choice for the management of presumed group A streptococcal infections as the streptococci are exquisitely sensitive to penicillin, and penicillin resistance in these microorganisms has never been reported. Cefazolin/cephalexin can be used when it is unclear whether a skin or soft tissue infection is caused by *S. aureus* or *S. pyogenes*. In fact, these agents should remain as the mainstay of therapy for uncomplicated skin and soft tissue infections because of their proven efficacy and cost advantage. It is important to note that cephalexin has been used as a comparator in clinical trials evaluating an expanded spectrum quinolone with the results demonstrating comparable efficacy for both agents [38].

From the data presented above, it would appear that the quinolones are comparable in efficacy to the conventional anti-staphylococcal and anti-streptococcal agents. The quinolone's broad spectrum and increased cost may not justify their use for uncomplicated skin and soft tissue infections, furthermore, based upon the MICs of ciprofloxacin, it may be prudent to avoid this agent for skin and soft tissue infections as other more appropriate agents exist, specifically the β-lactam agents (cephalexin/cephazolin, cloxacillin), and non-β-lactam agents such as clindamycin. In areas of high MRSA endemnicity, consideration may be given to the use of vancomycin or linezolid for the management of skin and soft tissue infections caused by the Gram-positive cocci. The potential advantage, however, of these new quinolones in the management of uncomplicated infections would be for use in individuals where adherence with dosing regimens involving multiple administrations may be a concern. Another potential advantage would be in those individuals where β-lactam allergies exists. The true potential benefit of the new quinolones is for the management of complicated skin and soft tissue infections because of their broad spectrum, encompassing activity against Gram-positive, Gram-negative, and anerobic microorganisms, without the need for the co-administration of other agents, infrequent dosing (frequently, once a day), lack of appreciable nephrotoxicity, and excellent oral bioavailability allowing either for immediate oral therapy or a rapid parenteral to oral stepdown [39]. The ideal positioning of these new expanded spectrum quinolones would therefore be for the management of polymicrobial infections particularly for those of the foot of persons with diabetes, pressure ulcerations or perineal processes such as perirectal abscesses. While the potential benefits of the expanded spectrum quinolones has been speculated in the preceding material, the data from the current and future clinical trials will have to be evaluated before making a firm recommendation with regards to their use.

Future direction – skin and soft tissue infections

Ciprofloxacin and ofloxacin have been extensively evaluated for the management of both complicated and uncomplicated skin and soft tissue infections, using a variety of oral and parenteral comparators. It may be prudent that the currently available expanded spectrum quinolone agents undergo the same rigorous evaluation as these earlier compounds. It would also be of benefit to determine whether there is any therapeutic advantage between the newer expanded spectrum quinolone agents as the studies to date have not been direct comparisons but rather comparisons to agents whose therapeutic spectra may be somewhat limited.

Bone infections

Osteomyelitis may be divided into several categories, specifically: hematogenous, arising from blood-borne organisms, most frequently seen in children; or contiguous spread from a surrounding area of skin and soft tissue infection such as in the diabetic foot, pressure ulcer, or from surgical inoculation or trauma [39–42]. Osteomyelitis may also be acute, occurring most frequently in children and following hematogenous spread; or chronic, which is associated with infected, dead bone, within a compromised soft tissue envelope [41, 42]. Several excellent reviews exist with regards to the role of the quinolones for the management of osteomyelitis [41–44]. Unlike the studies for the evaluation of new agents for the management of skin and soft tissue infections, which consider groups of essentially homogeneous patients (cellulitis, erysipelas, abscesses) and which are generally standardized and easily comparable, similar studies do not exist for the evaluation of antimicrobial agents in the management of osteomyelitis. Although a multitude of case reports exist documenting the success of various quinolones for the management of osteomyelitis, the surgical management, or lack thereof, dose, duration of therapy and location of the bone infection make direct comparisons between these studies difficult. A number of issues complicate the studies evaluating the role of antimicrobial agents for the management of osteomyelitis. Some of these parameters include significant differences in the patient populations being evaluated, and methodological variations, specifically open labeled *versus* blinded controlled clinical trials. Other factors that make comparisons between these studies difficult is that in some cases, the use of the antimicrobial agent was either singly or in combination, and the study endpoints and clinical outcomes varied [45]. It is difficult to know whether osteomyelitis is ever truly healed as relapses may occur years after the infection has presumably been treated, thus, the therapeutic endpoints considered in these studies are actually those for the induction of a remission instead of a true "cure."

The management of osteomyelitis whether acute or chronic is frequently associated with initial surgical debridement followed by postoperative antibiotics for a defined period of time. The rationale for this approach is to allow for bony reconstitution in a "clean" environment thus preventing reinfection of the freshly debrided bone [40].

Although data exists with regards to the use of ofloxacin, and other early quinolone agents, the majority of the data from randomized comparative studies for the management of osteomyelitis, particularly chronic osteomyelitis arises from studies comparing ciprofloxacin to other agents. Unfortunately, as previously mentioned, a comparison between the studies is difficult as the duration of therapy and dose of agent used in these studies varied. To further complicate comparisons, the patient numbers in these studies were small [46–49]. In these studies, the enterobacteraciae were the most frequently recovered microorganism with a frequent representation of *Pseudomonas auriginosa* and *S. aureus*. The duration of therapy with the oral agents ranged between 28–75 days. With the outcome of treatment for those receiving oral therapy ranging between 71–100% *versus* 84–100% for those treated with parenteral therapy [46–49]. It is difficult to make sweeping conclusions about these studies as the patient population was heterogeneous, treatment durations and follow-up were variable. These early studies do, however, suggest that oral quinolone therapy was usually successful and feasible. It is important to note that in these studies, the success of treatment was greatest with individuals with osteomyelitis caused by the Gram-negative microorganisms compared to those caused by *S. aureus* which is likely a reflection of the antibacterial spectrum of these agents.

Although there are numerous uncontrolled reports of the use of the new quinolone agents for the treatment of osteomyelitis, there have been remarkably few controlled studies assessing the efficacy of these agents for the treatment of chronic osteomyelitis in humans. In one prospective, randomized, non-blinded clinical trial, evaluating ciprofloxacin, lomefloxacin and levofloxacin for the treatment of chronic osteomyelitis, it was noted that levofloxacin achieved a cure rate of 60% (nine of 15 patients), lomefloxacin was effective in 71% (five of seven patients) and ciprofloxacin was effective in 40% (two of five patients) [50]. It is difficult to draw significant conclusions from this study as the patient numbers were small and duration of therapy and follow-up variable. The average duration of therapy was 60.6 days with an average follow-up of 11.8 months. In recent animal studies, oral levofloxacin and oral gatifloxacin have been compared to parenteral nafcillin [51, 52]. Both of these animal studies were performed using similar methodology. These authors report that levofloxacin showed a significant reduction in *S. aureus* infections compared to the non-treated, infected controls, however, it was inferior to that of parenteral nafcillin. Oral gatifloxacin was, however, as effective as parenteral nafcillin for the treatment of experimental *S. aureus* induced osteomyelitis in rabbits. These two studies provide important animal data about the potential management of osteomyelitis with oral antimicrobial therapy. Such data is lacking for the other new quinolones.

From this review, it would appear that data exists, albeit from a variety of controlled and uncontrolled studies suggesting that oral ciprofloxacin may be a consideration for the management of osteomyelitis. It may be ideal to target the use of ciprofloxacin for the management of osteomyelitis caused by Gram-negative microorganisms in light of the MIC's of the Gram-positive aerobic cocci to ciprofloxacin. Animal data is also available for some of the other quinolones, however, at this time since formal human studies have not been conducted, using the new quinolones for the management of osteomyelitis. Their use can, therefore not be recommended nor endorsed for the management of osteomyelitis particularly when concern has been raised about the cardiovascular safety of some of the newer agents since a prolonged duration of therapy is required for the treatment of osteomyelitis, specifically when using oral quinolone therapy.

Future direction – bone infections

Before agents other than ciprofloxacin and ofloxacin can be endorsed for the treatment of osteomyelitis, formal human studies are necessary. Prior to the performance of these studies, however, long-term safety data for the other quinolones such as levofloxacin, moxifloxacin, gatifloxacin and garenoxacin is necessary, particularly in light of toxicities encountered with some of the other quinolone agents. It would also be ideal if standardized controlled clinical trials for the treatment of acute and chronic osteomyelitis could be performed. The optimal positioning for the extended spectrum quinolones with expanded activity against the Gram-positive, Gram-negative and anaerobic microorganisms would be for the management of polymicrobial diabetic foot osteomyelitis, or osteomyelitis complicating pressure ulcerations. The quinolones would be ideal as oral alternatives to parenteral therapy for the management of these chronic infections, as the duration of therapy is prolonged and the oral route would be most convenient. It must be remembered, however, that for many of these infections the antimicrobial therapy is only one part of the management, and adjunctive measures such as debridement and pressure relief are also critical.

Prosthetic joint infections

Infections in prosthetic joints can be classified as "early" postoperative infections which become apparent within 1 month of the time of surgery or as "late" chronic infections presenting anytime after the first month of surgery [53]. The aerobic Gram-positive cocci particularly *S. epidermidis* and *S. aureus* are the most frequently recovered microorganisms in prosthetic joint infections [54, 55]. It is the goal of perioperative antimicrobial prophylaxis to decrease the risk of perioperative wound and deep infections with skin microorganisms. This, of course, does not preclude hematogenous infection arising from the urinary tract, vascular access devices and other sites such as pressure ulcerations in the postoperative period.

The optimal techniques for diagnosis and management of acute prosthetic joint infections has not been well defined and is deeply entrenched in tradition. For early postoperative infections, soft-tissue debridement in conjunction with antimicrobial therapy and retention of the prosthesis has a successful outcome in approximately 70% of cases [54, 56, 57]. Although these studies indicate high degrees of success, the data must be interpreted with caution as formal rigorous comparative studies do not exist comparing the type of surgery, duration and route of antimicrobial therapy and duration of follow-up.

In individuals who develop late chronic prosthetic joint infection, the diagnosis and management is also not standardized. The traditionally accepted approaches include either a one-step procedure with removal of the preexisting prosthesis, debridement and reimplantation of a new prosthesis in conjunction with periprocedure antimicrobial therapy, or, alternatively a two-stage procedure with removal of the infected hardware and debridement, implantation of an antibiotic spacer followed by 4–6 weeks of parenteral therapy and reimplantation of a new prosthesis [58–60]. Although infection in joint replacements occurs in approximately 4% of patients over the lifetime of the joint, it would be anticipated that a large body of data would exist surrounding the management of these infections, however, this is not the case [61, 62]. Several studies have demonstrated that if a prosthetic joint infection is detected early, debridement in conjunction with antimicrobial therapy may allow for prosthesis retention [63–65]. In these studies, it is suggested that for patients with a short duration of infection and stable orthopedic implants, debridement and antimicrobial therapy may lead to salvage of the prosthesis. Unfortunately, the patient numbers for these studies were small ranging from 18 to 69, study designs varied, bacteriology and antibiotic regimens differed as did the definitions of "cure."

Two studies have prospectively considered the role of the quinolones ofloxacin or ciprofloxacin in conjunction with rifampin for the management of *Staphylococcus* spp. or *S. aureus* infections [64, 66]. The addition of rifampin in conjunction with the quinolone appears to have beneficial effects in leading to preservation of the infected stable joint prosthesis, however, once again, caution is urged with the interpretation of this result as the number of study participants was small [64, 66].

These preliminary data provide hope that stable prosthesis may be retained if the infection is detected early and a limited debridement combined with a quinolone-rifampin regimen. It is important to note, however, that the protocols considering a quinolone-rifampin regimen have only considered staphylococcal prosthetic joint infections.

While the two studies [64, 66] of quinolone-rifampin regimen offer an alternative to the management of infected prosthetic joints, these studies must be interpreted with great caution as they only evaluated a small number of patients.

Future direction – prosthetic joint infection

Before more wide-sweeping conclusions can be drawn as to the role of oral quinolone therapy for the management of prosthetic joint infections can be made, formal prospective randomized controlled studies must be undertaken with a significant number of study subjects. These studies, however, will be difficult to conduct as they must address a number of factors such as the type of prosthesis (knee, hip) duration of initial infection, microbiology, surgical intervention at the time the infection was recognized, the duration of parenteral followed by oral antimicrobial therapy and antibiotic free interval after the initial treatment and the time a "cure" is established. Clearly, oral antimicrobial therapy is limited to individuals with stable prosthesis and for whom a definitive one- or two-stage procedure may not be indicated or those who decline a more aggressive approach.

Conclusions

In the preceding review, it is clear that the fluoroquinolones, particularly the newer agents with expanded activity against Gram-positive microorganisms are agents which may provide an alternative for the management of skin and soft tissue, and bone infections, particularly in those who are allergic to the β-lactam agents. It is important to recall that other well established agents currently exist for the management of the infections that have been reviewed and these agents should not be forgotten. These agents include cloxacillin and cefazolin/cephalexin for the management of uncomplicated skin and soft tissue infections where the rates of endemic MRSA do not preclude the use of these agents. Piperacillin/tazobactam or other β-lactam and non-β-lactam combinations for complicated skin and soft tissue infections such as clindamycin and gentamicin or cefazolin and metronidazole, are also considerations. While it is necessary to accept new agents such as the quinolones into the armamentaria for the management of skin and soft tissue and bone infections the other agents must not be completely replaced as they still offer significant therapeutic and economic benefits. The quinolones, particularly those with expanded antimicrobial activity, will be ideal agents for the management of the diabetic foot or infected pressure ulcerations. While it would be ideal to recommend these newer agents for the management of the polymicrobial diabetic foot infection, current safety data does not exist to support the use of these agents for prolonged periods of time. If formal studies are performed addressing long-term oral quinolone therapy for the management of osteomyelitis, then these newer agents can be embraced. Until that time, the conventional agents should be used. The treatment of infected orthopedic implants is far more complicated than merely using an antibiotic. The implant must be stable, debridement may be necessary, and long-term parenteral or oral antimicrobial therapy will be necessary. The quinolones, ofloxacin and ciprofloxacin have been used in combination with rifampin for the treatment of staphylococcal infections of stable prosthetic joints. These studies form the foundation from which future prospective studies should be undertaken to formally evaluate the role of parenteral or oral quinolone based regimens with or without rifampin for the management of staphylococcal infections. An appropriately focussed use of the quinolone agents will help maintain their viability into the future.

Acknowledgments
The author acknowledges the excellent secretarial assistance of Ms. Carolyn Schlippert in the preparation of this review.

References

1 Owens RC Jr, Ambrose PG (2000) Clinical use of the fluoroquinolones. *Med Clin North Am* 84: 1447–1469

2 Bongaerts GP, Hoogkamp-Korstanje JA (1993) *In vitro* activities of BAY Y3118, ciprofloxacin, ofloxacin, and fleroxacin against Gram-positive and Gram-negative pathogens from respiratory tract and soft tissue infections. *Anitmicrob Agents Chemother* 37: 2017–2019

3 Bauernfeind A (1997) Comparison of the antibacterial activities of the quinolones Bay 12-8039, gatifloxacin (AM 1155), trovafloxacin, clinafloxacin, levofloxacin, and ciprofloxacin. *J Antimicrob Chemother* 40: 639–651

4 Critchley IA, Sahm DF, Thornsberry C, Blosser-Middleton RS, Jones ME, Karlowsky JA (2002) Antimicrobial susceptibilities of *Streptococcus pyogenes* isolated from respiratory and skin and soft tissue infections: United States LIBRA surveillance data from 1999. *Diagn Microbiol Infect Dis* 42: 129–135

5 Goldstein EJ, Citron DM, Hudspeth M, Hunt Gerardo S, Merriam CV (1997) *In vitro* activity of Bay 12-8039, a new 8-methoxyquinolone, compared to the activities of 11 other oral antimicrobial agents against 390 aerobic and anaerobic bacteria isolated from human and animal bite wound skin and soft tissue infections in humans. *Antimicrob Agents Chemother* 41: 1552–1557

6 Goldstein EJ, Citron DM, Merriam CV, Tyrrell K, Warren Y (1999) Activity of gatifloxacin compared to those of five other quinolones *versus* aerobic and anaerobic isolates for skin and soft tissue samples of human and animal bite wound infections. *Antimicrob Agents Chemother* 43: 1475–1479

7 Goldstein EJ, Citron DM, Merriam CV, Warren YA, Tyrrell KL, Fernandez H (2002) *In vitro* activities of the des-fluoro (6) quinolone BMS – 284756 against aerobic and anaerobic pathogens isolated from skin and soft tissue animal and human bite wound infections. *Antimicrob Agents Chemother* 46: 866–870

8 Barry AL, Fuchs PC, Brown SD (2001) *In vitro* activities of three nonfluorinated quinolones against representative bacterial isolates. *Antimicrob Agents Chemother* 45: 1923–1927

9 Yan SS, Fox ML, Holland SM, Stock F, Gill VJ, Fedorko DP (2000) Resistance to multiple fluoroquinolones in a clinical isolate of *Streptococcus pyogenes*: identification of *gyrA* and *parC* and specification of point mutations associated with resistance. *Antimicrob Agents Chemother* 44: 3196–3198

10 Perez-Trallero E, Fernandez-Mazarrasa C, Garcia-Rey C, Bouza E, Aguilar L, Garcia-de-Lomas J, Baquero F (2001) Antimicrobial susceptibilities of 1,684 *Streptococcus pneumoniae* and 2,039 *Streptococcus pyogenes* isolates and their ecological relationships: results of a 1-year (1998–1999) multicenter surveillance study in Spain. *Antimicrob Agents Chemother* 45: 3334–3340

11 Barry AL, Jones RN (1987) *In vitro* activity of ciprofloxacin against Gram-positive cocci. *Am J Med* 82 (Suppl 4A): 27–32

12 Smith SM (1986) *In vitro* comparison of A-56619, A-56620, amifloxacin, ciprofloxacin, enoxacin, norfloxacin, and ofloxacin against methicillin-resistant *Staphylococcus aureus*. *Antimicrob Agents Chemother* 29: 325–326

13 Hooper DC (2001) Emerging mechanisms of fluoroquinolone resistance. *Emerg Infect Dis* 7: 337–341

14 Acar JF, Goldstein FW (1997) Trends in bacterial resistance to fluoroquinolones. *Clin Infect Dis* 24 Suppl 1: S67–S73

15 Santos S, Mato R, de Lencastre H, Tamasz A (2000) Patterns of multidrug resistance among methicillin-resistant hospital isolates of coagulase-positive and coagulase-negative staphylococci collected in the international multicenter study RESIST in 1997 and 1998. *Microb Drug Resist* 6: 199–211

16 Tacconelli E, Tumbarello M, Donati KG, Bettio M, Spanu T, Leone F, Sechi LA, Zanetti S, Fadda G, Cauda R (2001) Glycopeptide resistance among coagulase-negative staphylococci that cause bacteremia: epidemiological and clinical findings from a case- control study. *Clin Infect Dis* 33: 1628–1635

17 McCloskey L, Moore T, Niconovich N, Donald B, Broskey J, Jakielaszek C, Rittenhouse S, Coleman K (2000) *In vitro* activity of gemifloxacin against a broad range of recent clinical isolates from the USA. *J Antimicrob Chemother* 45 (Suppl 1): 13–21

18 Monsen T, Ronnmark M, Olofsson C, Wistrom J (1999) Antibiotic susceptibility of staphylococci

isolated in blood cultures in relation to antibiotic consumption in hospital wards. *Scand J Infect Dis* 31: 399–404

19 Greenberg RN, Kennedy DJ, Reilly PM, Luppen KL, Weinandt WJ, Bollinger MR, Aguirre F, Kodesch F, Saeed AM. 1987. Treatment of bone, joint, and soft-tissue infections with oral ciprofloxacin. *Antimicrob Agents Chemother* 31: 151–155

20 Mulligan ME, Ruane PJ, Johnston L, Wong P, Wheelock JP, MacDonald K, Reinhardt JF, Johnson CC, Statner B, Blomquist I, McCarthy J, O'Brien W, Gardner S, Hammer L, Citron DM (1987) Ciprofloxacin for eradication of methicillin-resistant *Staphylococcus aureus* colonization. *Am J Med* 82: 215–219

21 Piercy EA, Barbaro D, Luby JP, Mackowiak PA (1989) Ciprofloxacin for methicillin-resistant *Staphylococcus aureus* infections. *Antimicrob Agents Chemother* 33: 128–130

22 Peterson LR, Quick JN, Jensen B, Homann S, Johnson S, Tenquist J, Shanholtzer C, Petzel RA, Sinn L, Gerding DN (1990) Emergence of ciprofloxacin resistance in nosocomial methicillin-resistant *Staphylococcus aureus* isolates. Resistance during ciprofloxacin plus rifampin therapy for methicillin-resistant *S. aureus* colonization. *Arch Intern Med* 150: 2151–2155

23 Blumberg HM, Rimland D, Carroll DJ, Terry P, Wachsmuth IK (1991) Rapid development of ciprofloxacin resistance in methicillin- susceptible and -resistant *Staphylococcus aureus*. *J Infect Dis* 163: 1279–1285

24 Bergeron MG (1989) The pharmacokinetics and tissue penetration of fluoroquinolones. *Clin Invest Med* 12: 20–27

25 MacGregor RR, Graziani AL (1997) Oral administration of antibiotics: a rational alternative to the parenteral route. *Clin Infect Dis* 24: 457–467

26 Blondeau JM (1999) Expanded activity and utility of the new fluoroquinolones: a review. *Clin Ther* 21: 3–40

27 Mueller M, Brunner M, Hollenstein U, Joukhadar C, Schmid R, Minar E, Ehringer H, Eichler HG (1999) Penetration of ciprofloxacin into the interstitial space of inflamed foot lesions in non-insulin dependent diabetes mellitus patients. *Antimicrob Agents Chemother* 43: 2056–2058

28 Tarshis GA, Miskin BM, Jones TM, Champlain J, Wingert KJ, Breen JD, Brown MJ (2001) Once-daily oral gatifloxacin *versus* oral levofloxacin in treatment of uncomplicated skin and soft tissue infections: double-blind, multicentre, randomized study. *Antimicrob Agents Chemother* 45: 2358–2362

29 Liu HH, Bolash NK, McAnany ME, Lynch RA (1995) Susceptibility of bacterial isolates from complicated skin and skin structure infections to cefazolin, imipenem-cilastatin, ciprofloxacin and ofloxacin. *Drugs* 49 (Suppl 2): 215–218

30 Ramirez-Ronda CH, Saavedra S, Rivera-Vazquez CR (1987) Comparative, double-blind study of oral ciprofloxacin and intravenous cefotaxime in skin and skin structure infections. *Am J Med* 82 (suppl 4A): 220–223

31 Perez-Ruvalcaba JA, Quintero-Perez NP, Morales-Reyes JJ, Huitron-Ramirez JA, Rodriguez-Chagollan JJ, Rodriguez-Noriega E (1987) Double-blind comparison of ciprofloxacin with cefotaxime in the treatment of skin and skin structure infections. *Am J Med* 82 (suppl 4A): 242–246

32 Gentry LO, Ramirez-Ronda CH, Rodriguez-Noriega E, Thadepalli H, del Rosal PL, Ramirez C (1999) Oral ciprofloxacin *versus* parenteral cefotaxime in the treatment of difficult skin and soft tissue structure infections. A mulit-centre trial. *Arch Intern Med* 149: 2579–2583

33 Gentry LO, Rodriguez-Gomez G, Zeluff BJ, Khoshdel A, Price M (1989) A comparative evaluation of oral ofloxacin *versus* intravenous cefotaxime therapy for serious skin and skin structure infections. *Am J Med* 87 (suppl 6C) 57–60

34 Lipsky BA, Baker PD, Landon GC, Fernau R (1997) Antibiotic Therapy for Diabetic Foot infections: comparison of two parenteral-to-oral regimens. *Clin Infect Dis* 24: 643–648

35 Nichols RL, Smith JW, Gentry LO, Gezon J, Campbell T, Sokal P, Williams RR (1998) Multicentre, randomized study comparing levofloxacin and ciprofloxacin for uncomplicated skin and skin structure infections. *South Med J* 90: 1193–1200

36 Nicodemo AC, Robledo JA, Jasovich A, Neto W (1998) A multicentre, double-blind, randomized study comparing the efficacy and safety of oral levofloxacin *versus* ciprofloxacin in the treatment of uncomplicated skin and skin structure infections. *Int J Clin Pract* 52: 69–74

37 Graham DR, Talan DA, Nichols RL, Lucsti C, Corrado N, Morgan N, Fowler CL (2002) Once-daily, high-dose levofloxacin *versus* ticarcillin-clavulanate alone or followed by amoxicillin-clavulanate for complicated skin and skin-structure infections. A randomized open-labeled trial. *Clin Infect Dis* 35: 381–389

38 Parish LC, Routh HB, Miskin B, Fidelholtz J, Werschler P, Heyd A, Haverstock D, Church D

(2000) Moxifloxacin *versus* cephalexin in treatment of uncomplicated skin infections. *Int J Clin Pract* 54: 497–503
39 Karchmer AW (1999) Fluoroquinolone treatment of skin and skin structure infections. *Drugs* 58 (suppl 2): 82–84
40 Rissing JP (1997) Antimicrobial Therapy for chronic osteomyelitis in adults: role of the quinolones. *Clin Infect Dis* 25: 1327–1333
41 Haas DW, McAndrew MP (1996) Bacterial osteomyelitis in adults: evolving considerations in diagnosis and treatment. *Am J Med* 101: 550–561
42 Cierny G, Mader JT (1984) Adult chronic osteomyelitis. *Orthopedics* 7: 1557–1564
43 Cole WG (1984) Acute osteomyelitis overview. *Orthopedics* 7: 1553–1556
44 Lew DP, Waldvogel FA (1995) Quinolones and osteomyelitis: state-of-the-art. *Drugs* 49 (suppl 2): 100–111
45 Lew DP, Waldvogel FA (1999) Use of quinolones in osteomyelitis and infected orthopedic prosthesis. 58 (suppl 2): 85–91
46 Greenberg RN, Tice AD, Marsh PK, Craven PC, Reilly PM, Bollinger M, Weinandt WJ (1987) Randomized trial of ciprofloxacin compared with other antimicrobial therapy in the treatment of osteomyelitis. *Am J Med* 82 (Suppl 4A): 266–269
47 Gentry LO, Rodriguez GG (1990) Oral ciprofloxacin compared with parenteral antibiotics in the treatment of osteomyelitis. *Antimicrob Agents Chemother* 34: 40–43
48 Gentry LO, Rodriguez-Gomez G (1991) Ofloxacin *versus* parenteral therapy for chronic osteomyelitis. *Antimicrob Agents Chemother* 35: 538–541
49 Trujillo IZ, Valladares G, Nava A (1993) Ciprofloxacin and the treatment of chronic osteomyelitis in adults. *Drugs* 45 (suppl 3) 454–455
50 Greenberg RN, Newman MT, Shariaty S, Pectol RW (2000) Ciprofloxacin, lomefloxacin, or levofloxacin as treatment for chronic osteomyelitis. *Antimicrob Agents Chemother* 44: 164–166
51 Shirtliff ME, Calhoun JH, Mader JT (2001) Comparative evaluation of oral levofloxacin and parenteral nafcillin in the treatment of experimental methicillin-susceptible *Staphylococcus aureus* osteomyelitis in rabbits. *J Antimicrob Chemother* 48: 253–258
52 Shirtliff ME, Calhoun JH, Mader JT (2002) Gatifloxacin efficacy in treatment of experimental methicillin-sensitive *Staphylococcus aureus*-induced osteomyelitis in rabbits. *Antimicrob Agents Chemother* 46: 231–233
53 Estrada R, Tsukayama D, Gustilo R (1993) Management of THA infections: a prospective study of 108 cases. *Orthop Trans* 17: 1114–1115
54 Tsukayama DT, Estrada R, Gustilo R (1996) Infection after total hip arthroplasty: a study of the treatment of one hundred and six infections. *J Bone Joint Surg Am* 78: 512–523
55 Whiteside LA (1994) Treatment of infected total knee arthroplasty. *Clin Orthop* 299: 169–172
56 Hartman MB, Fehring TK, Jordan L, Norton HJ (1991) Periprosthetic knee sepsis: the role of irrigation and debridement. *Clin Orthop* 273 113–118
57 Burger RR, Basch T, Hopson CN (1991) Implant salvage in infected total knee arthroplasty. *Clin Orthop* 273: 105–112
58 Garvin KL, Hanssen AD (1995) Infection after a total hip arthroplasty: past, present, and future. *J Bone Joint Surg Am* 77: 1576–1588
59 Hanssen AD, Rand JA, Osmon DR (1994) Treatment of infected total knee arthroplasty with insertion of another prosthesis. The effect of antibiotic-impregnated bone cement. *Clin Orthop* 309: 44–55
60 Ivarrson I, Wahlstrom O, Djerf K, Jacobsson SA (1994) Revision of infected hip replacement. Two-stage procedure with a temporary gentamicin spacer. *Acta Orthop Scand* 65: 7–8
61 Gillespie WJ (1997) Prevention and management of infection after total joint replacement. *Clin Infect Dis* 25: 1310–1317
62 Keating MR, Steckelberg JM (1999) Editorial response: orthopedic prosthesis salvage. *Clin Infect Dis* 29: 296–297
63 Brandt CM, Sistrunk WW, Duffy MC, Hanssen AD, Steckelberg JM, Ilstrup DM, Osmon DR (1997) *Staphylococcus aureus* prosthetic joint infection treated with debridement and prosthesis retention. *Clin Infect Dis* 24: 914–919
64 Zimmerli W, Widmer AF, Blatter M, Frei R, Oschner PE, For the Foreign-Body Infection (FBI) Study Group (1998) Role of rifampin for treatment of orthopedic implant-related staphylococcal infections. A randomized controlled trial. *JAMA* 279: 1537–1541
65 Tattevin P, Cremieux AC, Pottier P, Huten D, Carbon C (1999) Prosthetic joint infection: when can

prosthesis salvage be considered? *Clin Infect Dis* 29: 292–295
66 Drancourt M, Stein A, Argenson JN, Zannier A, Curvale G, Roult D (1993) Oral rifampin plus ofloxacin for treatment of *Staphylococcus*-infected orthopedic implants. *Antimicrob Agents Chemother* 37: 1214–1218

Fluoroquinolone Antibiotics
ed. by A.R. Ronald and D.E. Low

The role of fluoroquinolones in the therapy and prophylaxis of neutropenic patients with cancer

Helen Giamarellou and Anastasia Antoniadou

Athens University School of Medicine, 4th Department of Internal Medicine, Sismanoglio General Hospital, 1 Sismanogliou St., 15126 Maroussi, Athens, Greece

Introduction

Patients with cancer who become severely neutropenic (<500 cells/mm^3) as a result of intensive myelosuppressive chemotherapy are at high risk of developing life-threatening infections which can progress to sepsis and death in a few hours, unless they are treated presumptively at the first sign of infection. This has led to the consensus that empiric therapy, while awaiting culture results, must be initiated promptly with the first evidence of a probable infection [1, 2]. Combinations of antibiotics, preferably an antipseudomonal beta-lactam plus an aminoglycoside provide wide coverage, bactericidal activity, and potential synergistic effects. While combination therapy may also prevent emergence of resistance. To avoid the nephrotoxic and ototoxic potential of the aminoglycosides, antibiotic monotherapy regimens such as ceftazidime, cefepime, cefpirome, cefoperazone-sulbactam and piperacillin/tazobactam as well as imipenem and meropenem have been administered with results that appear to be equivalent [2, 3].

Since 1988 the fluoroquinolones have been evaluated both as monotherapy and in combination with other agents in a number of studies [4–18]. The role of the quinolones for infection prophylaxis in the neutropenic host remains in dispute despite two recent meta-analysis [19–20].

In this review, the current role of the quinolones for both therapy and prophylaxis in the neutropenic patient is critically analyzed.

The role of fluoroquinolones in the therapy of the febrile neutropenic cancer patient

In-patient therapy

The fluoroquinolones, particularly ciprofloxacin, possess some advantages that could benefit the neutropenic host. These include bactericidal activity against Gram-negative agents ciprofloxacin being particularly effective against *Pseudomonas aeruginosa*; bioavailability both as oral and parenteral formulations; a favorable pharmacokinetic profile, relative safety, lacking ototoxicity and nephrotoxicity; and a limited need to monitor blood levels since drug dosing need not be individualized.

Over the past 15 years a shift in the etiology of infections in neutropenic patients has occurred. In most cancer centers, the predominant pathogen has shifted from Gram-negatives to coagulase-negative staphylococci and streptococci [2]. Even though the Gram-positive pathogens are usually less virulent, disseminated intravascular coagulation and the adult respiratory distress syndrome can occur. Predisposing conditions that have been incriminated for the reported increase in Gram-positive pathogens include aggressive chemotherapy and radiotherapy that injure the oral and gastrointestinal mucosa; increased use of intravascular access lines and other invasive interventions; and the use of quinolone prophylaxis during neutropenia which selects Gram-positive bacteria from the gastrointestinal flora. However, Gram-negative infections remain a major concern since they are responsible for a mortality in the range of 20–30% and are frequently fulminant. Also, Gram-negatives have re-emerged in centres where quinolone prophylaxis has been abandoned [21]. Therefore, therapy appropriately directed against the Gram-negative bacteria must remain the cornerstone of empiric treatment in the febrile neutropenic patient.

Ciprofloxacin is the most active fluoroquinolone against *P. aeruginosa* and has been studied most thoroughly as a single agent for febrile neutropenic patients. Studies using other quinolones are few and reported mostly as abstracts. Between 1989 and 1992, 13 studies were published in the English literature. In five, ciprofloxacin was used as a single agent; in eight, ciprofloxacin was evaluated in combination with other agents (Tab. 1) [14–18].

The success of ciprofloxacin in combination with another antimicrobial agent appears to be equivalent to that of the "standard" combination regimens. In contrast the five studies of ciprofloxacin as a single agent vary widely with reported success rates, from 14% to 82%. These differences may be attributed to the variability in the proportion of patients with profound neutropenia; differences in the proportion of bacteremic patients; variation in the timing of outcomes, i.e., at 48 h, 72 h, or the end of therapy; the previous use of antimicrobial prophylaxis; the maldistribution of underlying conditions; and differences in the definition of the outcome "failure." The main definitions now used in clinical studies are those of the National Cancer Institute (NCI), the European Organization for the Research and Treatment of Cancer (EORTC) and the Immunocompromised Host Society (ICHS) [2]. Pizzo et al. introduced the term "success with modification" defined as survival during the febrile episode despite the requirement for other antibacterial, antifungal, or antiviral agents [2]. According to this NCI definition, success requires survival throughout the febrile episode and until neutrophil recovery occurs. Failure equates with death. In contrast, EORTC and ICHS criteria differ mainly in that the "success with modification" outcome is not accepted.

Table 1. Comparative clinical effectiveness of ciprofloxacin monotherapy or in combination to established regimens in febrile neutropenia

Regimen	*n*	Ciprofloxacin regimen	Successful clinical response[a]	Refs
Ciprofloxacin	30	200 mg i.v. t.i.d	73%	[4]
Ciprofloxacin + vancomycin	35	400 mg i.v. b.i.d	77%	[5]
Ciprofloxacin + piperacillin	47	200 mg i.v. b.i.d.	61%	[6]
Ciprofloxacin + ceftazidime	106	400 mg i.v. b.i.d.	57.5%[b]	[7]
Ciprofloxacin vs. ceftazidime	21 vs. 25	200 mg i.v. b.i.d.	14% vs.21% [c]	[8]
Ciprofloxacin vs. ceftazidime	28 vs. 31	300 mg i.v. b.i.d.	82% vs. 58%	[9]
Ciprofloxacin vs. amikacin + piperacillin	63 vs. 91	200 mg i.v. b.i.d.	65% vs. 91%	[10]
Ciprofloxacin vs. netilmicin + azlocillin	73 vs. 70	300 mg i.v. b.i.d.	34% vs. 40%	[11]
Ciprofloxacin vs. ceftazidime + amikacin	124 vs. 122	400 mg i.v. b.i.d	50% vs. 50.8%[d]	[12]
Ciprofloxacin + netilmicin vs. netilmicin + piperacillin	115 vs. 99	200 mg i.v. b.i.d.	59% vs. 62%[e]	[13]
Ciprofloxacin + azlocillin vs. amikacin + ceftazidime	25 vs. 24	300 mg i.v. b.i.d.	32% vs. 50%[f]	[14]
Ciprofloxacin + azlocillin vs. gentamicin + azlocillin	80 vs. 67	200 mg i.v. b.i.d.	57.5% vs. 63%	[15]
Ciprofloxacin + azlocillin vs. netilmicin + azlocillin	37 vs. 36	200 mg i.v. b.i.d.	54% vs. 36%	[16]
Ciprofloxacin + penicillin G vs. netilmicin + piperacillin	51 vs. 46	200 mg i.v. b.i.d.	65% vs. 65%	[17]
Ciprofloxacin + teicoplanin vs. gentamicin + piperacillin	36 vs. 35	200 mg i.v. b.i.d.	78% vs. 49%	[18]

[a] Cure plus improvement.
[b] Success defined as survival through the neutropenic period; results refer to success without modification; another 41.5% responded successfully after modification.
[c] After modification with the addition of vancomycin success was achieved in 72% vs. 64%.
[d] Results expressed as success without modification; in 82 patients switch to oral ciprofloxacin (750 mg b.i.d) after at least 72 h of i.v. ciprofloxacin.
[e] Both groups converted to oral ciprofloxacin (500 mg b.i.d.) after 72 h.
[f] Oral ciprofloxacin was given to complete treatment that was started in hospital.

The borderline *in vitro* efficacy of ciprofloxacin against *Streptococcus* spp. and MRSA is of concern. In the EORTC study, patients with solid tumors and lymphomas had an overall success rate of 65% when treated with 200 or 300 mg of I.V. ciprofloxacin twice daily, whereas the overall success rate for patients treated with piperacillin plus amikacin was 91% (Tab. 1) [10]. Patients with Gram-positive coccal bacteremia had particularly poor outcomes. In six of eight patients therapy with ciprofloxacin failed, whereas no failure occurred in the corresponding four patients in the comparator arm. These poor results caused premature discontinuation of the trial. Also, an outbreak of bacteremia due to resistant *Escherichia coli* occurred in neutropenic patients during ciprofloxacin therapy [22]. To exploit the pharmacokinetics/pharmacodynamics of ciprofloxacin, a study was designed in which monotherapy with I.V. ciprofloxacin was prescribed with a dose of 400 mg thrice daily and compared to the conventional regimen of ceftazidime plus amikacin in 263 adult febrile neutropenic patients, most of whom had acute leukemia (79%) with neutrophils <100 cells/mm^3 (69%) [12]. Only one-half the patients in each group exhibited a successful clinical response "without modification." Both regimens were more effective against bacteremias due to Gram-negative (56.2% for the ciprofloxacin group *versus* 66.7% for the ceftazidime/amikacin group) compared to those due to Gram-positive organisms where only 35.7% and 23.1% respectively responded. Ciprofloxacin was as effective as ceftazidime plus amikacin against *P. aeruginosa* infections (71.4% *versus* 66.7%). Mortality was similar (5%) in the two treatment groups either during treatment or during the follow-up period. The authors concluded that monotherapy with ciprofloxacin may be recommended in centres in which: (i) infections caused by Gram-positive cocci are less frequent, (ii) where prophylaxis with quinolones is not routine, and (iii) where susceptibility to ciprofloxacin for the vast majority of Gram-negative pathogens is assured. However, the Infectious Diseases Society of America in the 2002 guidelines for "The Use of Antimicrobial Agents in Neutropenic Patients with Unexplained Fever" do not recommend "quinolone monotherapy" for routine initial empiric therapy [3].

In order to improve activity against Gram-positives, a beta-lactam or a glycopeptide (vancomycin or teicoplanin) has been added and the results support their use with ciprofloxacin [17, 18]. In a randomized trial in which ciprofloxacin was compared to ceftazidime, teicoplanin was added whenever catheter-related infection was suspected [9]. Despite the fact that cure rates were not significantly different, eight episodes of breakthrough bacteremias due to resistant, Gram-positive organisms occurred in the patients who received ciprofloxacin monotherapy.

Recently Antabli et al. [7] replaced amikacin in the conventional regimen of ceftazidime plus amikacin with ciprofloxacin, I.V. 400 mg twice daily. They reported a success rate of 99% in 106 patients treated with this regimen. However success was defined as survival through the neutropenic period and only 61 patients responded without regimen modification.

Among the newer broad-spectrum fluoroquinolones with enhanced *in vitro* activity against a wide range of Gram-positives including MRSA, MRSE and Pen-R *Streptococcus pneumoniae*, only clinafloxacin has been studied for patients with febrile neutropenia. Clinafloxacin retains the activity of ciprofloxacin against *P. aeruginosa* and other Gram-negative bacilli but is more active against Gram-positives and anaerobes. In a double-blind multicentre trial, 541 patients with febrile neutropenia were randomized to receive either I.V. clinafloxacin (200 mg twice daily) or I.V. imipenem (500 mg four times daily) as empiric monotherapy [23]. More baseline pathogens were susceptible to clinafloxacin (99%) compared to imipenem (95%). An initial favorable clinical response occurred in only 32% of patients treated with clinafloxacin and only 33% of those treated with imipenem but overall response with the addition of other antimicrobial agents (mostly vancomycin or an aminoglycocide) were similar at 95% and 93% respectively. The authors discuss the low initial response rates and accept that in many patients, modifications were made despite negative culture results and in the absence of clinical deterioration. Although death rates were low at 5% and 7% respectively, it should be noted that more Gram-negative infections in the imipenem group (15) were associated with death during the study than in the clinafloxacin group (5%; $p = 0.06$). Also more Gram-positive infections were associated with death in the imipenem group (13%) than in the clinafloxacin group (0%) ($p = 0.003$). Drug-related skin rash occurred more often with clinafloxacin (11% *versus* 6%) whereas nausea, *Clostridium difficile*-associated diarrhea and seizures occurred more often with imipenem.

Oral fluoroquinolones for empiric therapy in the febrile neutropenic "low-risk" patient

Febrile neutropenic patients have usually been hospitalized in order to start empiric broad-spectrum, intravenous, antimicrobial therapy. However, the concept of "risk-assessment" at the initial presentation with a febrile illness has been introduced. In several studies it has been demonstrated that the duration and depth of neutropenia as well as the rate at which the neutrophil count recovers, correlates with the frequency of infectious complications. Patients with hematologic malignancies and bone marrow transplants in whom the duration of severe neutropenia often exceeds 15 days, are at greatest risk. Talcott et al. [24] were among the first to recognize well-defined risk groups among febrile neutropenic patients. Their model identified the medical risk by applying clinical criteria available on the first day of fever and categorizing patients into four risk groups as follows: Group 1 included patients with hematologic disorders and bone marrow transplants who were hospitalized when they developed their febrile neutropenic episodes. They were considered as "high risk" and had substantial morbidity and an overall mortality rate of 13%. Group 2 included febrile patients with concurrent comorbidity (hypotension, altered mentation, respiratory failure, uncontrolled bleeding, dehydration, hypercalcemia, cord compression, etc.). Serious complications occurred in 40% and the overall mortality was 12%. Group 3 included febrile patients who had no concurrent comorbidity, but had ongoing poorly controlled cancer. Serious complications occurred in 25% of these patients and 18% died. Group 4 was composed of clinically stable outpatients with responsive tumor, and no concurrent comorbidity in whom only 3% developed serious complications and none died. Pizzo et al. defined "low risk" patients as those who were anticipated to have <10 days of neutropenia, were hemodynamically stable, and had no new pulmonary infiltrates, abdominal pain, nausea, vomiting or mental status changes [25]. These criteria encompass essentially the same patient population as that of Talcott et al. in their group 4 [24].

More recently Klastersky and co-workers [26] published a scoring system known as the MASCC score ("Multinational Association for Supportive Care in Cancer"), which was validated on 756 patients and based on (i) severity of symptoms, (ii) blood pressure and fluid status, (iii) comorbidities, (iv) status of the neoplasm, (v) age. A score of ≥ 21 allowed identification of "low risk" patients with a positive predictive value of 91%, specificity of 68% and sensitivity of 71%. In the "low risk" patients new therapeutic strategies are nowadays being evaluated to include: (i) hospital-based oral antibiotic therapy; (ii) outpatient antibiotic therapy using parenteral and/or oral regimens; (iii) initial hospital-based parenteral antibiotic therapy followed by oral therapy with discharge [27]. This approach except of cost effectiveness has the advantage of enhanced quality of life for patients, greater convenience for caregivers, and less risk of nosocomial superinfections with multiresistant microorganisms.

The bioavailability and broad-spectrum activity of the fluoroquinolones, particularly ciprofloxacin and ofloxacin made them attractive for oral use in febrile "low risk" neutropenic patients. In Table 2 details of representative studies treating febrile "low risk" neutropenic patients, either as inpatient or as outpatients, with oral fluoroquinolone monotherapy or in combination with another oral antibiotic active against Gram-positives is outlined [26–39]. "Low-risk" patients with cancer who are febrile and neutropenic can be safely prescribed appropriate empiric oral therapy. It is as effective as intravenous therapy with response rates of about 95% if the neutropenic episode lasts less than 7 days.

A switch from inpatient parenteral to outpatient oral therapy with oral ciprofloxacin (500 mg thrice daily) was studied in 56 febrile neutropenic patients who had defervesced within 72 h of parenteral therapy [27]. They were eligible for oral therapy if they were able to ingest oral medication, had no evidence of organ failure, and were hemodynamically stable. Solid tumors accounted for about half of the underlying diseases and the mean duration of neutropenia in both groups was 10 days. No significant difference in the response rate was observed between patients who continued parenteral antibiotics (either ceftazidime or imipenem/cilastatin) and patients managed as outpatients with ciprofloxacin (89% *versus* 76%). However the high rate of recur-

Table 2. Summary results of clinical trials with oral fluoroquinolones in "low-risk" neutropenic febrile patients

Design	Patients	Regimen	Results	Refs
Nonrandomized; outpatients; adults	111; Talcott group 4; solid tumors	Oral ofloxacin (400 mg b.i.d)	83% response rate; 14% hospitalized;3% death rate	[28]
Prospective, randomized; in patients vs. outpatients; adults	169; modified Talcott group 4; 70% solid tumors	Oral ofloxacin (400 mg b.i.d.)	Documented infection response rate: 62% inpatient; 65% oupatient;FUO: response rate 82% inpatient;85% outpatient;3% death rate	[29]
Non-randomized; outpatients; children	45; "low-risk"; 69% leukemia and lymphoma	Oral ciprofloxacin (200 mg/kg/24 h)[a]	89% response rate; 9% hospitalized[b]; 0% death rate	[30]
Non randomized; oupatients; adults	68; lymphomas	Oral perfloxacin (400 mg b.i.d.) plus amoxicillin/clavulanate	87% response rate; 12% hospitalized[b]; 1% death rate; 88% response rate PO	[31]
Prospective randomized; outpatients; children	73;modified Talcott group 4; 70% non leukemics	Oral ciprofloxacin (12,5 mg/kg b.i.d.) vs. IV ceftazidime	80% response rate PO; 94% response rate IV; 0% death rate	[32]
Prospective randomized; outpatients; adults	183; "low-risk"	Oral ciprofloxacin (750 mg b.i.d) vs. IV ceftriaxone	82% response rate PO; 75% response rate IV; 1% death rate	[33]
Prospective randomized; outpatients; mostly children	138; short neutropenia; solid tumors and stage I-II non Hodgkin lymphomas	Oral ciprofloxacin (12.5 mg/kg b.i.d) vs. IV ceftriaxone	83% response rate PO; 75.4% response rate IV; 7% vs 4% hospitalized[b]; 0% death rate	[34]
Prospective randomized; outpatients; children	93 febrile episodes; "low-risk"; 55% solid tumors	Oral ciprofloxacin (200 mg/kg b.i.d) vs. IV ceftriaxone plus IV amikacin[c]	100% response rate PO; 97.8% response rate IV; 0% death rate	[35]
Prospective, randomized; outpatients; adults	83; modified Talcott group 4; primarily solid tumors	Oral ciprofloxacin (750 mg b.i.d) plus clindamycin vs. IV aztreonam plus clindamycin	88% response rate PO; 95% response rate IV; 21% hospitalized[b];	[36]
Prospective, randomized; outpatients; adults	179; modified Talcott group 4; primarily solid tumors	Oral ciprofloxacin (500 mg b.i.d.) plus amoxacillin/clavulanate vs. IV aztreonam plus clindamycin	90% response rate PO; 87% response rate IV; 0% death rate	[27]

(Continued on next page)

Table 2. (Continued)

Design	Patients	Regimen	Results	Refs
Randomized double-blind, placebo-controlled; inpatients; adults + children	232;short neutropenia without comorbidities; 73% solid tumors	Oral ciprofloxacin (30 mg/kg/24 h) plus amoxicillin-clavulanate; vs. IV ceftazidime	71% response rate PO;67% response rate IV; 0% death rate	[37]
Prospective randomized; inpatients; mostly adults	312;short neutropenia without comorbidities; 68% solid tumors	Oral ciprofloxacin (750 mg b.i.d) plus amoxicillin-clavulanate vs. IV ceftriaxone plus amikacin	86% response rate PO; 84% response rate IV; 2% death rate	[38]

[a] A single dose of IV ceftazidime preceded ciprofloxacin administration
[b] Started therapy as outpatients but because of unexpected events they were admitted to hospital
[c] After 24 h of ceftriaxone and amikacin in both groups

rent fever (24%) in the oral ciprofloxacin group at a mean of 3 days after discharge, may be due to the fact that patients were not selected for short-duration neutropenia. Similarly Giamarellou et al. [12] treated 124 febrile neutropenic patients following at least 72 h of I.V. ciprofloxacin (400 mg, t.i.d.) and then switched therapy to inpatient oral ciprofloxacin (750 mg, b.i.d.) in 82 patients, with a "successful" outcome in 62 (74.4%). On the other hand, serum ciprofloxacin levels after p.o. intake in patients who did not suffer from mucositis were found by the same group of investigators to be in the expected range, but with rather delayed and prolonged peaks.

In five studies [30, 32, 34, 35, 37] pediatric cancer patients were admitted mostly as "low-risk" patients, with encouraging results (Tab. 2). The issue of cartilage injury was studied at a trial at NCI in pediatric cancer patients and changes were minimal and reversible and probably unrelated to ciprofloxacin therapy [39].

The most effective oral regimen studied in adults with febrile neutropenia with the least toxicity appears to be the combination of ciprofloxacin plus amoxicillin/clavulanate. In the published series most patients were being treated for solid tumors and the main prerequisite to enter the study was the prediction of less than seven days of neutropenia. Further studies are needed including redefinition of the "low-risk" model.

The role of fluoroquinolones for infection prophylaxis in the neutropenic patient with cancer

The majority of patients undergoing intensive chemotherapy develop an infection with neutropenia, partially as a result of cytostatic drug-induced lesions in the oropharyngeal and intestinal mucosa that serve as portals of entry for the "normal GI tract flora" [20]. Due to improved management, mortality has been dramatically decreased in these patients. However, persisting infection related morbidity has prompted studies with a variety of antimicrobial prophylaxis regimens. Aims of successful prophylaxis are the reduction of (i) numbers of proven infections; (ii) infection related mortality; (iii) the frequency of febrile neutropenia; and (iv) the empiric use of antimicrobials administered for febrile episodes.

Non-absorbable orally administered agents such as aminoglycosides, polymyxins and vancomycin were initially used for prophylaxis. Their benefit was marginal. Trimethoprim/sulfamethoxazole (TMP/SMX) replaced the latter regimens in the 1980s with reduction of the frequency of bacterial infections [40]. However, TMP/SMX did not prevent *P. aeruginosa* infections and it was associated with emergence of resistant bacterial and fungal overgrowth. As well, it prolonged myelosuppression and caused allergic reactions while not improving overall survival.

The advent of the fluoroquinolones in the early 1980s with their oral bioavailability and tolerance plus their activity against Gram-negatives, including *P. aeruginosa*, made them possible agents for prophylaxis in the neutropenic host. In addition, these agents achieved appreciable levels in serum and tissues as well as in the lumen of the colon, selectively eliminating aerobic Gram-negatives while leaving anaerobes intact and preserving "colonization resistance."

Since 1987 the preventive efficacy of various fluoroquinolones has been studied in several trials (Tab. 3) almost all of which were published before 1995 [41–57]. In most, including the two in which the prophylactic effect of a fluoroquinolone was compared to a placebo, a statistically significant reduction in the incidence of Gram-negative bacteremias was shown. However, neither the incidence of febrile episodes nor infectious mortality was decreased in neutropenic patients given ciprofloxacin, ofloxacin, norfloxacin or enoxacin. In eight studies, when compared to TMP/SMX, fluoroquinolone prophylaxis prevented Gram-negative bacteremia but it did not show an impact on other end points such as the incidence of fever, time to first febrile episode, incidence of microbiologically and clinically documented infections, fever of undetermined origin or mortality [48–55]. On the other hand, differences in study size, regional epidemiology, patient characteristics and study design made the interpretation of the published results controversial.

Two meta-analysis on fluoroquinolones effectiveness for preventing bacterial infection in neutropenic cancer patients have been published [19, 20]. In the first, Cruciani et al. [19] conducted a two part meta-analysis. Overall, 19 randomized studies met selective criteria and 2112 patients were included. In the first part 13 studies (1155 patients) that compared fluoroquinolones alone with control regimens (i.e., TMP/SMX, oral non-absorbable antibiotics or placebo) were analyzed. It was statistically confirmed that fluoroquinolones decreased the incidence of Gram-negative bacteremia (overall odds ratio [OR] 0.09; 95% confidence interval [CI] 0.05–0.16; $p < 0.001$) but not Gram-positive bacteremia (OR, 1.05; 95% CI, 0.76–1.45; $p = 0.7$), fever-related morbidity (OR, 0.76; 95% CI, 0.56–1.04; $p = 0.09$), infection-related morbidity (OR, 0.79; 95% CI, 0.47–1.34; $p = 0.4$) and use of empirical antibiotics.

In the second meta-analysis 18 trials of quinolone prophylaxis in patients undergoing chemotherapy for malignancy were included [20]. All studies combined evaluated 1408 subjects in total [707 subjects who received prophylaxis with a quinolone (ciprofloxacin, enoxacin, norfloxacin and ofloxacin), 334 with TMP/SMX and 367 with no prophylaxis]. In agreement with the Cruciani et al. meta-analysis [19], it was confirmed that, compared with those who received no prophylaxis, or with those who received TMP/SMX, patients on quinolones experienced 79% fewer Gram-negative infections (relative risk, 0.21; 95% CI, 0.12–0.37) translated into decreases of 35% in microbiologically documented infections and 46% in total infections as well as 77% fewer Gram-negative bacteremias. However, prophylaxis did not affect the incidence of febrile episodes or the frequency of Gram-positive, fungal or clinically documented infections, the use of empirical antibiotics or infection-related deaths. Norfloxacin appears to be the least effective prophylactic regimen.

Table 3. Randomized studies of a single fluoroquinolone *versus* no prophylaxis, placebo, oral non-absorbable antibiotics, trimethoprim-sulfamethoxazole or another quinolone for infection prophylaxis in neutropenic cancer patients

Study drugs	No. of episodes – Underlying disease	Days with neutropenia[a]	Fever development	MDI [Gram (+) vs. Gram (–)]	CDI	Mortality due to infection	Refs
Ciprofloxacin vs. control (no prophylaxis)	90 Ovarian cancer[b]	NR	33.3% vs.27.3%[c]	13% (13% vs. 0%) vs. 13% (7% vs. 7%)	NR	0% vs. 0%	[41]
Norfloxacin vs. control (no prophylaxis)	182 Acute leukemia (33%) Lymphomas (31%)	NR	80% vs. 86%	22% (18% vs. 8%) vs. 32% (14% vs. 15%)	NR	1% vs. 1%	[42]
Norfloxacin vs.placebo	68 Acute leukemia	32	100% vs. 100%	57% (46% vs. 11%) vs. 79%(39% vs. 39%[c])	NR	17% vs. 9%	[43]
Enoxacin vs. placebo	119 Acute leukemia	14	77% vs. 81%	35% (19% vs. 3%) vs. 53% (28% vs. 33%[c])	61% vs. 72%	2% vs. 3%	[44]
Norfloxacin vs. vancomycin + polymyxin	66 Acute leukemia (95%)	21	44% vs.63%[c]	33% (25% vs. 0%) vs. 50% (13% vs. 17%[c])	33% vs. 30%	8% vs. 13%	[45]
Ofloxacin vs. vancomycin + polymyxin	62 Acute leukemia	25	93% vs. 100%	27% (20% vs. 0%) vs. 47%(25% vs. 16%[c])	41% vs. 12%	7% vs. 9%	[46]
Ciprofloxacin vs. neomycin + polymyxin B + nalidixic acid	105 Acute leukemia	21	92% vs. 97%	40% (41% vs. 2%) vs. 67% (58% vs. 15%[c])	NR	0% vs. 9%[c]	[47]

(Continued on next page)

Table 3. (Continued)

Study drugs	No. of episodes – Underlying disease	Days with neutropenia[a]	Fever development	MDI [Gram (+) vs. Gram (–)]	CDI	Mortality due to infection	Refs
Ciprofloxacin vs. TMP – SMX + colistin	94 Acute leukemia	40	79% vs. 91%	10% (8% vs. 0%) vs. 30% (15% vs. 15%)	NR	0% vs. 4%	[48]
Ciprofloxacin vs. TMP – SMX + colistin	230 Acute leukemia (70%)	22	70% vs. 61%	14% (14% vs. 0%) 11% (7% vs. 4%)	31% vs. 24% vs.	3.4% vs. 0%	[49]
Ciprofloxacin vs. TMP-SMX	145 Solid tumors (36%) Acute leukemia (14%)	29	82% vs. 75%	22% (14% vs. 0%) vs. 31% (7% vs. 5.6%[c])	14% vs. 8%	4% vs. 0%	[50]
Norfloxacin vs. TMP – SMX	63 Acute leukemia	25	67%	32% (29%[c] vs. 0%) vs. 25% (6% vs. 13%)	13% vs. 16%	3% vs. 3%	[51]
Norfloxacin vs. TMP-SMX	44 Acute leukemia; (91% children)	20	43% vs. 87%[c]	19% (5% vs. 14%) vs. 26% (4% vs. 22%)	17% vs. 19%	NR	[52]
Norfloxacin vs. TMP – SMX	59 Acute leukemia	19	65% vs. 73%	8% (1% vs. 7%) vs. 10% (4% vs. 6%	2% vs. 1%	1% vs. 1%	[53]
Ofloxacin vs. TMP – SMX	102 Acute leukemia (62%)	15	22% vs. 48%[c]	8% (0% vs. 4%) vs. 21% (0% vs. 17%[c])	NR	4% vs. 8%	[54]
Ofloxacin vs. TMP – SMX	194 Acute leukemia	32	58% vs. 73%	14% (19% vs. 4%) vs. 29% (22% vs. 26[b]%	24% vs. 20%	9% vs. 5%	[55]

(Continued on next page)

Table 3. (Continued)

Study drugs	No. of episodes – Underlying disease	Days with neutropenia[a]	Fever development	MDI [Gram (+) vs. Gram (–)]	CDI	Mortality due to infection	Refs
Ofloxacin vs. norfloxacin	71 Leukemia (79%)	14	45% vs. 74%[c]	17% (17% vs. 0%) vs. 42% (28% vs. 14%[c])	0% vs. 11%	0% vs. 3%	[56]
Ciprofloxacin vs. norfloxacin	294 Acute leukemia (92%)	24	66% vs. 75%[c]	17% (11% vs. 4%) vs. 24% (12% vs. 9%)	13% vs. 14%	5% vs. 5%	[57]

[a] mean or median
[b] eligible patients received paclitaxel
[c] $p < 0.05$
NR: not reported
MDI: microbiologically documented infections
CDI: clinically documented infections
TMP – SMX: Trimethoprim – sulfamethoxazole

Despite the well established conclusion that the incidence of Gram-negative infections was decreased, several investigators consider this finding to be of marginal value. Over the last decade, Gram-positive microorganisms have come to predominate in febrile neutropenic infections. Breakthrough Gram-positive infections, especially streptococcal bacteremias have been reported during therapy or prophylaxis [58]. The efficacy of prophylaxis using the combination of a fluoroquinolone with a narrow spectrum anti-Gram-positive agent was evaluated in seven studies published since 1994 (Tab. 4) [59–65]. In the Cruciani et al. [19] second part metanalysis (six trials including 957 patients) the addition of penicillin V, oral vancomycin, or a macrolide significantly reduced the occurrence of Gram-positive infections including bacteremia (OR, 0.46; CI, 0.33–0.63; $p < 0.001$), especially of streptococci, without effecting the incidence of infection-related mortality (OR, 0.74; 95% CI, 0.40–1.38; $p = 0.3$) or fever-related morbidity (OR, 0.83; 95% CI, 0.62–1.13; $p = 0.2$). In three trials ciprofloxacin or ofloxacin was combined with rifampin [60, 63, 65]. In two rifampin reduced Gram-positive infections significantly, but in the third, the addition of rifampin did not improve the efficacy of ciprofloxacin [65]. More studies are obviously required.

The encouraging results of the initial trials in the late 1980s and early 1990s made fluoroquinolone prophylaxis a common practice for patients with predictable "long duration" neutropenia. The drawback of this strategy became apparent with the emergence of fluoroquinolone-resistant *Escherichia coli* and coagulase-negative staphylococci. Carratalá et al. [66] described 35 episodes of *E. coli* bacteremia in neutropenic patients with cancer. Thirteen episodes were due to quinolone-resistant strains with MICs of norfloxacin ranging from 16 to 128 µg/ml and of ciprofloxacin from 8 to 64 µg/ml. Among the variables analyzed, prophylaxis with norfloxacin was the only factor significantly associated with the development of quinolone-resistant *E. coli* bacteremia ($p < 0.001$). The results of the latter study suggested that quinolones used as prophylactic agents act as an important selective force to quinolone-resistant *E. coli* in the GI tract. These investigators isolated quinolone-resistant *E. coli* from the feces of 10 of 25 patients with cancer after a mean of 10 days of prophylaxis with norfloxacin [66].

Cometta et al. [67] reported that in 11 of 40 bacteremic *E. coli* isolates, the MICs of all currently available fluoroquinolones were >16 µg/ml. These strains were isolated from neutropenic patients receiving a fluoroquinolone as prophylaxis, whereas a 60% resistant rate to fluoroquinolones in coagulase-negative staphylococci isolated from the same population of patients was noted. Similarly Kern et al. [22] reported an increasing incidence of fluoroquinolone-resistant *E. coli* bacteremia in patients with leukemia (59%) most of whom had received prophylaxis with ofloxacin. The latter strains proved to be of four distinct genotypes, suggesting both the emergence of *de novo* resistance and the spread of specific resistant clones among patients.

Sustained selective pressure on the endogenous gut flora has resulted in the discontinuation of fluoroquinolone prophylaxis in many centres. In a recent

Table 4. Randomized studies of single fluoroquinolone prophylaxis *versus* combination of a fluoroquinolone plus an antibiotic with antigram – positive activity

Study drug	No. of episodes/ underlying disease	Days of neutropenia[a]	Fever development	MDI [Gram (+) vs.Gram (–)]	CDI	Mortality due to infection	Refs
Ofloxacin vs. ofloxacin + roxithromycin	131 Acute leukemia (86%)	28	64% vs. 70%	33% (30% vs.3%) vs. 25% (11%[b] vs. 12%)	NR	1% vs. 3%	[59]
Norfloxacin vs. ofloxacin vs. ofloxacin + rifampin	127 Acute leukemia (72%)	17	71% vs. 82% vs.77%	47% (24% vs. 5%) vs. 24%[b] (3%[b] vs. 3%) vs. 9%[b] (3%[b] vs. 0%)	8% vs. 5% vs. 20%	2% vs. 2% vs. 2%	[60]
Pefloxacin vs. pefloxacin + penicillin V	551 Acute leukemia (81%)	22	80% vs. 71%[b]	26% (18% vs. 2%) vs. 20% (13% vs. 1%)	15% vs. 11%	4% vs. 4%	[61]
Ciprofloxacin vs. ciprofloxacin + amoxicillin	53 Acute leukemia 82%)	19	74% vs. 76%	40% (33% vs. 6%) vs. 25% (23% vs. 12%)	0% vs. 8%	0% vs. 8%	[62]
Ciprofloxacin vs. ciprofloxacin + rifampin	40 Solid tumors (95%)	8.8	85% vs. 85%	50% (50% vs. 0%) vs. 20% (0%[b] vs. 20%)	NR	NR	[63]
Ciprofloxacin vs. ciprofloxacin + vancomycin	84 Solid tumors (45%) Acute leukemia 18%)	14	NR	29% (24%–5%) vs. 28% (16%–5%)	NR	0% vs. 0%	[64]
Ciprofloxacin vs. ciprofloxacin + rifampin	123 Solid tumors (95%)	9	87% vs. 79%	22% (13% vs. 6%) vs. 8% (3% vs. 3%)	13% vs. 10%	0% vs 0%	[65]

[a] mean or median; [b] $p < 0.05$; MDI: microbiologicalli documented infections; CDI: clinically documented infections

study, Delarive et al. [21], reviewed 112 consecutive episodes of prolonged neutropenia (median 17 days, range 14–52 days; 62% acute leukemia, 34% lymphoma) in Lausanne, before and after discontinuation of prophylaxis in adult patients with haematological malignancies at high risk of infection. Prophylactic ciprofloxacin and penicillin V was used in 41 episodes of neutropenia, whereas no prophylaxis was given in 71 episodes. After discontinuation of prophylaxis, the proportion of Gram-negative bacteremias rose from 25% to 85% of all bloodstream infections. However, the incidence of bacteremic and clinically documented infections, FUO, median time to first fever, duration of fever, antibiotic treatment, length of hospital stay, rate of ICU admission, incidence of serious complications and mortality were similar in patients with or without antimicrobial prophylaxis. The observed striking rebound in the proportion of Gram-negative bacteremias followed by concomitant decrease of Gram-positive bacteremias, supports the view that fluoroquinolone prophylaxis was a critical determinant in the shift to Gram-positive infections in the late 1980s and early 1990s. Supplementary to the above is the study of Martino et al. [42] who have reported that after the abrupt discontinuation of norfloxacin prophylaxis a rapid increase in the rate of fluoroquinolone-susceptible infections caused by enterobacteriaceae was observed.

Although the use of fluoroquinolone prophylaxis is associated with a significant reduction in the incidence of Gram-negative infections in neutropenic patients, the lack of benefit with regard to morbidity and mortality and their association with the emergence of resistance has made their use controversial. The 2002 IDSA Guidelines note that the efficacy of prophylaxis would warrant a rating of A-I from the standpoint of efficacy alone but concerns about emerging resistance and the failure to consistently reduce mortality rates leads to the recommendation that routine prophylaxis be avoided [3].

The newest generation fluoroquinolones like moxifloxacin, which possess promising Gram-positive activity, may be studied for future infection prophylaxis regimens. However, any study design should weight the risk of selection of resistant pathogens and the probable accelerated loss of these important agents from our armamentarium. In the meantime, the identification of subgroups which may possibly benefit from quinolone prophylaxis should be further defined in future studies.

References

1 Schimpff SC (1986) Empiric antibiotic therapy for granulocytopenic cancer patients. *Am J Med* 80(Suppl 5c): 13–20

2 Giamarellou H, Antoniadou A (2001) Infectious complications of febrile neutropenia. *Infect Dis Clin N Amer* 15: 457–482

3 Hughes WT, Armstrong D, Bodey GP, Bow EJ, Brown AE, Calandra T, Feld R Pizzo P, Rolston KVI, Shenep JL, Young LS (2002) Guidelines for the use of antimicrobial agents in neutropenic patients with cancer. *CID* 34: 730–751

4 Rolston KVI, Haron E, Cunningham C, Bodey GP (1989) Intravenous ciprofloxacin for infections in cancer patients. *Am J Med* 87(Suppl 5A): 261–265

5 Smith GM, Leyland MJ, Farrell ID, Geddes AM (1988) A clinical, microbiological and pharmacokinetic study of ciprofloxacin plus vancomycin as initial therapy of febrile episodes in neutropenic patients. *J Antimicrobial Chemother* 21: 647–655

6 Samuelsson J, Nilsson PG, Wahlin A, Lerner R, Winqvist I, Palmblad J (1992) A pilot study of piperacillin and ciprofloxacin as initial therapy for fever in severely neutropenic leukemia patients. *Scan J Infect Dis* 24: 467–475

7 Antabli BA, Bross B, Siegel RS, Small CD, Tabbara IA (1999) Empiric antimicrobial therapy of febrile neutropenic patients undergoing haematopoietic stem cell transplantation. *Int J Antimicrob Agents* 13: 127–130

8 Bayston KF, Want S, Cohen JA (1989) A prospective randomized comparison of ceftazidime and ciprofloxacin as initial empiric therapy in neutropenic patients with fever. *Am J Med* 87(Suppl 5A): 269–273

9 Lim SH, Smith MP, Goldstone AH, Machin SJ (1990) A randomized prospective study of ceftazidime and ciprofloxacin with or without teicoplanin as an empiric antibiotic regimen for febrile neutropenic patients. *Br J Haematol* 76(Suppl 2): 41–44

10 Meunier F, Zinner SH, Gaya H, Calandra T, Viscoli C, Klastersky J, Glauser M (1991) Prospective randomized evaluation of ciprofloxacin *versus* piperacillin plus amikacin for empiric antibiotic therapy of febrile granulocytopenic cancer patients with lymphomas and solid tumors. *Antimicrob Agents Chemother* 35: 873–878

11 Johnson PRE, Liu Yin JA, Tooth JA (1992) A randomized trial of high-dose ciprofloxacin *versus* azlocillin and netilmicin in the empirical therapy of febrile neutropenic patients. *J Antimicrob Chemother* 30: 203–214

12 Giamarellou H, Bassaris HP, Petrikkos G, Busch W, Voulgarelis M, Antoniadou A, Grouzi E, Zoumbos N (2000) Monotherapy with intravenous followed by oral high-dose ciprofloxacin *versus* combination therapy with ceftazidime plus amikacin as initial empiric therapy for granulocytopenic patients with fever. *Antimicrob Agents Chemother* 44: 3264–3271

13 Chan CC, Oppenheim BA, Anderson H, Swindell R, Scarffe JH (1989) Randomized trial comparing ciprofloxacin plus netilmicin *versus* piperacillin plus netilmicin for empiric treatment of fever in neutropenic patients. *Antimicrob Agents Chemother* 33: 87–91

14 Flaherty JP, Waitley D, Edlin B, George D, Arnow P, O'Keefe P, Weinstein RA (1989) Multicentre randomized trial of ciprofloxacin plus azlocillin *versus* ceftazidime plus amikacin for empiric treatment of febrile neutropenic patients. *Am J Med* 87(Suppl 5A): 278–282

15 Philpott-Howard JN, Barker KF, Wade JJ, Kaczmarski RS, Smedley JC, Mufti GJ (1990) Randomized multicentre study of ciprofloxacin and azlocillin *versus* gentamicin and azlocillin in the treatment of febrile neutropenic patients. *J Antimicrob Chemother* 26(Suppl F): 89–99

16 Hyatt DS, Roger TRF, McCarthy DM, Samson DS (1992) A randomized trial of ciprofloxacin plus azlocillin *versus* netilmicin plus azlocillin for the empirical treatment of fever in neutropenic patients. *J Antimicrob Chemother* 28: 324–325

17 Kelsey SM, Wood ME, Shaw E, Jenkins GC, Newland AC (1990) A comparative study of intravenous ciprofloxacin plus benzylpenicillin *versus* netilmicin plus piperacillin for the empirical treatment of fever in the neutropenic host. *J Antimicrob Chemother* 25: 149–157

18 Kelsey SM, Weinhardt B, Collins PW, Newland AC (1992) Teicoplanin plus ciprofloxacin *versus* gentamicin plus piperacillin in the treatment of febrile neutropenic patients. *Eur J Clin Microbiol Infect Dis* 11: 509–514

19 Cruciani M, Rampazzo R, Malma M, Lazzarini L, Todeschini G, Messori A, Concia E (1996) Prophylaxis with fluoroquinolones for bacterial infections in neutropenic patients: A meta-analysis *CID* 23: 795–805

20 Engels EA, Lau J, Barza M (1998) Efficacy of quinolone prophylaxis in neutropenic cancer patients: a meta-analysis. *J Clin Oncol* 16: 1179–1187

21 Delarive P, Baumgartner JD, Glauser MP, Cometta A (2000) Evaluation de la prophylaxie antibiotique chez les patients neutropeniques avec hémopathie maligne. *Schweizerische Medizinische Wochenschrift* 130: 1837–1844

22 Kern WV, Andriof E, Oethinger M, Kern P, Hacker J, Marre R (1994) Emergence of fluoroquinolone-resistant *Escherichia coli* at a cancer center. *Antimicrob Agents Chemother* 38: 681–687

23 Winston DJ, Lazarus HM, Beveridge RA, Hathorn JQ, Gucalp R, Ramphal R, Chow AW, Ho WG, Horn R, Feld R et al (2002) Randomized, double-blind, multicenter trial comparing clinafloxacin with imipenem as empirical monotherapy for febrile granulocytopenic patients *CID* 32: 381–390

24 Talcott JA, Siegel RD, Finberg R, Goldman L (1992) Risk assessment in cancer patients with fever and neutropenia: A prospective, two-center validation of a prediction rule. *J Clin Oncol* 10: 316–322
25 Freifeld A, Pizzo P (1997) Use of fluoroquinolones for empirical management of febrile neutropenia in pediatric cancer patients. *Pediatr Infect Dis J* 16: 140–146
26 Klastersky J, Paesmans M, Rubenstein EB, Bayer M, Elting L, Feld R, Gallagher J, Herrstedt J, Paoport B, Rolston K et al (2000) The Multinational Association for Supportive Care in Cancer risk index: a multinational scoring system for identifying low-risk febrile neutropenic cancer patients *J Clin Oncol* 16: 3038–3051
27 Rolston KVI, Rubenstein EB, Freifeld A (1996) Early empiric antibiotic therapy for febrile neutropenia patients at low risk. *Infect Dis Clin N Am* 10: 223–237
28 Malik IA, Khan WA, Aziz Z, Karim M (1994) Self-administered antibiotic therapy for chemotherapy-induced low-risk febrile neutropenia patients with non-hematologic neoplasms *CID* 19: 533–527
29 Malik IA, Khan WA, Karim M, Aziz Z, Khan MA (1995) Feasibility of outpatient management of fever in cancer patients with low-risk neutropenia: Results of a prospective randomized trial. *Am J Med* 98: 224–231
30 Aquino VM, Herrera L, Sandler ES, Buchanan GR (2000) Feasibility of oral ciprofloxacin for the outpatient management of febrile neutropenia in selected children with cancer. *Cancer* 88: 1710–1714
31 Gardembas-Pain M, Desablens B, Sensebe L, Lamy T, Ghandour C, Boasson M (1991) Home treatment of febrile neutropenia: An empirical oral antibiotic regimen *Ann Oncol* 2: 485–487
32 Mullen CA, Petropoulos D, Roberts WM, Rytting M, Zipf T, Chan KW, Culbert ST, Danielson M, Jeha SS, Kuttesch JF et al (1999) Outpatient treatment of fever and neutropenia for low risk pediatric cancer patients *Cancer* 86: 126–134
33 Minotti V, Gentile G, Bucaneve G, Jori AP, Micozzi A, Cavicchi F, Barbabietola G, Landonio G, Menichetti F, Martino P et al (1999) Domiciliary treatment of febrile episodes in cancer patients: a prospective randomized trial comparing oral *versus* parenteral empirical antibiotic treatment. *Support Care Cancer* 7: 124–139
34 Petrilli AS, Dantas LS, Campos MC, Tanaka C, Ginani VC, Seber A (2000) Oral ciprofloxacin *versus* intravenous ceftriaxone administered in an outpatient setting for fever and neutropenia in low-risk pediatric oncology patients: Randomized prospective trial. *Medic Pediatr Oncol* 34: 87–91
35 Paganini H, Rodriguez-Brieschske T, Zubizarreta P, Latella A, Firpo V, Casimir L, Armada A, Fernandez C, Caceres E, Debbag R (2001) Oral ciprofloxacin in the management of children with cancer with lower risk febrile neutropenia *Cancer* 91: 1563–1567
36 Rubenstein EB, Rolston KVI, Benjamin RS, Loewy J, Escalante C, Manzullo E, Hughes P, Moreland B, Fender A, Kennedy K et al (1993) Outpatient treatment of febrile episodes in low-risk neutropenic patients with cancer. Cancer 71: 3640–3646
37 Freifeld A, Marchigiani D, Walsh T, Chanock S, Lewis L, Hiemenz J, Hiemenz S, Hicks J, Gill V, Steinberg SM et al (1999) A double-blind comparison of empirical oral and intravenous antibiotic therapy for low-risk febrile patients with neutropenia during cancer chemotherapy. *N Engl J Med* 341: 305–311
38 Kern WV, Commetta A, de Bock R, Langenaeken J, Paesmans M, Gaya H for the International Antimicrobial Therapy Cooperative Group of the European Organization for Research and Treatment of Cancer (1999) Oral *versus* intravenous empirical antimicrobial therapy for fever in patients with granulocytopenia who are receiving cancer chemotherapy. *N Engl J Med* 341: 312–318
39 Freifeld A, Pizzo P (1997) Use of fluoroquinolones for empirical management of febrile neutropenia in pediatric cancer patients. *Pediatr Infect Dis* 16: 140–146
40 EORTC International Antimicrobial Therapy Project Group (1984) Trimethoprim-sulfamethoxazole in the prevention of infection in neutropenic patients *J Infect Dis* 150: 372–379
41 Carlson JW, Flower JM, Mitchell SK, Carson LF, Mayer AR, Copeland LJ (1997) Chemoprophylaxis with ciprofloxacin in ovarian cancer patients receiving paclitaxel: A randomized trial. Gynecol Oncol 65: 325–329
42 Martino R, Subira M, Altés A, López R, Sureda A, Domingo-Albós A, Pericas R, Brunet S (1998) Effect of discontinuing prophylaxis with norfloxacin in patients with hematologic malignancies and severe neutropenia. *Acta Haematol* 99: 206–211

43 Karp JE, Merz WG, Hendricksen C, Laughon B, Redden T, Bamberger BJ, Bartlett JG, Saral R, Burke PJ (1987) Oral norfloxacin for prevention of Gram-negative bacterial infections in patients with acute leukemia and granulocytopenia. *Ann Intern Med* 106: 1: 7
44 Talbot GH, Cassileth PA, Paradiso L, Correa-Coronas R, Bond L (1993) The enoxacin prophylaxis study group. Oral enoxacin for infection prevention in adults with acute non-lymphocytic leukemia. *Antimicrob Agents Chemother* 37: 474–482
45 Winston DJ, Winston GH, Nakao SL, Gale RP, Champlin RE (1986) Norfloxacin *versus* vancomycin/polymyxin for prevention of infections in granulocytopenic patients. *Am J Med* 80: 884–890
46 Winston DJ, Winston GH, Bruckner DA, Gale RP, Champlin RE (1990) Ofloxacin *versus* vancomycin/polymyxin for prevention of infections in granulocytopenic patients. *Am J Med* 88: 36–42
47 Jansen J, Cromer M, Akard L, Back JR, Wheat J, Allen SD (1994) Infection prevention in severely myelosuppressed patients: A comparison between ciprofloxacin and a regimen of selective antibiotic modulation of the intestinal flora. *Am J Med* 96: 335–341
48 Dekker AW, Rozenberg-Arska M, Verhoef J (1987) Infection prophylaxis in acute leukemia: a comparison of ciprofloxacin and trimethoprim-sulfamethoxazole and colistin. *Ann Intern Med* 106: 7–12
49 Donnelly JP, Maschmeyer G, Daenen S (1992) Selective oral antimicrobial prophylaxis for the prevention of infection in acute leukemia – ciprofloxacin *versus* cotrimoxazole plus colistin. *Eur J Cancer* 28A: 873–878
50 Lew MA, Kehoe K, Ritz J, Antman KH, Nadler L, Kalish LA, Finberg R (1995) Ciprofloxacin *versus* trimethoprim/sulfamethoxazole for prophylaxis of bacterial infections in bone marrow transplant recipients: a randomized, controlled trial. *J Clin Oncol* 13: 239–250
51 Bow EJ, Rayner E, Louie TJ (1988) Comparison of norfloxacin with cotrimoxazole for infection prophylaxis in acute leukemia. *Am J Med* 84: 847–854
52 Cruciani M, Concia E, Navarra A, Perversi L, Bonetti F, Arico M, Nespoli L (1989) Prophylactic cotrimoxazole *versus* norfloxacin in neutropenic children – perspective randomized study. *Infection* 17: 65–69
53 Orlandi E, Navarra A, Cruciani M, Caldera D, Morra E, Castagnola C, Concia E, Bernasconi C (1990) Norfloxacin *versus* cotrimoxazole for infection prophylaxis in granulocytopenic patients with acute leukemia. A prospective randomized study. *Haematologica* 75: 296–298
54 Liang RHS, Yung RWH, Chan TK, Chau PY, Lam WK, So SY, Todd D (1990) Ofloxacin *versus* co-trimoxazole for prevention of infection in neutropenic patients following cytotoxic chemotherapy. *Antimicrob Agents Chemother* 34: 215–218
55 Kern WV, Kurrie E (1991) Ofloxacin *versus* trimethoprim-sulfamethoxazole for prevention of infection in patients with acute leukemia and granulocytopenia. *Infection* 19: 73–80
56 D'Antonio D, Jacone A, Fioritoni G, Betti S, Di Girolamo A, Piccolomini R, Torluteno G (1991) Antibacterial prophylaxis in granulocytopenic patients: a randomized study of ofloxacin *versus* norfloxacin. *Cur Ther Res* 50: 304–311
57 The GIMEMA Infection Program (1991) Prevention of bacterial infection in neutropenic patients with hematologic malignancies. *Ann Intern Med* 115: 7–12
58 Bochud PY, Eggiman P, Calandra T, Van Melle G, Saghafi L, Francioli P (1994) Bacteremia due to viridans streptococcus in neutropenic patients with cancer: clinical spectrum and risk factors. *CID* 18: 25–31
59 Kern WV, Hay B, Kern P, Marre R, Arnold R (1994) A randomized trial of roxithromycin in patients with acute leukemia and bone marrow transplant recipients receiving fluoroquinolone prophylaxis. *Antimicrob Agents Chemother* 38: 465–472
60 Bow EJ, Mandell LA, Louie TJ, Feld R, Palmer M, Zee B, Pater J (1996) Quinolone-based antibacterial chemoprophylaxis in neutropenic patients: effect of augmented Gram-positive activity on infectious morbidity. *Ann Intern Med* 125: 183–190
61 The EORTC International Antimicrobial Therapy Cooperative Group (1994) Reduction of fever and streptococcal bacteremia in granulocytopenic patients with cancer. JAMA 272: 1183–1189
62 Fanci R, Leoni F, Bosi A, Guidi S, Ciolli S, Longo G, Donnini E, Rossi-Ferrini P (1993) Chemoprophylaxis of bacterial infections in granulocytopenic patients with ciprofloxacin *versus* ciprofloxacin plus amoxicillin. *J Chemother* 5: 119–123
63 Hidalgo M, Hornedo J, Lunbrecas C, Trigo JM, Gómez C, Perea S, Ruiz A, Hilt R, Cortés-Funes H (1997) Lack of ability of ciprofloxacin-rifampin prophylaxis to decrease infection related mor-

bidity in neutropenic patients given cytotoxic therapy and peripheral blood stem cell transplants. *Antimicrob Agents Chemother* 41: 1175–1177

64 Ford CD, Reilly W, Wood J, Classen DC, Burke PJ (1998) Oral antimicrobial prophylaxis in bone marrow transplant recipients: randomized trial of ciprofloxacin *versus* ciprofloxacin-vancomycin. *Antimicrob Agents Chemother* 42: 1402–1405

65 Gómez-Martin C, Solà C, Hornedo J, Perea S, Lumbreras C, Valenti V, Arcediano A, Rodriguez M, Salazar R, Cortés-Funes H et al (2000) Rifampin does not improve the efficacy of quinolone antibacterial prophylaxis in neutropenic cancer patients: results of a randomized clinical trial. *J Clin Oncol* 18: 2126–2134

66 Carratalá J, Fernández-Sevilla A, Tuban F, Callis M, Gudiol F (1995) Emergence of quinolone-resistant *Escherichia coli* bacteremia in neutropenic patients with cancer who have received prophylactic norfloxacin. *CID* 20: 557–560

67 Cometta A, Calandra T, Bille J, Glauser MP (1994) *Escherichia coli* resistant to fluoroquinolones in patients with cancer and neutropenia. *N Engl J Med* 330: 1240–1241

Fluoroquinolone Antibiotics
ed. by A.R. Ronald and D.E. Low

Less usual indications: Mycobacterial, Brucella, Yersinia, Francisella and other infections

Ziad A. Memish[1] and Manuel W. Mah[2]

[1] *Departments of Medicine and Infection Prevention and Control, King Fahad National Guard Hosptal, P.O. Box 22490, Riyadh 11426, Saudi Arabia*
[2] *Infection Prevention and Control, Peter Lougheed Centre, 3500-26th Avenue NE, Calgary, AB, T1Y 6J4, Canada*

Treatment of mycobacteria with fluoroquinolones

The fluoroquinolones possess *in vitro* activity against several clinically important mycobacterial species, as well as desirable pharmacokinetic and pharmacodynamic characteristics. Furthermore, recent clinical trials have clarified the role of the fluoroquinolones in the treatment of mycobacterial diseases. Although currently available fluoroquinolones are not regarded as first-line agents, they remain valuable alternative agents for these indications in special circumstances.

Mycobacterium tuberculosis

Drug-susceptible tuberculosis

Desirable pharmacokinetic and pharmacodynamic properties of the fluoroquinolones include good oral bioavailability, penetration into macrophages, and concentration-dependent killing allowing once-a-day dosing [1]. Their adverse effect profile and long-term safety in the treatment of tuberculosis in adults is also favorable [2], but fluoroquinolones should not be used in children because of potential injury to growing cartilage. Clinical experience with the fluoroquinolones in tuberculosis has been greatest with ofloxacin, ciprofloxacin, levofloxacin, and sparfloxacin. The *in vitro* activity of fluoroquinolones does not exceed that of standard first-line agents such as isoniazid or rifampin.

Three randomized, comparative trials reported during the 1990s provide insight into the efficacy of fluoroquinolone-containing treatment regimens for tuberculosis. In an open, randomized trial of 200 patients in Tanzania with sputum smear-positive pulmonary tuberculosis, a regimen of isoniazid plus rifampin plus ciprofloxacin (HRC) was compared with the standard regimen of isoniazid plus rifampin plus pyrazinamide plus ethambutol (HRZE) [3].

The duration of therapy was 6 months in both groups, and the difference in the proportion of HIV-infected patients in the HRC group (32% of 82) and the HRZE group (37% of 86) was not statistically significant. After 6 months of therapy, all patients in the HRC and HRZE trial arms had negative smears and cultures, but among the HIV-infected patients, the HRC regimen took significantly longer to achieve sputum smear and culture conversion ($p = 0.02$ for smear conversion and $p = 0.001$ for culture conversion). The overall bacteriologic relapse rate 6 months after completion of chemotherapy was 9.3% in the HRC group and 0% in the HRZE group ($p = 0.005$); differences in the relapse rate of the HIV-infected and non-HIV-infected groups were not significant. Thus this study demonstrated that the sterilizing activity of ciprofloxacin was not equivalent to that of pyrazinamide plus ethambutol in HIV-infected patients.

Ciprofloxacin was also evaluated in a double-blind, randomized trial of 60 patients with pulmonary tuberculosis in India [4]. The first regimen was 2 months of isoniazid plus pyrazinamide plus streptomycin plus rifampin, followed by 4 months of isoniazid plus rifampin. The second regimen was 2 months of isoniazid plus pyrazinamide plus streptomycin plus ciprofloxacin, followed by 4 months of isoniazid plus ciprofloxacin. In the 24 months after completion of chemotherapy, the bacteriologic relapse rate of 16.6% (ciprofloxacin-containing regimen) vs. 5.9% (rifampin-containing regimen) was not significantly different ($p > 0.10$), but this small study may have lacked adequate statistical power to detect a difference in outcome.

A third randomized trial assessed the effect of adding levofloxacin to a standard induction regimen of isoniazid plus rifampin plus pyrazinamide plus ethambutol (HRZE) in HIV-infected patients at 21 centres in the United States [5]. The 8-week sputum culture conversion rate was 97.3% for the HRZE group and 95.8% for the HRZE plus levofloxacin group ($p = 1.00$). This suggests that levofloxacin does not improve the sterilizing ability of a standard induction regimen composed of first-line agents.

Overall, these clinical trials suggest that currently-available fluoroquinolones do not enhance the efficacy of existing first-line regimens and may have inferior sterilizing activity in immunocompromised patients. Neither does current evidence support the use of fluoroquinolones as first-line therapeutic agents for tuberculosis. However, they do have a role as second-line agents with a good safety profile, and can be used to treat patients with multidrug-resistant tuberculosis or adverse reactions to first-line agents (Tab. 1).

Multidrug-resistant tuberculosis

The efficacy of fluoroquinolones in the treatment of multidrug-resistant tuberculosis (MDR TB) is difficult to assess because there are no controlled trials and these drugs are typically added to regimens containing five to six agents. Nonetheless, in a retrospective series of 63 MDR TB patients in Hong Kong, resistance to ofloxacin was independently associated with bacteriologic failure ($p < 0.05$) in a multiple logistic regression analysis [6]. This finding is corrob-

Table 1. Principles of fluoroquinolone use in tuberculosis

Principle	Rationale
Always administer fluoroquinolones as part of a multidrug regimen containing at least three drugs to which the organism is susceptible	Fluoroquinolones have less potent sterilizing action than first-line agents, so they should be added to at least two other agents
Do not administer a fluoroquinolone when resistance to other fluoroquinolones is known or suspected	Cross-resistance between members of the fluoroquinolone class of agents has been documented
Use once-a-day high dose administration of fluoroquinolones	Fluoroquinolones exhibit concentration-dependent killing; simplifies treatment regimen
Test serum or urine levels of fluoroquinolone	Gastrointestinal absorption is variable; killing of mycobacteria is concentration-dependent

orated by a second retrospective series from Turkey of 158 MDR TB patients in which successful treatment outcome, defined as negative smears and cultures on follow-up, was independently associated with absence of previous treatment with ofloxacin ($p = 0.005$) [7].

Latent tuberculosis infection

There are no data to support the efficacy of fluoroquinolones, alone or in combination, in the treatment of latent tuberculosis infection (LTBI). Current evidence-based regimens for LTBI in HIV-negative or HIV-positive patients are isoniazid for 9 months, or rifampin and pyrazinamide for 2 months, or rifampin for 4 months [8]. However, for patients infected with multidrug-resistant strains resistant to isoniazid and rifampin, and at high risk of developing active tuberculosis, the recommended special regimens based on expert opinion are pyrazinamide and ethambutol, or pyrazinamide and a fluoroquinolone (levofloxacin or ofloxacin) for 6–12 months. Immunocompetent patients are administered therapy for at least 6 months and immunocompromised patients are treated for 12 months [8].

Concerns have been raised about a higher frequency of adverse events (hepatitis and gastrointestinal intolerance) in patients taking the pyrazinamide plus fluoroquinolone combination [9, 10], so the pyrazinamide plus ethambutol combination offers a potential advantage. However, there are again no data on the efficacy of these special regimens. Fluoroquinolone-based regimens for treatment of LTBI are not recommended in children because of concern about potential harmful effects on bone growth.

Mycobacterium leprae

Considerable progress has been made towards the global eradication of leprosy. The 10–12 million cases of leprosy in the 1980s were reduced to 1.15 million cases by 1997 [11]. Because current standard treatment regimens for leprosy require prolonged drug administration and undesirable side-effects such as clofazimine-induced hyperpigmentation (which discloses the patient's diagnosis to others), there is ongoing interest in finding new therapeutic regimens to address these concerns.

Paucibacillary leprosy

A major advance occurred in 1997 with the WHO Expert Committee's acceptance of single-dose multidrug therapy for single-lesion paucibacillary leprosy [11]. This oral regimen composed of rifampin 600 mg plus ofloxacin 400 mg plus minocycline 100 mg (ROM) administered as a single dose resulted in cure rates equivalent to the standard 6-month WHO paucibacillary regimen (rifampin 600 mg monthly plus dapsone 100 mg daily for 6 months) in a randomized, double-blind, comparative trial of 1483 patients [12]. Hence the costs of therapy for single-lesion paucibacillary leprosy are lowered and compliance with treatment is enhanced. The WHO 6-month regimen of rifampin plus dapsone remains the preferred treatment for paucibacillary leprosy with two to five skin lesions.

Multibacillary leprosy

Currently, there are insufficient data on the efficacy of fluoroquinolones in the treatment of multibacillary leprosy (more than five skin lesions). Therefore, the WHO Expert Committee continues to recommend a 12–24 month regimen of rifampin plus clofazimine plus dapsone. However, the WHO Expert Committee also endorses the use of ofloxacin in combination regimens for patients with multibacillary leprosy who cannot take first-line drugs [11]. An adult multibacillary patient unable to take clofazimine may be treated with monthly administration of rifampin 600 mg plus ofloxacin 400 mg plus minocycline 100 mg (ROM) for 24 months. In addition, an adult multibacillary patient unable to take rifampin may be treated with daily administration of clofazimine 50 mg plus ofloxacin 400 mg plus minocycline 100 mg for 6 months, followed by daily administration of clofazimine 50 mg plus ofloxacin 400 mg or minocycline 100 mg for at least an additional 18 months.

Non-tuberculous mycobacteria

According to recent evidence-based guidelines for the treatment of nontuberculous mycobacteria, ciprofloxacin has proven clinical utility for *Mycobacterium fortuitum* pulmonary infections, and should be used as part of a two-drug oral regimen for 6–12 months. For serious non-pulmonary *M. fortuitum* infections, the combination of parenteral amikacin and high-dose cefoxitin is recommended [13]. For most other infections due to nontuberculous mycobacteria, the clinical efficacy of fluoroquinolones remains uncertain.

Mycobacterium avium complex

On the basis of short-term monotherapy trials, ciprofloxacin is considered a "second-line" agent for the treatment of *Mycobacterium avium* complex disease in patients with AIDS, and may be added to more efficacious agents such as macrolides (clarithromycin or azithromycin) and ethambutol [14]. Indications for the addition of ciprofloxacin include adverse reactions or failure to respond to first-line agents. In a randomized comparative trial, a regimen containing clarithromycin plus rifabutin plus ethambutol was superior to a regimen containing ciprofloxacin plus rifampin plus ethambutol plus clofazimine in terminating AIDS-related *Mycobacterium avium* complex bacteremia and enhancing survival [15].

Research priorities

There are several important unanswered questions for clinicians who use fluoroquinolones to treat mycobacterial infections. First, further comparative clinical trials are required to determine which of the available fluoroquinolones are the most active agents against mycobacteria. Second, as new fluoroquinolone agents are discovered, they need to be evaluated against existing agents. Possibly, future agents with enhanced bactericidal and sterilizing activity will qualify as first-line therapeutic agents.

Third, the efficacy of fluoroquinolone-containing regimens in the treatment of active or latent multidrug-resistant tuberculosis needs to be verified in randomized, comparative trials. Such studies are also needed for the treatment of multibacillary leprosy.

Brucellosis

Brucellosis is a zoonosis caused by facultative intracellular bacteria of the genus brucella. From *in vitro* animal and clinical studies three principles of brucellosis therapy has emerged [16–18]. Firstly, clinical efficacy in treating brucellosis could not be predicted by the *in vitro* sensitivity to different antimicrobial agents. Second, the treatment of brucellosis, like tuberculosis, requires prolonged therapy and with two agents, and thirdly, one of the two agents used to treat brucellosis needs to have good intracellular penetration.

Fluroquinolones, has excellent oral bioavailability, high tissue concentration, excellent intracellular penetration, and documented *in vitro* activity against infections caused by intracellular organisms including brucella spp. Most quinolones including ciprofloxacin, ofloxacin, lomefloxacin, and pefloxacin have moderate *in vitro* bacterial activity against brucella. Even recently produced quinolone like sitafloxacin and clinafloxacin possess excellent bactericidal activity against brucella spp *in vitro* but like the other quinolones continue to lack comparative clinical efficacy [19, 20].

In experimental animal models, studies have shown failure when ciprofloxacin, ofloxacin were used for as long as 21 days [21] and a lack of synergy was noted when streptomycin was combined with ciprofloxacin [22].

Clinical trials in human employing quinolones monotherapy have yielded unacceptably high failure rates ranging from 16% to 66%. These high failure rates may be attributed to the two- to 16-fold reduction of the efficacy of quinolones against brucella in acidic pH inside the macrophage [23]. Studies have shown as well that the use of monotherapy can lead to development of resistance and cross-resistance.

This led investigators to look into the possibility of combining a quinolone with another efficacious agent like rifampin. Two clinical trials have been performed to date utilizing a quinolone (ciprofloxacin or ofloxacin) in combination with rifampin in treatment of brucellosis. The first study by Akova et al. compared standard therapy of doxycycline and rifampin for 6 weeks in 30 patients against another group of 30 patients who received ofloxacin and rifampin for the same duration. The relapse rate in both groups was around 3% [24]. Agalar et al. compared the combination of ciprofloxacin/rifampin fro 6 weeks in 20 patients with doxycycline/rifampin for the same duration in another 20 patients. The relapse rate in the quinolone combination group was 15% vs. 10% in the standard therapy group [25].

In summary, fluoroquinolones must not be considered for use as a primary regimen for the treatment of brucellosis and until further data are available quinolones should not replace the standard two-drug regimen in the management of brucellosis.

Plague

Yersinia pestis is a Gram-negative coccobacillus, the causative agent of plague. The most common mode of transmission of *Y. pestis* to human is by the bite of infectious fleas, which cause bubonic plague. However, pneumonic plague also occurs.

Historically, Amikacin has been the preferred treatment for plague. Gentamicin, tetracycline and doxycycline are recommended as acceptable alternatives. The fluroquinolones has demonstrated efficacy *in vitro* and in animal studies. *In vitro* data revealed equal or greater activity of ciprofloxacin, levofloxacin, and ofloxacin against *Y. pestis* when compared to aminoglycosides or tetracyclinee [26, 27]. Ciprofloxacin as well demonstrated superior efficacy in animal studies when compared to doxycycline and aminoglycosides in pneumonic plague [28]. However, there is lack of published clinical trials on the use of fluoquinolones in human plague cases. Despite that Inglesby et al. recommended the use of intravenous ciprofloxacin (or other fluroquinolone) as an alternative to Amikacin in children/adults/pregnant women in a setting of contained casuality when plague is used as a biological weapon. And oral ciprofloxacin (or other fluroquinolone) in all the above groups in the setting of mass casuality and post-exposure prophylaxis when plague is used as a biological weapon [29].

Tularaemia

Tularemia is a rare zoonotic disease caused by *Francisella tularensis*, a fastidious, aerobic Gram-negative intracellular bacterium. The natural host includes rabbits, rodents and squirrels. Human contract the disease mostly through mosquito bites or by handling infected animals. Aminoglycosides (Streptomycin and gentamicin), tetracycline and chloramphenicol have been traditionally considered agents of choice for the treatment of tularemia since the 1940s. A drawback of the later two agents is an increased risk of relapse. Fluoroquinolones are attractive agents to treat *F. tularensis* because of its many unique properties. These properties include their high tissue levels, penetration into macrophages and PMNLs, their bactericidal activity; their stability within an acidic environment; and their minimal toxicity in adults. *In vitro*, experimental and clinical data suggest that quinolones may be useful for treating tularemia. Syrjala et al. demonstrated that 10 strains of *F. tularensis* have *in vitro* susceptibility to ciprofloxacin, norfloxacin, ofloxacin, and pefloxacin [30]. Ikaheimo et al. studied the *in vitro* antimicrobial susceptibility of 38 strains of type B *F. tularensis*. Ciprofloxacin, Levofloxacin, grepafloxacin, and trovafloxacin had similar low MIC_{90}s of less than 0.05 mg/ml [31]. Clinical data available to date suggest that quinolones are an excellent alternative for treating tularemia. Limaye et al. reviewed the English literature (1966–1998) and summarized 10 reports of tularemia patients all successfully cured with orally administered quinolones [32] in contrast to published relapse rates associated with gentamicin and tetracycline of 6% and 12% respectively.

Chocarro et al. challenged these results with a report of 7/14 patients failing oral ciprofloxacin. This poor outcome was related to clinical differences between the patient population studied and the fact that Choccarro used ciprofloxacin as primary therapy in fewer cases when compared to Limaye et al. (42% vs. 80%) [33]. The efficacy of quinolones in the treatment of adult tularemia was reaffirmed by Perez-Castrillon et al. when he compared the efficacy of three antibiotics (Streptomycin, Ciprofloxacin, and doxycycline) in treating 142 confirmed tularemia cases. Therapeutic failure among the 142 patients treated occurred in 32 patients (22.4%). Ciprofloxacin showed the lowest frequency of failure and with the fewest side-effects [34].

Children with tularemia are often subjected to parenteral treatment with aminoglycoside. This is because of the problem of administering tetracyclinee and the concern about quinolone causing arhtropathy in immature animals. Johnson et al. studied the efficacy of oral ciprofloxacin 15–20 mg/kg daily in two divided doses for 10–17 days in 12 children (median age, 4 years; range, 1 to 10) with ulceroglandular tularemia. In two cases, treatment was withdrawn after 3 days and 7 days because of rash. All children recovered without complications [35].

It can be concluded that quinolones should be considered efficacious alternate agents for treating tularemia in patients who do not require parenteral therapy or are intolerant of more standard treatment regimens.

Anthrax

Anthrax is a zoonotic disease caused by endopores of *Bacillus anthracis* Gram-positive soil organisms. Naturally occurring anthrax can be acquired through contact with an anthrax-infected animal or anthrax contaminated animal products. In humans three types of anthrax infection occur: inhalational, cutaneous and gastrointestinal. Anthrax has been recognized for years as a possible biological weapon and as recently as late 2001, 12 cases of documented anthrax was diagnosed in the United States as a bioweapon related incident with six inhalational and six cutaneous cases [36]. Naturally occurring *Bacillus anthracis* is rarely resistant to penicillin and doxycycline and both agents are FDA approved for treatment of the disease. Ciprofloxacin is active *in vitro*, effective in animal models of inhalational anthrax and also FDA approved for this indications [37]. Other fluoroqinolones like levofloxacin, trovafloxacin, gatifloxacin, and moxifloxacin are also active *in vitro* against anthrax and probably as effective as ciprofloxacin, but lacks the primate efficacy data and FDA approval. Despite concerns about recently engineered *B. anthracis* strains resistant to penicillin and doxycycline, no information has been published on engineering a quinolone-resistant strain.

The initial therapy for adults with clinically evident inhalational or severe cutaneous anthrax is 400 mg of ciprofloxacin given intravenously every 12 h to be switched to oral ciprofloxacin 500 mg taken every 12 h for 10 days in the case of naturally acquired anthrax and 60 days if the disease occurred in the context of bioterrorism [37].

References

1 Berning SE (2001) The role of fluoroquinolones in tuberculosis today. *Drugs* 61: 9–18 (*A comprehensive review of how to use fluoroquinolones for tuberculosis therapy. In addition to summarizing microbiologic and pharmacokinetic data, the author addresses practical issues such as administration regimens, drug reactions, and drug interactions.*)

2 Berning SE, Madsen L, Iseman MD, Peloquin CA (1995) Long-term safety of ofloxacin and ciprofloxacin in the treatment of mycobacterial infections. *Am J Respir Crit Care Med* 151: 2006–2009 *(Review of 7 years' experience with ofloxacin and ciprofloxacin in 103 patients. Both agents were well tolerated.)*

3 Kennedy N, Berger L, Curram J, Fox R, Gutmann J, Kisyombe GM, Ngowi FI, Ramsay AR, Saruni AO, Sam N et al (1996) Randomized controlled trial of a drug regimen that includes ciprofloxacin for the treatment of pulmonary tuberculosis. *Clin Infect Dis* 22: 827–833 *(Among the HIV-infected patients in this randomized trial, ciprofloxacin did not have equivalent steriliz-*

ing activity to pyrazinamide plus ethambutol at 6 months after completion of anti-tuberculous chemotherapy.)

4 Mohanty KC, Khamgaye TM (1993) Controlled trial of ciprofloxacin in short-term chemotherapy for pulmonary tuberculosis. *Chest* 104: 1194–1198 (*Twenty-four months after completion of anti-tuberculous chemotherapy, a ciprofloxacin-based regimen achieved an equivalent cure rate to a rifampin-based regimen. The sample size was small in this randomized study and statistical power to detect a difference in outcome was not stated.)*

5 El-Sadr WM, Perlman DC, Matts JP, Nelson ET, Cohn DL, Salomon N, Olibrice M, Medard F, Chirgwin KD, Mildvan D et al (1998) for the Terry Beirn Community Programs for Clinical Research on AIDS (CPCRA) and the AIDS Clinical Trials Group (ACTG). Evaluation of an intensive intermittent-induction regimen and duration of short-course treatment for human immunodeficiency virus-related pulmonary tuberculosis. *Clin Infect Dis* 26: 1148–1158 (*In this randomized study of HIV-infected patients, levofloxacin did not enhance the sterilizing activity of the standard 4-drug, first-line treatment regimen for tuberculosis.)*

6 Yew WW, Chan CK, Chau CH, Tam CM, Leung CC, Wong PC, Lee J (2000) Outcomes of patients with multidrug-resistant pulmonary tuberculosis treated with ofloxacin/levofloxacin-containing regimens. *Chest* 117: 744–751 *(A retrospective case series of 63 patients with multidrug-resistant tuberculosis. Cure rate was 81%. Adverse outcome was independently associated with lung cavitation, ofloxacin resistance, and poor adherence to therapy.)*

7 Tahaoglu K, Torun T, Sevim T, Atac G, Kir A, Karasulu L, Ozmen I, Kapakli N (2001) The treatment of multidrug-resistant tuberculosis in Turkey. *N Engl J Med* 345: 170–174 *(Review of a large series of multidrug-resistant tuberculosis cases. Successful treatment, achieved in 77% of cases, was independently associated with younger age and absence of previous treatment with ofloxacin. Demonstrates that multidrug-resistant tuberculosis can be successfully treated within the resource constraints of low-income nations.)*

8 American Thoracic Society (2000) Targeted tuberculin testing and treatment of latent tuberculosis infection. *Am J Respir Crit Care Med* 161: 5221–5247 *(No data support the efficacy of fluoroquinolones for treatment of latent tuberculosis infection. A pyrazinamide plus fluoroquinolone regimen may be useful for patients with latent infection due to multidrug-resistant strains.)*

9 Horn DL, Hewlett D, Alfalla C, Peterson S, Opal SM (1994) Limited tolerance of ofloxacin and pyrazinamide prophylaxis against tuberculosis. *N Engl J Med* 330: 1241

10 Ridzon R, Meador J, Maxwell R, Higgins K, Weismuller P, Onorato IM (1997) Asymptomatic hepatitis in persons who received alternative preventive therapy with pyrazinamide and ofloxacin. *Clin Infect Dis* 24: 1264–1265

11 WHO (1998) Seventh Report of the WHO Expert Committee on Leprosy. World Health Organization. *Tech Rep Ser* 874: 1–43 *(Outlines currently recommended antimicrobial regimens for leprosy. This report endorsed a single-dose multidrug regimen for treatment of single-lesion, paucibacillary leprosy.)*

12 Single-Lesion Multicentre Trial Group (1997) Efficacy of single dose multidrug therapy for the treatment of single-lesion paucibacillary leprosy. *Indian J Lepr* 69: 121–129 *(Describes a multicentre, double-blind, randomized, comparative trial of the standard 6-month WHO multidrug, paucibacillary regimen* vs. *a single-dose regimen of rifampin plus ofloxacin plus minocycline (ROM). Among the 1381 patients who completed the study (1483 enrolled), the relapse rate was equivalent in the 2 treatment groups.)*

13 American Thoracic Society (1997) Diagnosis and treatment of disease caused by nontuberculous mycobacteria. *Am J Respir Crit Care Med* 156: S1–S25 *(Comprehensive review of the treatment of infections due to nontuberculous mycobacteria. Ciprofloxacin is a proven first-line agent for combination therapy of* Mycobacterium *fortuitum lung infection. For most other infections, the available data do not support use of fluoroquinolones as first-line therapy.)*

14 Benson CA (1994) Treatment of disseminated disease due to *Mycobacterium avium* complex in patients with AIDS. *Clin Infect Dis* 18 Suppl 3: S237–242 *(This review paper states that new macrolides (clarithromycin or azithromycin) are more potent agents against* Mycobacterium avium *complex disease than ciprofloxacin, which can be used as an adjunctive agent.)*

15 Shafran SD, Singer J, Zarowny DP, Phillips P, Salit I, Walmsley SL, Fong IW, Gill MJ, Rachlis AR, LaLonde RG et al (1996) A comparison of two regimens for the treatment of *Mycobacterium avium* complex bacteremia in AIDS: rifabutin, ethambutol, and clarithromycin vs. rifampin, ethambutol, clofazimine, and ciprofloxacin. Canadian HIV Trials Network Protocol 010 Study Group. *N Engl J Med* 335: 377–383 (*Multicentre, randomized, comparative trial of treatments for*

AIDS-related Mycobacterium avium *complex bacteremia. Ciprofloxacin-based regimen is inferior to a clarithromycin-based regimen.)*

16 Hall WH (1990) Modern chemotherapy for brucellosis in humans. *Rev Infect Dis* 12: 1060–1099 *(A comprehensive review summarizing critically and selectively the medical literature on modern chemotherapy for Brucellosis in humans.)*

17 Solera J, Martinez-Alfaro E, Espinosa A (1997) Recognition and optimum treatment of Brucellosis. *Drugs* 53: 245–256 *(A comprehensive review of Brucellosis with emphasis on aetiology, epidemiology, clinical spectrum, diagnosis and treatment. Detailed review of in vitro, animal, and clinical studies on brucella treatment with different class of antimicrobial agents.)*

18 Solera J (2000) Treatment of human Brucellosis. *J Med Liban* 48: 255–263 *(A comprehensive review of how different classes of antimicrobial agent could be used in the treatment of Brucellosis with guide to the treatment of human Brucellosis.)*

19 Trujillano-Martin I, Garcia-Sanchez E, Martinez IM, Fresnadillo MJ, Garcia-Sanchez JE, Garcia-Rodriguez JA (1999) *In vitro* activities of six new fluroquinolones against *Brucella melitensis. Antimicrob Agents Chemother* 43: 194–195 *(In vitro activity of eight fluroquinolones were tested against 160* Brucella *melitensis strains. Sitafloxacin was the most active fluroquinolone tested. Other fluroquinolones tested including levofloxacin, trovafloxacin, and moxifloxacin had activities similar to or slightly greater than that of ciprofloxacin.)*

20 Gracia-Rodriguez JA, Garcia-Sanchez JE, Trujillano I, Garcia-Sanchez E, Garcia Garcia MI, Fresnadillo MJ (1995) Susceptibilities of *Brucella melitensis* isolates to clinafloxacin and four other new fluroquinolones. *Antimicrob Agents Chemother* 39: 1194–1195 *(In vitro activity of six fluroquinolones were tested against 120 clinical isolates of* Brucella *melitensis and three reference strains of the same species. Clinafloxacin was the most active compound tested. The activity of ciprofloxacin and the other four agents were less than clinafloxacin.)*

21 Shasha B, Lang R, Rubinstein E (1992) Therapy of Experimental Murine Brucellosis with streptomycin, co-trimoxazole, ciprofloxacin, ofloxacin, pefloxacin, doxycycline, and rifampin. *Antimicrob Agents Chemother* 36: 973–976 *(*Brucella *infected mice were treated with streptomycin, co-trimoxazole, ciprofloxacin, doxycycline, and rifampin intraperitoneally and with ciprofloxacin, ofloxacin, pefloxacin, doxycycline, and rifampin orally for 14 to 21 days. Therapy failure was noted in all mice treated with ciprofloxacin, ofloxacin, and pefloxacin administered orally as well as in mice treated intraperitoneally with ciprofloxacin.)*

22 Lang R, Shasha B, Rubinstein E (1993) Therapy of experimental Murine brucellosis with streptomycin alone and in combination with ciprofloxacin, doxycycline, and rifampin. *Antimicrob Agents Chemother* 37: 2333–2336 *(In vivo efficacy of streptomycin, doxycycline, rifampin, ciprofloxacin, and their combination was evaluated for a* Brucella *melitensis experimental infection in a mouse model. Therapy failure was noted in streptomycin and ciprofloxacin treated animals. Also none of the animals receiving the streptomycin-ciprofloxacin combinations was cured.)*

23 Akova M, Gur D, Livermore DM, Kocagöz T, Akalin HE (1999) *In vitro* activities of antibiotics alone and in combination against *Brucella* melitensis at neutral and acidic PHs. *Antimicro Agents Chemother* 43: 1298–1300 *(Azithromycin, streptomycin, and quinolones were active against* Brucella *melitensis at PH 7.0 but not at PH 5.0, rifampin and doxycycline retained activity at PH 5.0. Regardless of PH, azithromycin-rifampin and ofloxacin-rifampin showed less synergy than established standard combination.)*

24 Akova M, Uzun O, Akalin HE, Hayran M, Unal S, Gür D (1993) Quinolones in treatment of Human Brucellosis: Comparative trial of ofloxacin-rifampin vs. doxycycline-rifampin. *Antimicrob Agents Chemother* 37: 1831–1834 *(A prospective randomized study comparing the efficacy of ofloxacin plus rifampin with doxycyline plus rifampin both combination given for 6 weeks against Brucellosis. Thirty patients were enrolled in each arm with relapse rates of 3.3% and 3.2% respectively.)*

25 Aglar C, Usubutun S, Turkylmaz R (1999) Ciprofloxacin and rifampin vs. doxycycline and rifampin in the treatment of Brucellosis. *Eur J Clin Microbiol Infect Dis* 18: 535–538 *(Open randomized clinical trial comparing the efficacy of ciprofloxacin-rifampin* vs. *doxycycline-rifampicin both for 6 weeks in the treatment of brucellosis. Twenty (20) pateints were enrolled in each arm of the study and the relapse rate was 15% vs 10%.)*

26 Smith MD, Vinh SX, Nguyen TT, Wain J, Thung D, White NJ (1995) *In vitro* antimicrobial susceptibilities of strains of *Y. pestis. Antimicrob Agents Chemother* 39: 2153–2154 *(In vitro activities of 14 antimicrobial agents were determined for 78 strains of* Y. pestis*. The most active antibiotics were ceftriaxone and ciprofloxacin, followed by ofloxacin and ampicillin.)*

27 Frean JA, Arntzen L, Capper T, Bryskier A, Klugman KP (1996) *In vitro* activities of 14 antibiotics against 100 human isolates of *Yersinia pestis* from a Southern African plague focus. *Antimicrob Agents Chemother* 40: 2646–2647 *(In vitro activities of 14 antibiotics against 100 human isolates of* Y. pestis. *Among the injectable agents tested, cefotaxime was the most active, and among the oral agents, both levofloxacin and ofloxacin were highly active.)*

28 Russell P, Eley SM, Green M, Stagg AJ, Taylor RR, Nelson M, Beedham RJ, Bell DL, Rogers D, Whittington D, Titball RW (1998) Efficacy of doxycycline and ciprofloxacin against experimental *Y. pestis* infection in mice. *J Antimicrob Chemother* 41: 301–305 *(The efficacies of ciprofloxacin and doxycycline prophylaxis and therapy was assessed against experimental plague. Ciprofloxacin prophylaxis and therapy was successful for up to 24 h after challenge, but not after 48 h.)*

29 Inglesby TV, Dennis DT, Henderson DA, Bartlett JG, Ascher MS, Eitzen E, Fine AD, Friedlander AM, Hauer J, Koerner JF et al (2000) plague as a biological weapon: Medical and Public health management. *JAMA* 283: 2281–2290 (*This is a consensus statement of the working group on civilian biodefense. Describes the history, epidemiology, microbiology, pathogenesis and clinical manifestations, diagnosis and therapy for plague based on an extensive review of the scientific literature.)*

30 Syrjala H, Schildt R, Raisainen S (1991) *In vitro* susceptibility of Francisella tularensis to fluroquinolones, treatment of tularemia with norfloxacin, ciprofloxacin Eur JClin Microbial Infect Dis (1991) 10: 68–70 *(In vitro susceptibility was demonstrated in 10 strains of* F. tularensis *to ciprofloxacin, norfloxacin, ofloxacin and pefloxacin.)*

31 Ikaheimo I, Syrjala H, Karhukorpi J, Schildt R, Koskela M (2000) *In vitro* susceptibility of *Francisella tularensis* isolated from humans and animals. *J Antimicrob Chemother* 46: 287–290 *(The in vitro susceptibility of 38 strains fo* F. tularensis *was determined using E test. The quinolones examined had low* MIC_{90}*s including ciprofloxacin, levofloxacin, grepafloxacin and trovafloxacin.)*

32 Limaye AP, Hooper CJ (1999) Treatment of Tularemia with fluroquinolones: Two cases and review. *Clin Infect Dis* 29: 922–924 *(A description of two cases of acutely ill immunocompromised patients who had presumed atypical pneumonia and responded to treatment with levofloxacin. The diagnosis of tularemia confirmed in these two cases by positive blood culture, review of eight more cases of tularemia treated with quinolones with favourable clinical response was documented.)*

33 Chocarro A, Gonzalez A, Garcia I (2000) Treatment of Tularemia with ciprofloxacin. *Clinical Infect Dis* 31: 623 *(Out of 57 cases of tularemia, 14 patients were treated with ciprofloxacin, relapse was observed in 50%. Ciprofloxacin was used as primary therapy in <42%.)*

34 Perez-Castrillon JL, Bachiller-Luque P, Martin-Luquero M, Mena-Martin FJ, Herreros V (2001) Tularemia epidemic in northwestern Spain: clinical description and therapeutic response. *Clinical Infect Dis* 33: 573–576 *(Description of of the clinical characteristics and clinical response to an outbreak of tularemia (142 cases). The therapeutic failure rates was 22.5%. Ciprofloxacin was the antibiotic with the lowest resistance and therapeutic failure.)*

35 Johansson A, Berglund L, Gothefors L, Sjostedt A, Tarnvik A (2000) Ciprofloxacin for treatment of tularemia in children. *Pediatr Infect Dis J* 19: 449–453 *(A study on the clinical response of 12 children with ulcenoglandular tularemia to 10–14 drugs of oral ciprofloxacin. All children recovered without complications.)*

36 Swartz MN (2001) Recognition and management of Anthrax – An update. *New Eng J Med* 345: 1621–1626 *(An extensive up-to-date review of the literature on the bacteriology, pathogenesis, epidemiology, clinical features, diagnosis and treatment of anthrax if used as a biological war agent.)*

37 Inglesby TV, Henderson DA, Bartlett JG, Ascher MS, Eitzen E, Friedlander AM, Hayer J, McDade J, Osterholm MT, O'Toole T (1999) Anthrax as a biological weapon: Medical and Public Health Management. *JAMA* 281: 1735–1745 (*Consensus statement made by the working group on civilian biodefense based on review of the available literature with clear guidelines on medical and public management of anthrax if used as a bioweapon.*)

Fluoroquinolone Antibiotics
ed. by A.R. Ronald and D.E. Low

The quinolones: future prospects

Allan R. Ronald and Donald E. Low

It has been a remarkable journey. Nalidixic acid was first synthesized in 1961 as a 1,8 naphthyridine by-product of chloroquine production and found to have a limited Gram-negative antibacterial spectrum sufficient only for patients with urinary infection [1]. Now, four decades later, we have an array of agents which appear to be remarkably safe and well tolerated, readily administered through both oral and parenteral routes with wide distribution throughout the body, with surprising effectiveness for a wide range of bacterial infections. No one would have predicted this outcome during the first two decades of quinolone history. For those of us who have lived with these molecules through their therapeutic evolution, we continue to be surprised and delighted with the ability of the pharmaceutical industry to modify the basic molecule and manipulate it to achieve major changes in antibacterial activity and improve pharmacokinetics. With regard to changing structure and ensuing activity and adverse reactions, the basic molecule has proved to be very amenable in a way reminiscent of the beta-lactam molecule.

These substantial gains are not occurring without threats to the ongoing success of this story.

Real and possible adverse effects have altered the projections of use on several occasions. We still have lingering concerns about the effects of quinolones on cartilage development and long-term consequences to normal joint function. To date, there has been no evidence that this is important for human populations but studies continue. Poorly understood adverse reactions to several of the quinolones have led to their removal from routine use within months of their introduction. Both temafloxacin and trovafloxacin were promising agents until rare but occasionally fatal complications resulted in their restricted use or removal from the marketplace. Fortunately these idiosyncracies have not been widely shared among the fluoroquinolones and their use in tens of millions of individuals, have not identified other significant adverse reactions that result in fatal outcomes. However, vigilance and ongoing surveillance must be maintained. Their use in early pregnancy with the possibility of teratological consequences remains a concern as well as the alterations to QT intervals, tendon ruptures, hypoglycemia, and the acquisition of important allergies. However, the overall safety and tolerance of these agents remain one of the features that have led to their frequent choice as therapeutic agents throughout the world.

The emergence of resistance and its subsequent spread is beginning to pose a much more serious threat to their continued effective use. Resistance has appeared in almost every instance with widespread use of these agents. In particular, the spread of resistant clones among *N. gonorrhoeae* and *S. pneumoniae*, are beginning to limit the use of these agents for syndromic treatment of genitourinary and respiratory infections respectively. The emergence and spread of resistant *Pseudomonas aeruginosa* and now *Enterobacteriaceae* and methicillin-resistant staphylococci is creating obstacles to their use for institutionally-acquired infections. The emergence of resistance in enteric pathogens is now occurring and will almost certainly alter the importance of these agents for acute GI infectious illnesses.

Could we have prevented and controlled the emergence of resistance with widely accepted and implemented antimicrobial practices that would be realistic within the world in which we live? This remains a challenge for the World Health Organization and for all of us who worry that antimicrobial resistance will overwhelm our abilities to design, manufacture, and distribute new modified molecules.

Our understanding of pharmacokinetics and pharmacodynamics does encourage consideration of changes in the strategies we employ to treat patients with these drugs. Almost certainly we could use these agents for much shorter periods of time with the eradication of the pathogen in otherwise healthy hosts. Shorter courses of therapy will lead to less resistance emerging because of less antibacterial exposure. Also perhaps initial therapy should be routinely substantially increased with a loading dose in order to ensure that mutants within a population of microbes are either killed or reduced in numbers to that they do not become the predominant pathogen, and lead to the emergence of resistance. Studies that shorten the course of therapy, use dosing strategies that prevent emergence of resistance, and determine more precisely the adverse effects of these dosing changes, should be a priority.

Control of these agents likely should have been attempted with an agreement on and imposition of international guidelines. Their widespread use in animal feed for growth promotion has led to the emergence of resistance among several classes of bacteria and this is continuing. If we had known then what we know now about the evolution of resistance, we would never have approved their use in agriculture. Their use in humans for prophylaxis and formulations with low doses have also been associated with the emergence of resistance. As resistance emerges and more active agents are approved for use in humans, so will the prevalence of bacteria with first-step mutants that will be considered by *in vitro* susceptibility testing to be susceptible. If we determine that first step mutants are in themselves a contradiction to the use of this class of antimicrobials, their new testing procedures must be developed to detect these isolates. This will require a paradigm shift in our thinking of susceptibility testing, that is from testing for pharmacological reasons to testing for biological ones. Although our world has a very poor and inadequate history of useful regulatory measures that extend beyond national borders, these will become increasingly necessary and should be a priority. Studies, particularly from the Scandinavian countries, have definitively proven that antimicrobial misuse is mirrored by development of resistance.

The quinolones are also not readily destroyed biologically in the environment and may persist indefinitely. As a result, the increasing exposure within ecosystems to the quinolones may generate additional resistance. This is an area which requires further research.

In summary, what may the future look like?

- First of all, new molecules will continue to be identified and some of these will be effective against pathogens which have emerged as resistant to the currently available quinolones. We will need to learn how to use these in a way which will delay the process of the emergence and spread of resistant pathogens.
- We will use the quinolones differently. We will usually begin with a loading dose and prescribe them for a much shorter course that current routine use.
- We will develop more confidence in their use in areas where currently they are restricted because of concerns about long-term adverse consequences. Their general safety in children and in pregnancy will emerge over time.
- International and national guidelines for the use of the quinolones as well as for other important antimicrobial agents will emerge and their misuse will gradually decrease, but not without bureaucracies and impediments that will frustrate both the pharmaceutical companies and each of us as prescribers.
- Parenteral therapy will become less important as the current drugs and their successors will prove to be very effective when prescribed orally.

We predict that by 2010, we will have an additional five or six fluoroquinolones that will augment our current regimens. Hopefully if resistance has not emerged to unacceptable levels, these drugs will continue to be among the most frequently prescribed, most effective antibacterial agents available for the treatment of bacterial infections.

References

1 Ronald AR, Turck M, Petersdorf RG (1966) Nalidixic acid in the treatment of urinary tract infections. *N Engl J Med* 275: 1081–1089

Index

MIX
Papier aus verantwortungsvollen Quellen
Paper from responsible sources
FSC® C105338
FSC
www.fsc.org

If you have any concerns about our products,
you can contact us on
ProductSafety@springernature.com

In case Publisher is established outside the EU,
the EU authorized representative is:
Springer Nature Customer Service Center GmbH
Europaplatz 3, 69115 Heidelberg, Germany

Printed by Libri Plureos GmbH
in Hamburg, Germany